Chinese Bodywork

A Complete Manual of
Chinese Therapeutic Massage

Chinese Bodywork

A Complete Manual of
Chinese Therapeutic Massage

Editor-in-Chief
Sun Chengnan

Translator
Wang Qiliang, Research Fellow of TCM

Pacific View Press

Berkeley, California

Consultants: Zhou Fengwu, Lu Yongchang

Editor-in-Chief: Sun Chengnan

Deputy Editors: Bian Chunqiang, Qu Jingxi

Editorial Staff: Wang Zhiyi, Wang Qinglin, Luan Changye, Xue Jingyi

Writers: Tian Changying, Zhu Lixiang, Zhu Heting, Du Wenzun, Li Pinzhi, Zhang An, Zhang Sufang, Yang Yuru, Guo Zhengzhi, Zhou Chuanxing, Hou Yingxiang, Han Chuanming, Sheng Yongqi

Photography: Hao Wei

Illustrations: Liu Wenxue

Managing Editors: Wang Daoyin, Li Yu

Editor, North American Edition: Howard Pearlstein

Design, North American Edition: Jane Walsh

Cover Design: Rene Yung

Technical Consultant, North American Edition: Carl Dubitsky

Original edition published by Shandong Science and Technology Press of China in 1990.

This edition is printed with the permission of Shandong Science and Technology Press, and is only distributed in North America.

Library of Congress Catalog Number: 93-85293

ISBN 1-881896-06-4

Published in the United States of America by Pacific View Press

Printed in the United States of America

Contents

Foreword

The work of the Shandong Branch of Massage Committee (CTMA) is to preserve and develop the legacy of Traditional Chinese Medicine, as well as to make the full scope of Chinese Medical Massage more accessible and available. Toward these goals, we enjoined massage therapists of the entire province to summarize and systematize their own clinical experiences, as well as those of past masters of Traditional Chinese Medicine. These past masters include Xu Qianguang, Wei Zhixin, Li Guangxi, Sun Maocai, Li Dexiu, Sun Zhongsan, Zhang Hanchen, Gu Daifeng, Zhong Hongjiu, Liu Shaonan and others. Drawing from all this accumulated knowledge, techniques of various schools of massage were examined, selected and refined. The product of that extensive work is this book, which, if we remember that Shandong Province is originally the home of Confucius and Mencius, and the ancient states of Qi and Lu, represents a treasure-trove of the skills of Chinese Medical Massage.

This book was compiled in a series of steps. First, we brought dozens of massage specialists and medical experts together in conferences. Through detailed discussion and consultation, they determined the outline of contents and style of compilation, and defined assignments for each area. The next step was to produce preliminary drafts composed from widespread collections of data and careful selections. After this, a jury of experts and academicians was invited to examine and revise the drafts, and make recommendations for amendments. Then, a series of selected individuals refined and improved the manuscript. The entire process took three years.

The unwavering standard for this book was scientific accuracy and practicality. We sought truth from facts and did not confine ourselves to conventional procedures and limitations. We have taken great measures to retain the original techniques and clinical experiences of all the schools of massage.

It is our hope that this book will be a useful reference for clinicians, teachers and researchers of massage.

Sun Chengnan, Editor-in Chief
Autumn, 1989

Introduction to the
North American Edition

The origins of Oriental Bodywork stretch back into Chinese antiquity. The oldest written medical text still in existence, the *Huang Di Nei Jing Su Wen* (The Yellow Emperor's Internal Canon), is dated 100 B.C.. In it, the mythical First Emperor of China, Huang Di, asked his physician, Qi Bo, to describe the role of therapeutic massage and bodywork in oriental medicine. The Divine Healer replied:

> *In the spring and summer, when food is plentiful and humans tend to become lazy and slothful, finger pressure is used to increase digestive fire and restore vigor.*

When China was unified during the Qin Dynasty in the 3rd century B.C., bodywork was known as *Moshou* (hand rubbing). During the Han Dynasty (206 B.C. - 220 A.D.), Chinese therapeutic massage became known as *Anmo* (press and rub). By the 5th century, it had evolved to such a level that a Doctoral Degree was created for it at the Imperial College of Medicine in Xian, the ancient capital of the Tang Dynasty. (Later, during the Ming Dynasty [1368 - 1644], the term, *Tuina* [push and hold, was added].)

Chinese *Anmo* is the source of all forms of Oriental massage. During the 6th century, Chinese medicine spread to the Japanese archipelago and the Korean peninsula with the trade missions sent to open up routes of commerce. Japanese *Anma* developed directly from this presence, as did Korean *Amma* Therapy. Japanese *Shiatsu* is a modern combination (1915) of traditional *Anma* massage, Chinese abdominal manipulation, the acu-point system, Do-in exercises and Western anatomy and physiology. This combination is presented in a form that would today be called neuromuscular massage.

Additionally, there is apocryphal information that the Portuguese Jesuits who opened the first trade missions in China brought *Tuina* teaching manuals back to Europe in the seventeenth century. These manuals allegedly formed the basis of the Swedish Remedial Gymnastics and Movement Cure developed by Per Ling in the eighteenth century. If true, this suggests that Oriental bodywork is also the source of European massage.

Along with the rest of traditional medicine, therapeutic massage and bodywork fell out of favor during China's Republican Period (1911 - 1949). However, with the establishment of the People's Republic in 1949, the Chinese government recognized the basic genius of Traditional Chinese Medicine and made a massive effort to integrate it with modern Western medicine. By honoring the living masters of the healing arts and encouraging the study and integration of those arts into the medical mainstream of the world, medical practice in China has become a blend of traditional Chinese and Western medicine offered side-by-side in hospitals and clinics throughout the country. Today, depending on the sophistication of the region and local access to Western medicine, objective decisions based on clinical observation may point to the more effective therapies available in each case, regardless of their sources.

Therapeutic massage and bodywork has been a distinct medical specialty in every dynasty in China's history up to the present day, with medical schools and hospitals devoted exclusively to its practice, as well as departments for its study established in every school of traditional medicine and hospital. *Tuina-Anmo* is a doctoral discipline and requires 5 or 6 years of medical training, depending on the particular specialization. *Tuina* has developed primarily for the treatment of traumatic injury and pediatric care, while *Anmo* has become directed mainly towards the treatment of internal disease.

Mastery of bodywork has always been required of traditional physicians. It was integral to improvement of their digital sensitivity to help them develop the refined palpation skills necessary for competent diagnosis and practice of Chinese medicine.

The Chinese medical system is one of the oldest holistic paradigms of health in the world. Based on the naturalist observations of Taoist priests and refined by the Neo-Confucianists, the system includes a simple style of living based on moderation and attunement to natural cycles as the key to a long and harmonious life. The Chinese recognized that the highest ideals of human attainment — wisdom, serenity and compassion — accrue with age, and they venerated their elders. In a culture such as ours, which idealizes youth, this may be difficult to understand, but it is a significant and essential difference. In the Chinese medical view, the epitome of sophisticated refinement is learning the art of living in order to maintain vital clarity and health into old age. The medical arts focus on preventing disease, in addition to curing it.

In the Chinese view, preventive medicine requires more than curative arts. Of course, a practitioner must master subtle diagnostic skills and a comprehensive understanding of the sequence of patterns presented by various diseases in their stages of progression, as well as the treatment protocols necessary to re-establish a balanced, harmonious situation at any of those stages. These arts are essential and were brilliantly developed and embraced.

The diagnostic skills were incorporated into the Four Examinations: Looking, Asking, Listening/Smelling, and Touching. The Patterns of Disharmony were observed and described with a rich palette of discriminating filters: Eight Principles, Six Stages, Five Elements, Four Levels, Three Warmers, Yin and Yang, and Organ patterns. Treatment includes an exceptionally wide range of techniques, through herbs, diet, acupuncture and moxibustion, therapeutic massage and bodywork, exercise and mental discipline.

But the keystone of the system — the crown jewel of preventive medicine — was always moderate living — understanding how to live one's life skillfully to avoid the common degenerative diseases which rob life of its joy. The prescription for a long and happy life was clear, and included knowledgeable control of diet, appropriate exercise, meditation, adequate rest, moderation in all things and regular bodywork.

Because of this, Chinese physical medicine has evolved in a different climate than its Western counterpart. Bodywork has always been an integral and respected tool in the armamentarium of the Chinese physician. Physical manipulation has always been a medical discipline.

As a legitimate part of Chinese medicine, *Tuina* and *Anmo* have benefited from the use of TCM diagnostic methodology. Common injuries and illnesses are divided into various etiologies according to their symptoms. What is viewed by Western medicine as one and the same disease may have various causes, each of which presents itself in a slightly different fashion, and each of which requires a different treatment protocol. Tongue, Pulse and Differentiations According to the Eight Principles have been given, where applicable, to each condition under consideration in this book, which allows for precise, case-specific treatment.

Several thousand years of continuous development by countless handhealers of genius have given us an astonishing variety of hand techniques, and a sophisticated understanding of their technical use for the management of the flow of *Qi* in the human body. These techniques have all been classified by their various actions and prescribed according to the traditional Chinese understanding of anatomy and physiology.

Because the Chinese treat physical medicine as a single entity, the scope of practice of Therapeutic Massage and Bodywork includes all of the techniques we in the West usually divide into massage and bodywork, physical therapy and chiropractic. Spinal adjustments (called pulling or twisting here) are often used and clearly discussed in this text.

In order to use this book to its full potential, you should have a firm basic understanding of TCM. This will reveal the logic behind the selection and sequence of hand techniques and treatment locations. That logic, once clear, can be applied to any situation. For the expert practitioner and the student alike, the diagnostic differentiations and treatment protocols are an incredibly rich feast. Even if only learned by rote, the proper application of these techniques is a perfect way to learn the true heart of Oriental Bodywork, as well as a truly effective means of treating the conditions listed. Here are all the possibilities that have been revealed by a three thousand year inquiry into the art, distilled and reviewed by the modern masters of Shandong Province, China, and presented in well-written English.

All of them are here, as if handed to you on a silver platter — 45 different simple, complex and special hand techniques, presented in detail along with an analysis of their effects. More than 150 common medical, surgical, gynecological and traumatic conditions are discussed in detail, each with all their various etiologies and specific treatment protocols. There is also a succinct but thorough review of Chinese sports massage, as well as a section on self-massage, both for general health and maintenance, and for a variety of specific conditions, presented in detail.

You can't help learning Chinese Therapeutic Massage and Bodywork from this book. It's the best book on the subject ever written in the English language. It belongs in the library and curriculum of every Oriental bodywork therapist in the West.

Carl Dubitsky OBT, LMT, NCTMB
Boulder, Colorado, July 1993

Fundamentals

Principles of Therapeutic Massage

Principles of Therapeutic Massage

The principles of medical massage are the Theories of Yin-Yang, Five Elements, Yin and Yang Organs, Meridians and Collaterals, as well as Nutrient, Defense, Energy, and Blood Systems. The guidelines are the Four Methods of Examination, Eight Principles, Syndrome Differentiation and Therapy Selection. Through various techniques, massage may dredge Meridians and Collaterals, normalize Yin-Yang, harmonize the Nutrient and Defense Systems, rectify Vital Energy and Blood, and regulate the Yin and Yang Organs. As in other medical specialties, massage is inseparable from these fundamental theories of Traditional Chinese Medicine.

Relationship between Theories of Yin-Yang, Five Elements and Massage

Yin and Yang are general terms for the two opposite aspects of matter and energy in nature. They are interrelated to and contradicted by each other. They coexist in a dynamic state — an excess of one leads to a decrease in the other and vice versa. Under specific circumstances, Yin or Yang may be transmuted into its opposite. They are the source of the unceasing movement, variation and development of all things. Our ancestors pointed this out:

> Yin-Yang is the principle of Heaven and Earth, the guiding discipline of all things under the sun, the origin of change, the root and starting point of life and death, and the mansion of divinities. (Familiar Conversations, Ch. 5)

Every thing and every action belongs to either Yin or Yang. Generally speaking, matter and energy that are dynamic, external, upward, warm, obvious, increasing and hyperkinetic belong to the category of Yang. Those of the opposite belong to Yin. For example, the heavens would be Yang, the earth would be Yin; the sun would be Yang, the moon would be Yin; fire would be Yang while water is Yin; and warm is Yang while cold is Yin.

In the human body, the upper part is Yang, the lower is Yin; the back is Yang, the abdomen is Yin. The Six Hollow Organs are considered Yang, the Five Parenchymatous Organs, Yin. The Meridians of the Small Intestine, Triple Warmer, Large Intestine, Urinary Bladder, Gall Bladder, Stomach and Governor Vessel all are considered Yang, while those of Heart, Pericardium, Lung, Kidney, Liver, Spleen and Conception Vessel would be Yin.

The Eight Traditional Methods of Massage are also classified according to Yin and Yang. Techniques which require forceful actions and aggressive techniques such as nipping, grasping, dotting, etc., belong to Yang and produce purging effects. Those techniques which involve soft manipulation and gentle techniques such as stroking, round-rubbing, revolving, etc., belong to Yin and produce invigorating effect. Some techniques are directly named for this relationship, such as "Divide Yin-Yang, Combine Yin-Yang," etc.

In normal physiological conditions, the Yin and Yang of the human body maintain a state of active equilibrium. If this equilibrium is violated, there will be disharmony between Yin and Yang and diseases occur.

> *Fair Yin and firm Yang make a peaceful and orderly vitality. When Yin and Yang dissociate, vital essence and energy die out.* (Ibid., Ch. 3) *An excess of Yang brings about heat syndrome; an excess of Yin brings about cold syndrome.* (Ibid., Ch. 5)

Although clinical manifestations of diseases are multiple, complex and endlessly variable, they still must be included in the categories of Yin and Yang. The variations of disease conditions may also be regarded as the result of the waxing and waning of Yin-Yang, and well as of their mutual transformation. Ancient doctors pointed out that one should select a therapeutic method in line with the changing tendency of disease.

> *For evils which originate outside the skin, expel them with profuse sweating; for fierce and aggressive ones, press and restrain them; for those of Excess, disperse and discharge them. Examine the Yin-Yang attribute of the disease to determine the use of the gentle and the forceful. Treat Yin when Yang falls ill, treat Yang when Yin falls ill. Tranquilize Vital Energy and Blood — let each of them guard its post. When Blood is excessive, the patient ought to be bled; when Vital Energy is deficient, the patient ought to be massaged.* (Ibid.)

Traditional Chinese massage closely relates techniques with Meridians and Points. Massage may invigorate the patient's resistance, expel pathogenic factors and regulate the balance between Yin and Yang. For example, in treating hypertension due to deficiency of Liver-Kidney Yin, the therapeutic principle is to nourish the Yin and tranquilize the uprising of Liver Yang. Therefore, we select points of the Kidney Meridian and Knead Yaoyan (Ex-B 3), Sanyinjiao (Sp 6), Yongquan (K 1), etc., to nourish the Yin. Since Liver and Gall Bladder are related in an intra-extra manner, we may select Gall Bladder Meridian points, and grasp Fengchi (GB 20) and dot Huantiao (GB 30), to simultaneously purge the Liver Yang.

The Theory of Five Elements is an ancient philosophic concept explaining the composition of the natural world. Traditional Chinese doctors used this theory to describe the anatomical bases of the human body, the physiological functions of various systems and their pathological phenomena.

Ancient doctors matched the Five Yin Organs with the Five Elements and accepted them as the centers of the body. Additionally, they held that the human body corresponds with the variations of nature through the Five Directions, the Five Seasons, the Five Colors, etc., and that the integrity of the body is achieved through the functions of the Meridians and Collaterals. The relationship between the Five Yin Organs is found in the principles of the Five Elements Theory: Generation, Control, Invasion, Insult. Pathogenesis, prevention and treatment of diseases are explained on the basis of this theory.

> If the Energy of an Element is in excess, what it conquers is subdued, and what it does not conquer is insulted; if the Energy of an Element is deficient, what it does not conquer is insulted and subjugated, and what it conquers is despised and insulted. (Ibid., Ch. 67)

Traditional Chinese massage therapists obtain data through the Four Methods of Examination — Looking, Listening-Smelling, Asking, and Touching (Pulse Feeling and Palpation). By analyzing this data in accordance with Five Elements Theory, the origin, location and nature of a disease may be learned.

Treatment should be considered and selected according to the following principles:

> Seek those which exist and those which do not exist.
> Treat those in excess and those which are deficient.
> Purge the South — invigorate the North.
> Provide Water to nourish Wood.
> Assist Metal to control Wood.
> Invigorate Fire to generate Earth.
> Strengthen Water to quench Fire.
> Support Earth to inhibit Wood, etc.

In addition, specific therapeutic measures should be used, such as eliminating Vital Energy stagnation and Blood stasis. All these principles and procedures come from clinical practice and conform to the Theory of Five Elements. For instance, in treating insomnia due to dissociation of Heart and Kidney, we nip Shenmen (H 7), Lingdao (H 4), Tongli (H 5) and Shaohai (H 3); we grasp the armpit to quench Heart Fire; round-rub Yaoyan (Ex-B 3); push Yongquan (K 1); and knead Sanyinjiao (Sp 6) to nourish Kidney Water. This is the method of "Purge the South — invigorate the North."

In short, Yin-Yang and Five Elements Theory are fundamental metaphors from ancient times. They were the origins of Traditional Chinese Medicine, including Traditional Chinese massage, and are still effective in guiding our clinical practices. Of course, we must be aware there are also some elements in them reflecting their historical period of birth, and they should be studied and analyzed with discrimination, guided by the rationale of "One divides into two."

Relationship between Massage and Organs-Meridians

Organs and Meridians are important components of the human body. Theories of Yin and Yang Organs, and Twelve or Fourteen Meridians are the roots of Traditional Chinese Medicine. Our ancestors emphasized that if one fails to understand theories of Organs and Meridians, one will inevitably make mistakes as soon as talk or work begins.

There are Five Yin and Six Yang Organs, and several extraordinary internal organs within the human body. There are Twelve Regular Meridians, their related Collaterals, and, according to some schools of TCM, two Extra Meridians. They form a network connecting the entire body.

> *Internally, Twelve Meridians link up with every organ. Externally, they connect with all limbs and joints.*
> (Spiritual Pivot, Ch. 33)

Through the anatomical and physiological connection of Meridians and Collaterals, various tissues and organs comprise an integrated human body. In massage therapy, as in other areas of TCM, diseases may be analyzed, diagnosed and treated according to theories of Organs and Meridians.

It is said that what is in the interior must manifest itself in the exterior. Therefore, pathological changes within the body may be detected externally. On the basis of the organs' functions and the manifested symptoms and signs, we can determine the location and nature of the disease, and select appropriate areas, points and techniques for treatment. For instance, according to the principle that Spleen is related to the mouth, responsible for transportation and conversion, and the nourishment of muscles, we may infer that poor appetite, tastelessness in the mouth, pale lips, loose stool, muscular atrophy and the like are signs and symptoms of Spleen disease, bringing us to conclude that areas and/or points of Spleen and Stomach Meridians should be massaged.

Illness of internal organs may also exhibit their signs and symptoms along traveling routes of Meridians to which they are attached. Heart Meridian of Hand Shaoyin starts from Heart and branches off from Heart Network. Its chief offshoot leaves Heart Network for Lung, emerges out of the axilla, travels along the flexor side of the upper arm medially and posteriorly, and passes through the elbow and the forearm medially and posteriorly. Therefore, chest pain, rib cage distension and pain, back and interscapular pain, as well as pain on the medial sides of the arms are evidence of Heart disease. Accordingly, areas and/or points of the Heart Meridian should be massaged.

Diseases of one internal organ may influence or invade another internal organ, even harass the entire body through the Meridians. Under these circumstances, appropriate areas and points can only be selected after the various interrelations and interconnections have been fully considered. If Depressed Liver attacks Spleen, there will be poor appetite, belching, regurgitation, and such symptoms. In this case, we should massage areas and/or points of both Liver and Spleen. If Lung heat invades Large Intestine, there will be constipation and the like, and we should massage locales and/or points of both Large Intestine and Lung.

In Chapter 10 of *Spiritual Pivot*, there is such an account: "Branches of Kidney Meridian depart from Lung, connect with Heart, and terminate in the chest." This implies that Heart communicates with Kidney. Heart Fire descends to warm Kidney — Kidney Water ascends to irrigate Heart. Under normal conditions, they regulate each other to maintain the homeostasis of Yin and Yang. If Heart and Kidney dissociate, the symptoms will be vexation, insomnia, reddened tongue, thready and rapid pulse, etc. To treat this disorder, Heart Fire should be quenched by grasping the armpit, nipping Shenmen (H 7), etc., while Kidney Water must be replenished by pushing and kneading Yongquan (K 1), Sanyinjiao (Sp 6), etc. In order to promote the mutual communication between Heart and Kidney, and to secure harmony between Yin and Yang, multiple manipulations and techniques should be used.

Exogenous evils may also invade the body through the Meridians. "First, the invasion of exogenous evils starts at the skin. If the body fails to expel them at this stage, they take residence in the minute branches of the Collaterals. If the body fails to expel them at this stage, they go on to reside in the Collaterals. If the body still does not expel them at this stage, they inhabit the Meridians which connect with internal organs." *Familiar Conversations*, (Ch. 63) Massage therapy can dredge Meridians, harmonize Yin and Yang, regulate internal organs, and expel exogenous evils, because its techniques act on areas and points on Meridians. Sometimes massage therapy may elicit sensations of soreness, heaviness, numbness and distension, as those elicited in acupuncture.

It is important to bear in mind that Theories of Organs and Meridians were derived from clinical practice over a long period of time, and are still of great significance in massage today.

Descriptions of the Paths of Fourteen Commonly Used Meridians and Selected Points

The Lung Meridian of Hand Taiyin originates from the middle Energizer, connects with the Large Intestine, then turns upwards along the opening of the Stomach, passes through the diaphragm and links to the Lung. From there it emerges out of the armpit from the Lung Network, travels along the front of the inner side of the upper arm down to the elbow, then advances along the outside of the forearm, enters into the wrist, passes Yuji (Lu 10) and ends at the tip of the thumb. It has a branch which departs from it before reaching the wrist, and runs along the inner side of the index finger to its tip.

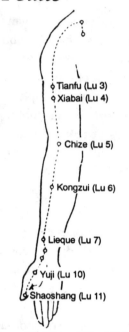

Lung Meridian of Hand Taiyin

The Large Intestine Meridian of Hand Yangming starts at the medial tip of the index finger, travels up the hand between the first and second metacarpal bones and two tendons, continues along the lateral anterior edge of the arm to the shoulder, the spine and Quepen (St 12). There it connects with the Lung and links to the Large Intestine. A branch of this Meridian rises from Quepen (St 12), passes through the neck and the cheek and ends in the gums. Its left and right branches emerge from the mouth, cross at Renzhong (GV 26) and end beside the nostrils.

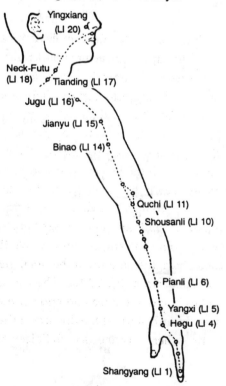

Large Intestine Meridian of Hand Yangming

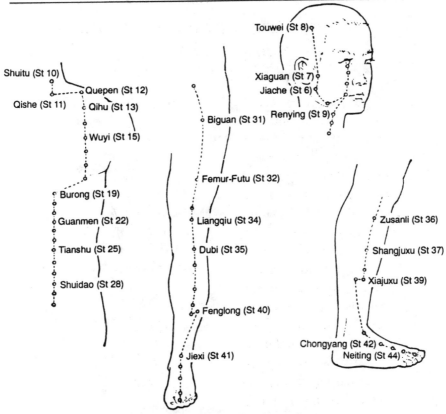

Stomach Meridian of Foot Yangming

The Stomach Meridian of Foot Yangming begins at the sides of the nose, enters the upper gums, emerges from the mouth, curves down around the lips where the branches intersect at Chengjiang (CV 24), then passes beneath the cheek to Daying (St 5), along the jaw line through Jiache (St 6) to Xiaguan (St 7), and up along the hair line to the forehead. At Daying (St 5), a branch descends through Renying (St 9) and the throat, enters Quepen (St 12), continues down through the diaphragm to enter the Stomach and connect with the Spleen. A straight branch descends from Quepen (St 12) travels down the chest, passes beside the navel and enters Qijie (St 30). Another straight branch begins at the opening of the Stomach, descends within the abdomen and joins the previous branch at Qijie (St 30) where the two become one and continue down through Biguan (St 31), Futu (St 32), the patella, the anterior of the tibia, the dorsal side of the foot and ends at the lateral tip of the 2d toe. There is another branch which starts 3 Body Inches below the knee and ends at the lateral tip of the middle toe. One more branch starts at the dorsum of the foot, enters the big toe and ends at its tip (where it connects with Spleen Meridian of Foot Taiyin).

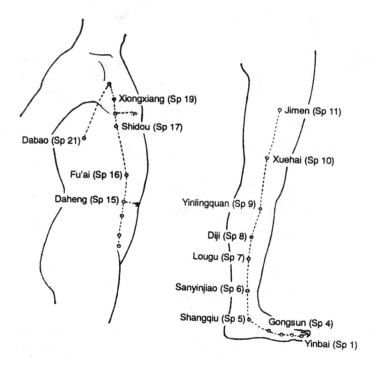

The Spleen Meridian of Foot Taiyin

The Spleen Meridian of Foot Taiyin begins at the medial tip of the big toe and travels along the junction of red and white skin, through the first metatarsal joint, rising forward of the malleolus medialis, then enters the calf and rises along the back of the tibia to the knee, continuing up along the front of the thigh to enter the abdomen. There it enters the Spleen, connects with the Stomach, passes through the diaphragm, through the pharynx, and the root of the tongue and ends on the underside of the tongue. There is also a branch which rises from the Stomach and passes through the diaphragm to the Heart, where it links with the Heart Meridian of Hand Shaoyin.

The Heart Meridian of Hand Shaoyin begins in the Heart, linking the Heart Network, and passes down through the diaphragm to connect with the Small Intestine. A branch rises from the Heart Network, passes through the throat and joins the Eye Network. Another branch rises from the Heart Network through the lung, passes out through the armpit, travels along the inner back of the arm through the palm along the inner side of the little finger to the tip where it ends, linking with the Small Intestine Meridian of Hand Taiyang. (See illlustration on next page.)

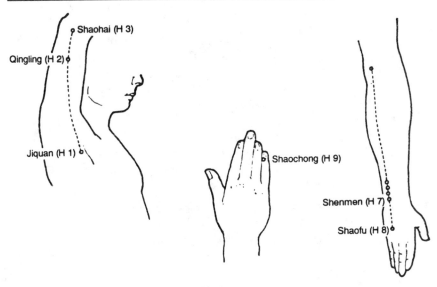

The Heart Meridian of Hand Shaoyin

The Small Intestine Meridian of Hand Taiyang begins at the ulnar side of the tip of the little finger, rises along the back of the hand, emerging at the ulnar joint and rises along the back of the fore- and upper arm to emerge at Jianjing (GB 21). It then winds around the scapula, crosses the shoulder, goes through Quepen (St 12), connects with the Heart, passes through the diaphragm, through the stomach and enters the Small Intestine. One branch of this Meridian goes from Quepen (St 12), rises along the neck to the cheek, to the outer corner of the eye, and then turns, ending in the ear. Another branch starts at the cheek, rises to the bottom of the orbit, to the inner corner of the eye (where it meets the Urinary Bladder Meridian of Foot Taiyang) and ends at the zygomatic arch.

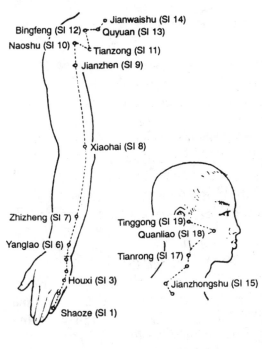

Small Intestine Meridian of Hand Taiyang

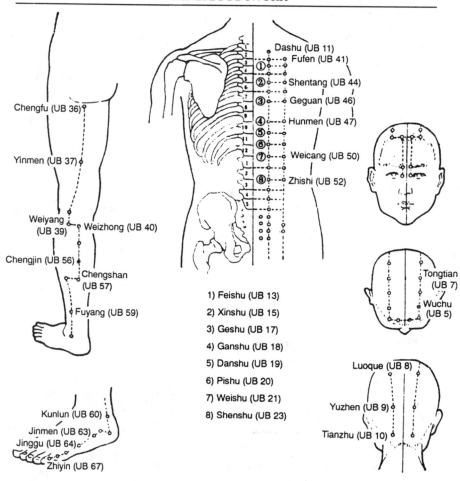

Chengfu (UB 36)

Yinmen (UB 37)

Weiyang (UB 39) Weizhong (UB 40)

Chengjin (UB 56)

Chengshan (UB 57)

Fuyang (UB 59)

Kunlun (UB 60)
Jinmen (UB 63)
Jinggu (UB 64)
Zhiyin (UB 67)

Dashu (UB 11)
Fufen (UB 41)
Shentang (UB 44)
Geguan (UB 46)
Hunmen (UB 47)

Weicang (UB 50)

Zhishi (UB 52)

1) Feishu (UB 13)
2) Xinshu (UB 15)
3) Geshu (UB 17)
4) Ganshu (UB 18)
5) Danshu (UB 19)
6) Pishu (UB 20)
7) Weishu (UB 21)
8) Shenshu (UB 23)

Tongtian (UB 7)
Wuchu (UB 5)

Luoque (UB 8)

Yuzhen (UB 9)

Tianzhu (UB 10)

Urinary Bladder Meridian of Foot Taiyang

The **Urinary Bladder Meridian of Foot Taiyang** begins at the inner corner of the eye, rises through the forehead to the crown. One branch descends from the crown to the temple. A straight branch descends from the crown, passes through the brain to emerge at the nape, traveling down the neck, shoulder and back parallel to the spine, to enter the abdomen through the back muscles, connects with the Kidney and joins the Urinary Bladder. A third branch descends from the lumbar region along the spine through the gluteal area to the popliteal fossa. A fourth branch begins at the inner side of the scapula, descends parallel to the spine, passing the hip cup, along the side and back of the thigh to join the previous branch at the popliteal fossa. This combined branch passes through the calf, emerging behind the lateral malleolus, traveling the fifth metatarsal past Jinggu (UB 64) to end at the outer tip of the little toe, where it links with the Kidney Meridian of Foot Shaoyin.

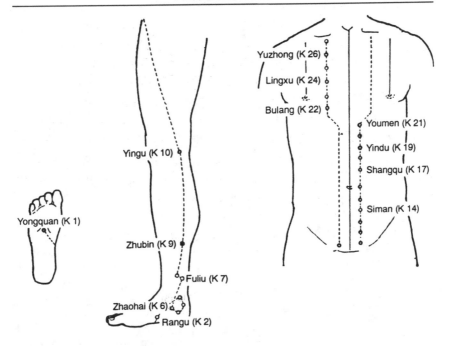

Kidney Meridian of Foot Shaoyin

The **Kidney Meridian of Foot Shaoyin** begins at the base of the little toe and runs obliquely to the arch, emerges from beneath Rangu (K 2), and passes along behind the medial malleolus (where a minute branch descends to the heel). The Meridian continues, rising within the calf to emerge at the inner popliteal fossa, up the back of the inner thigh, through the spine to connect with the Kidney and connect with the Urinary Bladder. It has a straight branch which extends from the Kidney past the Liver, through the diaphragm, through the Lung, along the throat to end at the root of the tongue. A second branch rises from the middle thigh to the perineum, to the lower abdomen, passing beside the midline, continues on the same line up to the upper abdomen and chest and ends at the lower edge of the clavicle. Another branch passes from the Lung to the Heart to the chest, where it links with the Pericardium Meridian of Hand Jueyin.

The **Pericardium Meridian of Hand Jueyin** begins in the center of the chest where it links the Pericardium and enters the Triple Warmer (Sanjiao). A branch of this Meridian begins in the chest and emerges 3 Body Inches below the armpit, ascends to the armpit, then travels along the inner upper arm between the Lung and Heart Meridians, extends between two tendons of the forearm, along the midline of the palm to end at the tip of the middle finger. A branch goes from the palm to the tip of the ring finger and links with the Triple Warmer Meridian of Hand Shaoyang. (See illlustration on next page.)

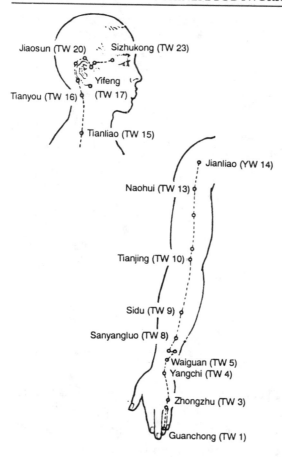

Triple Warmer Meridian of Hand Shaoyang

The **Triple Warmer Meridian of Hand Shaoyang** begins at the tip of the ring finger and goes up along the outside of the finger and the back of the hand. It crosses the wrist, runs between the ulna and radius, through the elbow, up the outside of the arm, crosses the Gall Bladder Meridian of Foot Shaoyang, enters Quepen (St 12), crosses over and enters the chest to connect with the Pericardium. From there it passes through the diaphragm and links the Upper, Middle and Lower Warmers. A branch comes out of the Pericardium, emerges at Quepen (St 12), rises along the nape, comes forward around and over the ear, then descends to the cheek and ends at the lower orbit. Another branch begins behind the ear, enters the ear and emerges at the front of it, ending at the outer corner of the eye, where it links with the Gall Bladder Meridian of Foot Shaoyang.

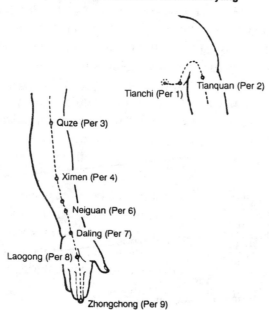

Pericardium Meridian of Hand Jueyin

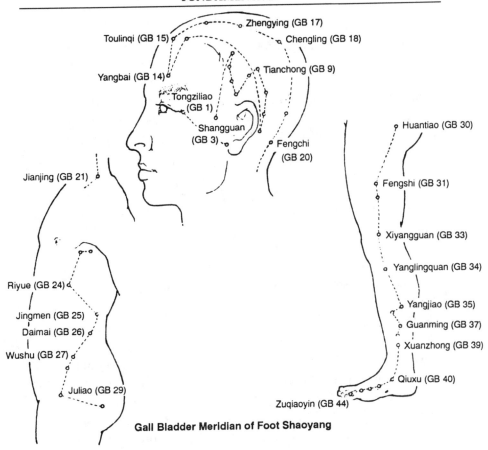

Gall Bladder Meridian of Foot Shaoyang

The Gall Bladder Meridian of Foot Shaoyang begins at the outer corner of the eye, rises to the corner of the forehead, descends behind the ear, down the neck to the shoulder to enter Quepen (St 12). A branch begins behind the ear, enters into the ear, emerging at the front and finishes just behind the outer corner of the eye. Another branch begins at the outer corner of the eye, descends to Daying (St 5), meets the Triple Warmer Meridian, passes to the lower orbit, then goes down to Jiache (St 6), along the neck, enters Quepen (St 12), passes through the chest and the diaphragm, connects with the Liver and links to the Gall Bladder. From there, it travels along the interior of the rib cage, emerges from Qichong (St 30), winds around above the external genitals to enter the hip cup transversely. A straight branch leaves Quepen (St 12), descends along the armpit and the flank to meet the previous branch at the hip cup. From there, the combined branch runs down the outer leg, to Xuanzhong (GB 39), passes the front of the lateral malleolus, across the top of the foot to end at the lateral tip of the fourth toe. Another branch comes from the top of the foot to the tip of the big toe, where it links with the Liver Meridian of Foot Jueyin.

The **Liver Meridian of Foot Jueyin** begins on the dorsum of the big toe, passes along the top of the foot and turns up 1 Body Inch before the medial malleolus. It rises to a spot 8 Body Inches above the medial malleolus and crosses the Spleen Meridian of Foot Taiyin, then rises along the leg, to the popliteal fossa and up the inner thigh to a point above the external genitals. It winds around the external genitals and enters the lower abdomen, links the Liver, connects with the Gall Bladder, passes along the side of the Stomach, then penetrates the diaphragm, branches out at the rib cage to the back of the throat, to the opening of the parotid gland and the Eye Network, emerging from the forehead to meet the Governor Vessel Meridian at the crown of the head. A branch comes from the Eye Network, passes down the inside of the cheek, and winds around inside the lips. Another branch extends from the Liver to pass through the diaphragm and end in the Lung.

The **Conception Vessel Meridian** begins inside the pelvis (lower part of Zhongji (CV 3), rises above the external genitals along the midline inside the abdomen past Guanyuan (CV 4) to the throat, where it divides into two branches, ascends along the cheeks and enters the eyes.

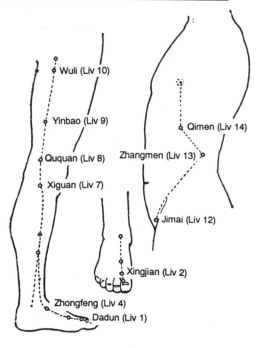

Liver Meridian of Foot Jueyin

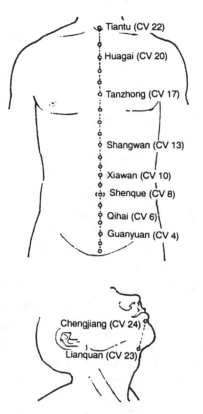

Conception Vessel Meridian

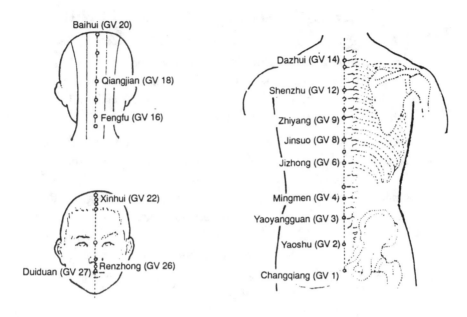

Governor Vessel Meridian

The **Governor Vessel Meridian** originates in the bottom of the lower abdomen. In females, it contacts the opening of the ureter, connects with the external genitals and the perineum, meets Foot Shaoyin, combines with the Collaterals of Taiyang, then passes up through the spine and links with the Kidney. It also starts at the inner corner of the eye with the Taiyang Meridian, rises along the forehead, crosses its opposite branch at the crown of the head, enters the skull and connects with the brain, then descends along the nape of the neck down both sides of the spine to the lumbar region, where it enters the body and connects with the Kidney. In males, the Governor Vessel Meridian's course is similar to that in females, with this addition: a branch rises straight from the lower abdomen, passes through the navel and the Heart, enters the throat, to the lower cheek, where it winds around the lips and ends between the eyes.

(This section is presented as a general overview of concepts. For a comprehensive examination of meridians and points, we recommend a dedicated text on the subject, such as Acupuncture, Meridian Theory, and Acupuncture Points *by Li Ding, Pacific View Press, 1992.)*

Relationship between Nutrient Energy (Ying), Defensive Energy (Wei), Vital Energy (Qi), Blood (Xue) and Massage

Nutrient Energy, Defensive Energy, Vital Energy and Blood are important constituents of the human body, and the substance of stimulating forces. They moisten, nourish, and warm the body, defend it against harm and maintain normal physiological activity.

Nutrient Energy and Defensive Energy are converted from the essence of food and drink. The former is the clear and gentle part of the essence, circulating through the vessels and nourishing the whole body. The latter is the fierce and aggressive aspect of the essence, traveling swiftly and smoothly outside the vessels. Ancient doctors pointed this out.

> *Mankind receives Vital Energy from grains. After having been taken into the Stomach, their essence is transported to the Lung, where it is distributed to various internal organs. The clear part of such essence is called Ying, the turbid part is called Wei.* (Spiritual Pivot, Ch. 18)
>
> *Nutrient Energy releases fluids and juices into the vessels which transform into Blood, nourishing the four limbs, Five Yin and Six Yang Organs. Defensive Energy warms the muscles, replenishes the skin, enriches the juncture between muscles and the skin, and commands the opening and closing of sweat pores.* (Ibid. Ch. 71)

Vital Energy is the commander of Blood — Blood is the mother of Vital Energy. Blood circulates because Vital Energy acts as its motive force. When Vital Energy stagnates, there will be stasis of Blood. When Vital Energy is uninhibited, the circulation of Blood will be helped. Vital Energy may be classified as both an inborn and post-partum element. The former refers to Kidney Energy and the latter refers to Spleen-Stomach Energy and Lung Energy. Vital Energy cannot be separated from the internal organs. If there are dysfunctions of the organs, the source of Vital Energy and Blood would be impaired and their circulation inhibited.

As we have noted, the generation, transportation and distribution of Nutrient Energy, Defensive Energy, Vital Energy and Blood are closely related to the Five Yin and Six Yang Organs. The Kidney stores essence which is converted into Blood; the Heart directs the Blood; the Liver stores the Blood, and the Spleen controls Blood. The Lung directs Vital Energy; the Kidney takes in Celestial Energy with the Lung and promotes breath; the Liver disperses energy, etc.

The crucial element of life is motion. "Ascending, descending, coming in and going out are fundamental patterns of Vital Energy motion; every internal organ participates in these motions." *Familiar Conversations* (Ch. 68) If these motions are inhibited, there will be pathological changes such as the depression of Liver Energy, the adverse rising of Stomach Energy, the sinking of Spleen Energy, the stasis and obstruction of Lung Energy, etc.

By acting on areas and/or points of the human body, through direct or indirect mechanisms of the Meridians, massage can promote the circulation of Vital Energy and Blood, and thereby regulate and normalize disorders of internal organs. For example, in treating depression and stagnation of Liver Energy, we rub and round-rub both rib cage regions from top to bottom, push Tanzhong (CV 17) to either side, and revolve Huantiao (GB 30) with the elbow. If a patient suffers from Deficiency of Spleen, there will be signs and symptoms of poor appetite, dyspepsia, emaciation, shortness of breath, pale complexion, pale tongue with white fur, slow and weak pulse, etc. We round-rub Zhongwan (CV 12), knead Zusanli (St 36) and Pishu (UB 20), pinch the spine, etc. In other words, we enrich the patient's Vital Energy and Blood through stimulation of Spleen and Stomach.

Since massage regulates the functions of the Meridians and internal organs, it may increase one's vitality. Clinical experiences have demonstrated that those who practice prophylactic massage are usually full of vigor, calm of mind, healthy and physically strong. Their eyesight and hearing are good and their reactions are quick and agile.

Relationship between Muscle, Tendon, Bone, Joints and Massage

Muscles, tendons, bones and joints are structures of locomotion. Bones establish the shape, while the others enable physical activity. Tendons are tough and sturdy and connect the bones and muscles. Bending and stretching, grasping and releasing, standing and walking — all these activities depend on the extension and contraction of muscles and tendons. Bones belong to the Extraordinary Yang Organs. In each joint cavity, there is synovial fluid which acts as a lubricant.

These structures of locomotion are all nourished by Vital Energy and Blood, and they are closely related to the internal organs. The exogenous evils which attack the body may also attack the locomotive structures. These structures are also prone to injury by trauma. In Essentials of Bone-Setting in *The Golden Mirror of Medicine*, there are instructive accounts:

> *All bones are not of the same type in a body. The arrangement*
> *and connections of the Twelve Tendon Meridians are also*

different. It is necessary for doctors to be well acquainted with their shapes, locations, and distribution. In clinical practice, we should be clever in selecting appropriate techniques and performing them with agile hands according to the various conditions and circumstances. Such techniques may include dragging to separate in order to reunite, pushing to approach a spot in order to reposition it, or putting right the oblique to perfect the flaw. The types of fractures (horizontal, oblique, shattered, etc.) and the condition of tendons (flaccid, cramped, turning over, separated, joined together, etc.) may be learned by palpation. Understanding these circumstances, the suffering of patients can be relieved after performance of the appropriate measures.

In treating diseases of the locomotive structures, one should distinguish Cold syndromes from Heat syndromes.

In Cold syndrome, the tendon is tense. In Heat syndrome, the tendon is flaccid. (A Collection of Traumatological Classics written by Hu Tingguan in the Qing Dynasty.)

If Dampness and Heat are not eliminated, the large tendon shrinks and becomes shortened; the small tendon stretches and becomes lengthened. Shrinking can cause permanent contraction. Stretching can cause atrophy. (Familiar Conversation Ch. 3)

The Paths and Branches of the Twelve Tendinomuscular Meridians

Taiyang Tendinomuscular Meridian of the Foot (Urinary Bladder) starts from the little toe, passes along the outside of the ankle, and rises obliquely to join the knee. Its lower branch passes along the outside of the ankle, joins the heel, and rises to the popliteal fossa. Another branch travels to the outside of the calf to rise and combine with the previous branch. The combined branch rises to the buttocks, and passes parallel to the spine to the nape of the neck. From here, a branch rises to join the root of the tongue, while a straight branch rises to the occiput, then to the crown of the head, then descends to the nose. Another branch spreads over the upper eyelid and ends just below the zygomatic arch. Still another branch rises from the back, passes transversely across the shoulder and joins Jianyu (Liv 15). A branch of this enters the armpit, emerges at Quepen (St 12) and rises to Wangu (GB 12); another branch departs from Quepen (St 12) and rises obliquely to the area below the zygomatic arch. (See illlustration on next page.)

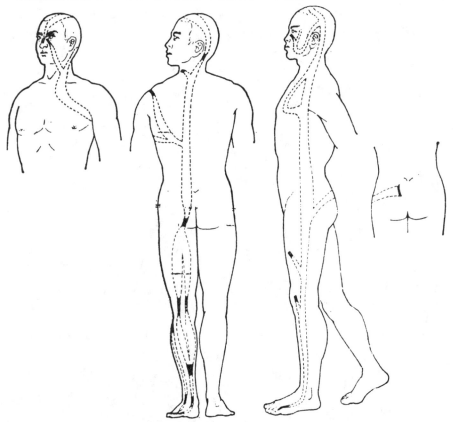

**Taiyang Tendinomuscular Meridian
of the Foot (Urinary Bladder)**

**Shaoyang Tendinomuscular Meridian
of the Foot (Gall Bladder)**

Shaoyang Tendinomuscular Meridian of the Foot (Gall Bladder) begins at the 4th toe and rises along the outside of the ankle, the tibia and the knee, to the upper part of the femur at Futu (St 32). Its branch rises from the fibula to the thigh and joins the hipbone. A straight branch rises along the flank, passes in front of the armpit, connecting the breast, and joins Quepen (St 12). Another straight branch rises from the armpit, passes through Quepen (St12), passes in front of Taiyang (UB) behind the ear to the corner of the forehead, crosses its opposite branch at the crown, then descends to the chin and rises to the zygomatic arch. A branch of this rises to the outside corner of the eye.

Yangming Tendinomuscular Meridian of the Foot (Stomach) rises from the 2d, 3rd, and 4th toes along the dorsum of the foot, passing obliquely across the bones of the lower leg to the outside of the knee, then rises straight to the hip cup and travels along the rib cage to link the spine. A straight branch rises along the shank to the knee, with its own branch which crosses the fibula to Shaoyang (GB). Another straight branch rises along the front of the thigh to the hipbone, curves into the external genitals, and spreads in the abdomen to join Quepen (St 12). From there it rises through

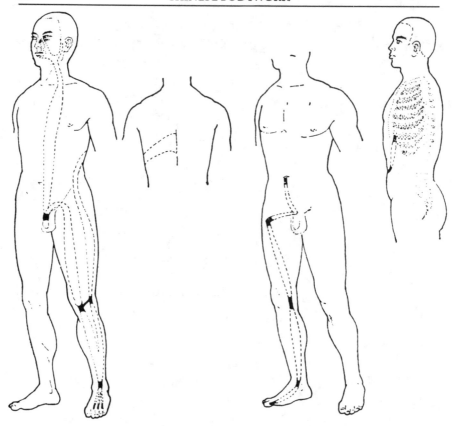

Yangming Tendinomuscular Meridian
of the Foot (Stomach)

Taiyin Tendinomuscular Meridian
of the Foot (Spleen)

the neck, passes by the mouth to just below the zygomatic arch, to the nose
to join with Taiyang (UB). Its branch extends from the neck to a spot in front
of the ear. (Taiyang [UB] extends over the upper eyelid. Yangming [St]
extends across the lower eyelid.)

Taiyin Tendinomuscular Meridian of the Foot (Spleen) rises from the
medial tip of the big toe to the inner ankle. Its straight branch rises along
the tibia to the medial of the knee, passes up the thigh to the hipbone, and
collects at the external genitals. From there, it rises across the abdomen to
join the navel, passes inside to join the rib cage and spreads in the chest.
When inside the body, it holds to the spine.

Shaoyin Tendinomuscular Meridian of the Foot (Kidney) starts at the
base of the little toe and passes obliquely under the inner ankle, to Taiyin
(Sp), to the heel, rises to join with Taiyang (UB), continues behind the tibia
along the inner thigh where it combines again with Taiyin (Sp), to the
external genitals, from which it rises inside the body, along the spine to the
nape of the neck to meet the occiput and unite again with Taiyang (UB).
(See illlustration on next page.)

Jueyin Tendinomuscular Meridian of the Foot (Liver) rises from the big toe to just forward of the inner ankle, along the shank, beneath the tibia, along the inner thigh to the external genitals and connects with the tendinomuscular Meridians there.

Taiyang Tendinomuscular Meridian of the Hand (Small Intestine) rises from the little finger to the wrist, along the inner forearm to a spot at the back of the elbow (where a sensation radiating back to the little finger may be induced when the spot is flicked). From there it rises to and enters the armpit. A branch passes behind the armpit, winds around the scapula, rises along the neck in front of Taiyang of the Foot (UB) and joins Wangu (GB 12) behind the ear. A branch leaves this spot and enters the ear. A straight branch emerges from the ear, descends to the chin and rises to the outer corner of the eye.

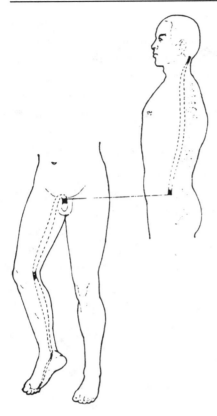

**Shaoyin Tendinomuscular Meridian
of the Foot (Kidney)**

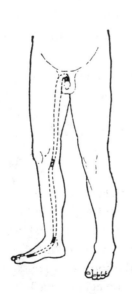

**Jueyin Tendinomuscular Meridian
of the Foot (Liver)**

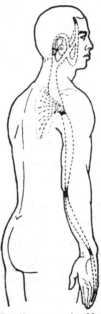

**Taiyang Tendinomuscular Meridian
of the Hand (Small Intestine)**

Shaoyang Tendinomuscular Meridian of the Hand (Triple Warmer) rises from the tip of the 4th finger to the wrist, along the forearm to the elbow, then rises along the outside of the upper arm to the shoulder and the neck, and unites with Taiyang of the Hand (SI). A branch rises through the mandibular joint to the root of the tongue. Another branch rises to Jiache (St 6), passes in front of the ear to link the outer corner of the eye and the chin, and ends above the ear.

Yangming Tendinomuscular Meridian of the Hand (Large Intestine) rises from the tip of the index finger through the wrist, along the forearm to the outside of the elbow, then rises along the upper arm to the tip of the shoulder. A branch winds around the scapula alongside the spine. A straight branch rises from the tip of the shoulder to the neck. Another branch rises to the cheek to just below the zygoma. Another straight branch rises in front of Taiyang of the Hand (SI), above the ear, across the crown and descends to the chin.

Taiyin Tendinomuscular Meridian of the Hand (Lung) rises along the thumb from its tip to the area behind the thenar mound, then continues along to the radial artery and forearm to the elbow. From there it passes along the inner upper arm, enters the armpit, emerges from Quepen (St 12) to pass along the front of the shoulder tip and returns to Quepen (St 12),

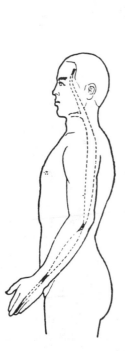

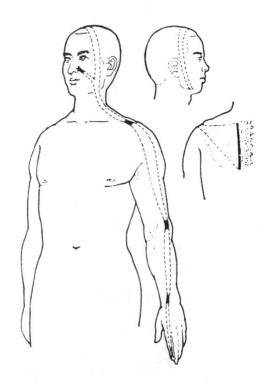

Shaoyang Tendinomuscular Meridian
of the Hand (Triple Warmer)

Yangming Tendinomuscular Meridian
of the Hand (Large Intestine)

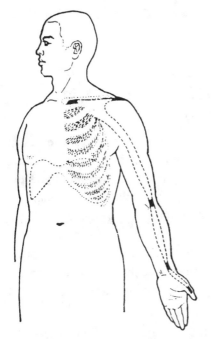

Taiyin Tendinomuscular Meridian
of the Hand (Lung)

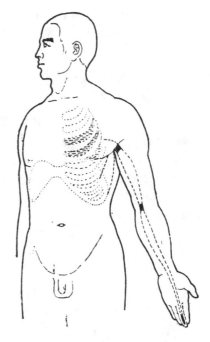

Jueyin Tendinomuscular Meridian
of the Hand (Pericardium)

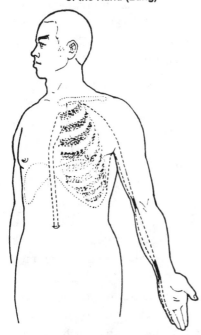

Shaoyin Tendinomuscular Meridian
of the Hand (Heart)

descends into the inner chest, spreads out through the upper opening of the Stomach (cardia), joins back together below, to the rib cage.

Jueyin Tendinomuscular Meridian of the Hand (Pericardium) rises from the middle finger beside the Taiyin tendinomuscular Meridian of the Hand (Lu) to the inner elbow, along the inner side of the upper arm to enter the armpit, where it descends and spreads out through both front and rear of the rib cage. A branch enters the armpit and spreads through the chest to the upper opening of the Stomach.

Shaoyin Tendinomuscular Meridian of the Hand (Heart) rises from the inner side of the little finger through the bone at the base of the palm to the inner side of the elbow, then continues upwards to enter the armpit. From there it crosses Taiyin (Lu) to join with the interior of the chest, passes along the upper opening of the stomach, then descends to the navel.

Relationship between Massage and Syndrome Differentiation/Therapy Selection

Syndrome Differentiation/Therapy Selection is the basic rule and most prominent feature of both TCM and Traditional Chinese Massage. By using the Four Methods of Examination (Looking, Listening-Smelling, Asking, and Touching [Pulse Feeling and Palpation]), we can obtain comprehensive information about various signs and symptoms. By applying the Eight Principles of Differentiation (Yin-Yang, External-Internal, Cold-Heat, Deficiency-Excess), we can analyze this information and determine the nature of the disease. Of course, the doctor must be completely attentive to the patient and observe these rules strictly, because an incorrect diagnosis will lead to incorrect treatment and adverse effects.

The Four Methods are interrelated and mutually complementary. The Eight Principles are also interdependent. In deciding between the External and the Internal, Cold-Heat and Deficiency-Excess must simultaneously be taken into account. In determining Cold or Heat, External-Internal and Deficiency-Excess are integral factors to the decision. And these six principles are all governed by the first two: Yin and Yang.

Manifestations of disease are complex and erratic. In clinical practice, the primary and secondary conditions, the branch and root of the pathogenesis, and the degree of severity and urgency must also be considered and appraised.

Once we learn the exact nature and correct diagnosis of a disease, we may select appropriate therapeutic measures, such as nourishing Yin, invigorating Yang, relieving the External, discharging the Internal, warming the Cold, cooling the Heat, strengthening the Deficiency, attenuating the Excess, etc. For instance, we see a patient suffering from headache, stiffness of the neck, with aversion to cold, fever and chills, white fur on the tongue, and superficial pulse. These are signs and symptoms of the External and Excess, caused by exogenous evils of Wind and Cold. In order to induce perspiration and expel these evils, we may select the following: Open Celestial Gate, revolve Taiyang (Ex-HN 4), knead and grasp Fengchi (GB 20), dot and knead Dazhui (GV 14), grasp Quchi (LI 11) and Hegu (LI 4). However, since people's constitutions vary from one to another, the areas and/or points chosen, techniques selected, and amount of force exerted are subject to discretion, and one should not be bound unnecessarily by convention.

To be a qualified massage therapist, it is necessary to master the theoretical system and the essence of TCM in a comprehensive manner. Since space does not permit us to pursue this subject at appropriate length, please refer to a textbook of TCM for details on the Four Methods of Examination and the Eight Principles of Differentiation.

The Relationship between Massage and the Natural Environment

Human beings live in nature, are inseparable from nature, and are part of nature. We rely on the Essence of heaven and earth for our existence. Changes in the natural environment influence our bodies directly or indirectly, resulting in corresponding adjustment of the functions of various organs and systems. The concept, Man, as a microcosm, is connected with the macrocosm is a guideline of TCM, and it is reflected in physiology, pathology, diagnosis, treatment and prevention. For instance, in the warm weather from Spring to Summer, Yang Vital Energy develops and prospers. The texture of the skin becomes loose and there will be more perspiration and less urination. In the cold weather from Autumn to Winter, Yang Vital Energy shrinks and wanes. Yin Energy begins to develop, the skin becomes tense, and there will be less perspiration and more urination. Moreover, the pulse changes as the season changes. It is stringy in Spring, full in Summer, hairy in Autumn, and stony in Winter. *(See Familiar Conversations, Ch. 17.)* Diurnal cycles of physiological and pathological conditions have also been noticed in our tradition:

> The Yang Vital Energy is in charge of the External by day. It grows at daybreak, thrives at noon, and becomes void at sunset — thus the Energy Gate is closed. (Ibid., Ch.3)

The places where people live also influence the body.

> "Those who reside in the highland live a long life, while those who dwell in the lowland die young. (Ibid., Ch. 70)

So, massage therapy varies from person to person, from time to time, and from place to place. For instance, in Winter when the Yang Vital Energy wanes, we should avoid nourishing Yin, such as kneading Sanyinjiao (Sp 6), nipping Xuehai (Sp 10), Yanglingquan (GB 34) and Yongquan (K 1), etc., so as not to impair the Yang Vital Energy. In Summer, when the Yang Vital Energy prospers and discharges into the outside environment, we should avoid opening the Celestial Gate, revolving Taiyang (Ex-HN 4), grasping Fengchi (GB 20), and nipping Dazhui (GV 14), so as not to deplete the body fluid and Energy. Although these are not absolute stipulations, we must bear them in mind in clinical practice. In another type of situation, in treating a patient suffering from rheumatoid arthritis, we should be aware of the humidity. When we are in an arid region, the technique should be somewhat gentle; in a humid environment, the technique should be appropriately more energetic, and the course of treatment should be longer.

Massage requires a quiet and comfortable environment, and this is especially important in treating diseases caused by emotional disturbances. In treating a disease which involves fever, it would be best to perform massage in a cool and refreshing environment. In treating a patient suffering from deficiency of Yang and Preponderance of Yin, the best environment for massage would be warm. While they may seem insignificant, environmental conditions have a great influence on the therapeutic effects of massage. The massage therapist should be flexible in approach and responsive to the condition of the patient, the time and the environment.

Commonly Used Herbal Preparations and Devices

Herbal Preparations for lubrication, friction and therapeutic stimulation.

These are preparations applied to the points or areas where techniques are to be performed. They are used to reduce friction, protect the skin, and improve the therapeutic effects of massage through their pharmacological actions. Herbal preparations are selected according to the condition of disease. For instance, in treating an External Syndrome, sudorifics may be useful; in treating Blood stasis, herbal preparations which activate Blood may be useful; in treating Cold Syndrome, herbal preparations of a hot nature may be helpful; in treating Heat Syndrome, preparations of a cold nature might be desired, etc. The appropriateness of each preparation's other characteristics, such as dryness, dampness, concentration, and lubricity, should also be considered. Generally, after massage, there is no need to wash them away immediately because they remain effective. According to forms of dosage, they may be classified as preparations of juice, water, alcohol, vinegar, oil, honey, powder; or as a decoction, medicated plaster, pill, etc.

Juice Preparations

These refer to undiluted juices obtained from fresh, uncooked substances. They may be changed into water preparations by adding a small amount of water.

1. Scallion (Allium fistulosum, Cong Bai)

After washing Chinese scallion stalks, crush them to obtain the juice. Properties are pungent and warm. It may induce perspiration, communicate Yang, and promote normal urination. Grasping and kneading Fengchi (GB 20), Dazhui (GV 14) and the nose with scallion juice on the fingers helps treat the common cold, headache, stuffy nose, etc. Applying scallion juice to Shenque (CV 8) and the lower abdomen may relieve abdominal pain, dysuria and other symptoms. Thick scallion juice is suitable for adults. Slightly diluted scallion juice is more suitable for children.

2. Ginger (Zingiber officinale, Sheng Jiang)

Pound the ginger into a pulp to obtain its juice. Its properties are pungent and slightly warm. It may relieve the External, disperse Cold, warm the Middle Warmer, and stop vomiting. It is useful in treating the common cold, stiff neck, headache, dyspnea, and cough due to retention of phlegm and fluids when applied to the neck and nape, and points such as Fengchi (GB 20), Dazhui (GV 14), Fengmen (UB 12) and others. Abdominal pain, diarrhea, vomiting and abdominal distention may be treated by application to Jiuwei (CV 15), Shangwan (CV 13), Zhongwan (CV 12), and Xiawan (CV 10), among others.

3. Garlic (Allium sativum, Da Suan)

Peel the skin from the garlic cloves and pound them to extract their juice. The properties of garlic juice are pungent and warm. It may detoxify evils, warm the Middle Warmer and invigorate the Stomach. When applied to Tanzhong (CV 17) and Feishu (UB 13), it is useful for the common cold and convulsive coughing. It may also be used to reduce swelling and stop itching when rubbed and kneaded locally on tinea or rash.

4. Peppermint (Mentha haplocalyx, Bo He)

Pound the leaves and stalks to extract the juice. Its properties are pungent and cool. It may disperse Wind, clear Heat, relieve depressed Energy, and expel pathogenic factors from the External. When applied to the forehead at Taiyang (Ex-HN 4), Yingxiang (LI 20), Jiache (St 6), and Tiantu (CV 22), it may treat an attack of Wind-Heat, headache, stuffy nose, sore throat and toothache due to Wind-Fire, etc.

5. Patchouli (Agastache rugosa, Huo Xiang)

Pound the leaves and stalks to squeeze out the juice. Properties are pungent and slightly warm. It helps clear Summer-Heat, resolve Dampness, rectify Vital Energy, and harmonize the Middle Warmer. When applied to Yintang (Ex-HN 2), Shenting (GV 24), Taiyang (Ex-HN 4), Fengfu (GV 16), and Fengchi (GB 20) it helps treat headache due to sunstroke and dizziness due to adhesion of Dampness. Nausea, vomiting, feelings of fullness and heaviness in the chest may be treated by rubbing and kneading it onto the upper abdomen. Applied locally, it may stop itching caused by mosquito bites or rubella.

6. Water chestnut (Eleocharis tuberosa, Bi Qi)

Wash and clean the chestnuts, then break them into pieces and wring the juice out. The properties are sweet and slightly cold. This can help to clear Heat, improve eyesight, eliminate stasis, and resolve Phlegm. The juice is slippery and greasy and is often used in massage of children. Fever due to Deficiency of Spleen, mass in the abdomen, jaundice and other childhood diseases may be treated by applying this juice to the forearms and abdomen coupled with point massage.

7. Lotus Leaf (Nelumbo nucifera, He Ye)

Pound to crush out the juice. Properties are bitter, astringent and placid. It can raise and disperse Clear Yang, clear away Summer-Heat, resolve stasis and stop bleeding. It is most commonly applied to the abdomen and the back. It is used in treating rubella, pox, purpura, etc.

8. Snakegourd (Trichosanthes kirilowii, Gua Lou)

Peel the skin of the fresh fruit, discard the seeds, and crush the fruit for its juice. Its properties are sweet and cold. It can moisten the Lung, Large Intestine and skin, resolve Phlegm, and eliminate Stagnation. When applied to Huagai (CV 20), Tanzhong (CV 17) and Rugen (St 18), it can treat cough due to Phlegm-Heat, choking pain and stuffiness in the chest, and swollen breasts. In local application, it is effective for chapped hands and feet, and can alleviate the pain of boils.

9. Dandelion (Taraxacum mongolicum, Pu Gong Ying)

Wash a bunch of the whole herb and crush it for the juice. Its properties are sweet, bitter and cold. It can clear Heat, detoxify evils, reduce swelling, and eliminate stagnation. When applied to the neck and nape, it is useful against scrofula, carbuncles, and cellulitis. When applied to the chest and breast, it may prevent and treat the swelling and pain of acute mastitis. When applied locally, it treats skin infections which produce pus.

10. Lotus (Nelumbo nucifera, Lian Fang)

Select thick and tender ones and wring them to extract the juice. Properties are sweet and cold. This may be used to clear Heat, promote production of body fluids, cool Blood and resolve stasis. The juice is slippery and greasy and often used to treat children for such ailments as dryness and itching of the skin, poxes and infections which produce pus.

11. Swine bile

Fresh bile is best. The dried preparation, ground in water, may be used as a substitute, as may chicken bile, which is also effective. Its properties are bitter and cold. It may be used to clear Heat, relax the bowels, reduce swelling, and eliminate stagnation. When applied to Shenque (CV 8), it may alleviate constipation, abdominal distension and jaundice. It is also effective against dizziness, hypertension, etc., when applied to Yongquan (K 1) with rubbing and kneading.

12. Egg White

Break the eggs and separate out the whites. Properties are sweet, salty, and placid. It may be used to strengthen Spleen-Stomach, moisten the skin, reduce swelling, and relieve pain. It is useful for toothache, gingivitis, parotitis, scrofula, sore throat and other such ailments when applied to cheeks and the sides of the neck. The use of cactus pulp in conjunction with the egg white will improve the results. Apply to the chest or abdomen to treat cough and fever in children, infantile malnutrition, etc. In local application, it is useful against pain and dry-itch of poxes and pus-producing skin infections.

13. Human milk

Obtain milk from a healthy woman, although fresh cow's milk may be used as a substitute. The properties are sweet, salty and placid. It is useful to invigorate the weak, benefit Vital Energy, clear Heat, moisten Dryness, supplement the Five Yin Organs, improve the functions of the gastrointestinal tract, nourish Blood, etc., and is commonly used in treating the diseases of children. To treat conjunctivitis, lachrymal excess, and tic caused by Wind evil, apply to Yintang (Ex-HN 2), Taiyang (Ex-HN 4), Fengchi (GB 20) and the area around the eye. When applied to the upper abdomen, the navel or lower abdomen, it is useful in treating weak flatulence, infantile malnutrition, abdominal pain, diarrhea, and anuresis in children. When applied locally to the skin, it may relieve the pain and itching caused by chapping or dryness. As a medium in massage, milk can invigorate the weak and clear Heat.

Water Preparations

Soak medical herbs in clear water (warm or hot). The time of soaking depends on the herb selected. Generally, pungent-warm and pungent-cool sudorifics such as Herba Ephedrae and Flos Chrysanthemi are soaked for 20 minutes. Herbs which clear Heat and detoxify evils, such as Radix Scutellariae and Rhizoma Coptidis are soaked for more than 30 minutes. The water should be stirred during soaking.

1. Herba Ephedrae (Ephedra sinica, Ma Huang)

Its properties are pungent, slightly bitter and warm. It may induce perspiration, relieve the External, quell asthma and promote normal urination. When applied to Fengchi (GB 20), Fengfu (GV 16), and Dazhui (GV 14), its sudorific qualities are heightened, and headache and bodily indisposition may be relieved. Ability to quell asthma and stop coughing may be increased by application to Tiantu (CV 22), Tanzhong (CV 17), and Feishu (UB 13). It is also effective in treating rubella.

2. Ramulus Cinnamomi (Cinnamomum cassia, Gui Zhi)

Properties are pungent, sweet and warm. It may relax muscles, induce perspiration, warm Meridians, and communicate Yang. It is useful for common cold and headache when applied to Baihui (GV 20), Fengfu (GV 16), and Fengchi (GB 20). When applied to the back along the Governor Vessel and Urinary Bladder Meridians, it may eliminate feeling of heaviness in the chest, dyspnea due to retention of phlegm, and pain and cold sensation of the back. When applied to the lower abdomen, it may promote normal urination.

3. Herba Schizonepetae and Radix Ledebourialle (Schizonopeta tenuifolia, Jing Jie; Ledebouriella sesloides, Fang Feng)

Soak these two herbs in equal parts. Properties are pungent and warm. They may relieve the External, expel Wind, resolve Dampness, and alleviate pain. When applied to Taiyang (Ex-HN 4), Fengchi (GB 20), and Dazhui (GV 14), they may treat headache accompanying common cold. When applied to the neck, they help relieve pain and swelling of the throat. When applied to the back and joints, they can alleviate cold sensations and relieve joint pains.

4. Coriander (Coriandrum sativum, Yan Sui Zi)

Its properties are pungent and slightly warm. It can induce perspiration, promote eruption, strengthen stomach, and aid digestion. In treating measles and poxes, it is often used to alleviate dry-itching of the skin and promote eruption, especially when there is fever without perspiration.

5. Flos Chrysanthemi (Chrysanthemum morifolium, Ju Hua)

Its properties are sweet, bitter and placid. It may expel wind, clear Heat and improve eyesight. It is often applied to the forehead, the center of the sole of the foot, and various points. It is useful in treating headache, fever, conjunctival congestion, swelling and pain of the eye, dizziness and hypertension.

6. Herba Lophatheri (Lophatherum gracile, Dan Zhu Ye)

Its properties are sweet, placid and cold. It may clear Heat from the Pericardium, relieve vexation, promote normal urination, relieve thirst, and is often used in the massage of children.

7. Moschus (Moschus moschiferus, She Xiang)

Grind it into extremely fine powder and soak in warm water. Its properties are pungent and warm. It is useful to open Apertures, ward off evils, activate Blood, and dispel stagnation. When applied to Yingxiang (LI 20), Tiantu (CV 22), and Tanzhong (CV 17), it is useful to treat coma, fright-induced epilepsy, unconsciousness, and cold limbs due to retention of Phlegm. When applied to Shenque (CV 8), it may treat abdominal pain and masses in the abdomen. Local application of Moschus is useful to treat bruises caused by trauma. Usually, it is incorporated in a compound prescription in the form of adhesive plaster. It is rarely used because of scarcity.

8. Tea

Properties are bitter, sweet and slightly cold. It may refresh the mind, improve eyesight, clear Heat, stop thirst, promote digestion, increase urination, and is often used with children to reduce fever.

9. Cold water

This is commonly used as a medium for massage with children to reduce fever.

Alcohol Preparations

Soak herbs in strong liquor or rice wine for 1-3 weeks. Stir occasionally. Herbs may also be soaked in a container for 1-3 days, then boiled indirectly by immersing the container in boiling water for several hours. Filter to remove the residue. There are a variety of alcoholic preparations for external application. Most of them contribute to activate Blood, resolve stasis, rectify Vital Energy, relieve pain, expel Wind, eliminate Dampness, soften Tendons and strengthen bones. The most common prescriptions follow:

1. For treating new or existing non-opened trauma.

Radix Angelicae Sinensis (Dang Gui)	9 gm
Radix Paeoniae Rubra (Chi Shao)	9 gm
Flos Carthami (Hong Hua)	9 gm
Radix Arnebiae seu Lithospermi (Zi Cao)	12 gm
Resina Olibani (Ru Xiang)	6 gm
Myrrha (Mo Yao)	6 gm
Caulis Milletti (Ji Xue Teng)	24 gm

Rhizome Cyperia (Xiang Fu)	9 gm
Fructus Auranti Immaturus (Zhi Shi)	6 gm
Radix Rubiae (Qian Cao)	9 gm
Rhizoma Corydalis (Yuan Hu)	9 gm
Herba Menthae [crystal] (Bo He)	0.9 gm (add afterwards)

Soak these herbs in a 60% alcohol solution or a strong liquor (1.5 kg) to prepare the infusion, or boil with steam. This may also be administered orally.

2. To eliminate Cold, dispel stasis, reduce swelling, and relieve pain, or for treating trauma of waist and legs.

Radix Angelicae Sinensis (Dan Gui)	9 gm
Rhizoma Ligustici Wallichi (Chuan Xiong)	9 gm
Flos Carthami (Hong Hua)	12 gm
Radix Aconiti (Fu Zi)	15 gm
Radix Aconiti Kusnezoffii (Wild root) (Cao Wu)	15 gm
Agkistrodon seu Bungaris (Bai Hua She)	12 gm
Herba Asari (Xi Xin)	9 gm
Rhizoma Curcuma Longae (Jiang Huang)	9 gm
Sanguis Draconis (Xue Jie)	12 gm
Ramulus Cinnamomi (Gui Zhi)	12 gm
Myrrha (Mo Yao)	12 gm
Fructus Auranti (Zhi Ke)	12 gm
Borneolum (Bing Pian)	3 gm (add afterwards)

Soak herbs in 1.5 kg of white spirit or boil them by steam to prepare the infusion.

3. For treating blockage syndrome in traumatized limbs, or for atrophy of extremities.

Radix Angelicae Sinensis (Dan Gui)	9 gm
Flos Carthami (Hong Hua)	9 gm
Myrrha (Mo Yao)	9 gm
Radix Angelicae Pubescentis (Du Huo)	12 gm
Rhizoma seu Radix Notopterygii (Qiang Huo)	12 gm
Ramulus Cinnamomi (Gui Zhi)	18 gm
Pericarpium Zanthoxyli (Hua Jiao)	9 gm
Lignum Pini Nodi (Song Jie)	15 gm
Herba Schizonepetae (Jing Jie)	9 gm
Radix Ledebouriellae (Fang Feng)	9 gm
Phryma leptostachya var. asiatica (Tou Gu Cao)	12 gm
Herba Lycopodii (Shen Jin Cao)	12 gm

Semen Strychnotis [processed] (Ma Qian Zi)	9 gm
Scolopendra (Wu Gong)	6 gm
Herba Ephedrae [unprocessed] (Ma Huang)	9 gm

Soak herbs in 1.5 kg white spirit, or boil with steam to obtain decoction.

4. An effective treatment for abdominal distension and pain when applied to Shenque (CV 8) with kneading.

Cortex Cinnamomi (Rou Gui)	9 gm
Flos Caryophylis (Ding Xiang)	6 gm
Fructus Illicium Verum (Ba Jiao Hui Xiang)	9 gm
Radix Angelicae Dahuricae (Bai Zhi)	6 gm
Fructus Evodiae (Wu Zhu Yu)	9 gm
Herba Asari (Xi Xin)	6 gm
Fructus Piperis Longi (Bi Ba)	9 gm
Rhizoma Alpiniae Officinari (Gao Liang Jiang)	9 gm
Radix Aucklandiae (Mu Xiang)	9 gm
Pericarpium Citri Reticulatae Viride (Qing Pi)	9 gm
Moschus (She Xiang)	0.3 gm (add afterwards)

Soak herbs in 1.5 kg white spirit to prepare infusion.

5. White Spirit (Alcohol may be used as a substitute.)

Its properties are pungent, sweet and warm. It is useful to disperse Cold, dredge Collaterals, resolve stasis and eliminate stagnation. White spirit or alcohol may be applied to various parts of the body. To increase the effects when dispersing Cold, rub the patient's back, waist and legs quickly with ignited spirit. Take extreme care to avoid burns. The main indicators for use are joint pains caused by Cold-Dampness, cold and numb sensation of the skin, swellings, bruises, dryness and itching of the skin.

Powder Preparations

Select herbs according to the disease condition, and grind them into extremely fine powder. Most powder preparations are made of powdered herbs and talcum, or mainly made of talcum, for instance, prickly-heat powder, face powder, dusting powder, etc. They may clear Heat, eliminate Dampness, lubricate the skin, prevent injuries and alleviate itching. In treating children with massage for epilepsy due to fright, Cinnabaris (Zhu Sha) powder is often applied to Yintang (Ex-HN 2), Shangen (nasal bridge), Inner Laogong (Per 8) with nipping and kneading in these areas. In treating unconsciousness, a small amount of Moschus (She Xiang) or Borneolum (Bing Piang) may be applied to Yingxiang (LI 20) and Renzhong (GV 26) to aid resuscitation.

Oil Preparations

This may be an infusion made by soaking herbs in oil (generally sesame oil), or an ointment prepared by mixing a powder or different kinds of powders with oil. Finished preparations of various oils such as liquid paraffin may also be used.

1. Sesame Oil

Its properties are sweet, placid and slightly warm, and may help invigorate the weak, strengthen Spleen, and moisten dryness. In treating malnutrition in children, Deficiency of Spleen-Stomach, or dry rough skin, it is often applied to the abdomen or back.

2. Flos Carthami Ointment

Soak a small amount of Flos Carthami (Hong Hua) in chicken oil and boil. After cooling, it may be applied to chapped skin.

3. Chinese Ilex Oil

It is useful to expel Wind, invigorate the weak, moisten and nourish skin. When used as a medium in massage, it can treat rubella, pain, itching, or swelling of the skin.

4. Turpentine Oil

This may be used to expel Wind or eliminate Dampness, and is often applied to skin surfaces at joints or injured muscles for joint pain and bruises.

5. Glycerine

This helps invigorate the weak and moisten dryness, and is often used in clinical practice to treat Deficiency of Spleen-Stomach and dry skin.

6. Menthocamphorate

It may expel Wind, relieve pain, reduce swelling and stop itching. When applied to the skin surface on the head, the neck or the abdomen, it aids treatment of headache caused by common cold, dizziness caused by sunstroke, nausea, vomiting, etc. Applied locally, it is also effective in stopping itching of mosquito bites.

7. Essential Balm

This may help expel Wind, relieve pain, refresh the mind, restore consciousness, clear Summer-Heat, and ward against evils. It may be applied to any part of the body. It is effective in treating common cold, dizziness, nasal congestion, headache, abdominal pain and distension, joint pain, and bites of mosquitoes or bedbugs.

8. Massage Emulsion

This may relax Tendons, activate Blood, reduce swelling and relieve pain. It is often used to treat swelling and pain from bruising during gymnastic competitions.

Vinegar Preparations

These are commonly used to treat traumatic injury. Soak the herbs or pills prescribed for trauma in high-quality vinegar, and grind into dilute paste. The paste is effective for reducing swelling and relieving pain. You may also mix a fine powder of unprocessed Cape Jasmine (Zhi Zi) with a little ginger juice and vinegar (enough to make a paste). In addition to reducing swelling and relieving pain, this paste helps clear Heat as well. Many different prescriptions may be soaked in vinegar, and these should soak for 7 days, after which the infusions may be used. Adding white spirit to vinegar may increase the effectiveness of the herbs. These are called spirit-vinegar preparations.

Devices

Massage Clubs

Massage clubs are simple, economical, supplementary devices for massage therapists. They are substitutes for the arm, and supplement the therapist's physical strength. The best material for making clubs is rubber, but other materials such as plastic, Bakelite, bamboo, mulberry wood, etc., may also be used. They are designed to simulate various parts of the arm and hand.

Finger Clubs

Fingertip Club

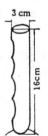

16 cm long with a diameter of 3 cm. Its tip is flattened. There are four indentations along its length to provide a firm grip.

Hold this club in one hand with its tip on a selected point or area. Move it in a revolving motion, increasing force gradually from mild to deep, to knead the underlying muscles. The skin should not be scratched.

Indications: Pain deep in gaps or openings of small joints. It helps relax spasm and relieve pain.

Finger-Pad Club

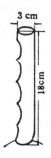

18 cm long by 3 cm diameter. It has a flexible tip and 4 finger indentations.

Hold the club in one hand with its tip on the chosen point or area, press and revolve to knead the underlying muscles until the patient feels warmth at the spot. The direction of the kneading should follow the principle of Meet-Follow Invigorate-Reduce.

Indications: Localized muscular pain or tenderness, numbness.

Palm-of-Hand Clubs

Thenar Mound Club

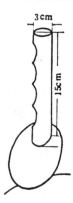

15 cm long by 3 cm diameter with 4 finger indentations.

Hold it in one hand, put the head of the club on the selected area, and proceed in the same manner as with the finger-pad club, until the patient feels warmth, choosing the direction by the same principle of Meet-Follow Invigorate-Reduce.

Indications: Muscular numbness, joint pain caused by Cold-Dampness, traumatic bone pain.

Palm Club

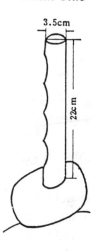

22 cm long by 3.5 cm diameter with 8 indentations for holding with both hands.

Hold this club with one or both hands on the selected area, follow the same procedure as above.

Indications: Large areas of muscular pain or tenderness, joint pain due to Wind-Cold-Dampness, traumatic bone pain.

Arm Clubs

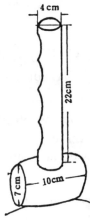

Short Club

The head of this club simulates full, round muscles, i.e., ulnar flexor. The head is 10 cm long by 7 cm diameter. The handle is 22 cm long by 4 cm diameter with 8 finger indentations. Use the same way as the previous club, but throughout a larger area. This technique is called Substitute Arm Revolving.

Indications: Wide-ranging areas of muscular pain and tenderness caused by Wind-Cold-Dampness, such as in back and waist or limbs, traumatic bone pain.

Long Club

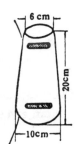

This simulates a forearm. It is a truncated cone, with a diameter 6 cm across at the small end and 10 cm at the other. Finger indentations are at both ends and on both sides for 2-hand use.

Hold both ends and place the club on an area with full and round muscles and a long concave area, such as the shoulder, back, waist or buttocks. Place the larger end in the concave area, with the smaller end on the raised muscles. Revolve as before until patient feels a warm sensation. Use the same guiding principle.

Indications: Pain or numbness of the shoulder, back, chest, abdomen, waist and limbs where muscles are full and round. It is effective in treating disease caused by Wind-Cold-Dampness and trauma.

Elbow Clubs

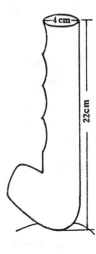

Pointed Elbow Club

The head is triangular and the tip should be blunt, and not too sharp. The handle is 22 cm long by 4 cm diameter with 8 finger indentations.

Hold this club with one or both hands and place the tip on an area of full, round muscles, such as Huantiao (GB 30) or Chengfu (UB 36). Press and revolve throughout a wide area, increasing pressure gradually from mild to deep, until the patient feels a numbness. Take care to avoid harsh or brusque movements. Follow the guiding principle.

Indications: Uprising of excessive Liver Yang, depression of Liver Energy, paralysis.

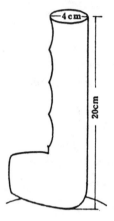

L-shaped Club

Also called Flat Protruding Elbow. The head forms a rounded triangle. The handle is 20 cm long by 4 cm diameter, with 8 finger indentations.

Hold the handle firmly with one or both hands, press and revolve where muscles are round and full. Motion should be gentle and slow, covering a wide area, and following the guiding principles.

Indications: Headache due to Excess Fire, toothache, pain in chest, ribs or hips, hypertension, numbness of legs.

Beating Clubs

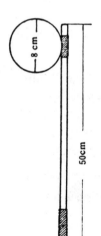

Large Ball Club

This features a thick-skinned hollow ball of 8 cm diameter attached to a 50 cm handle of rattan. The rattan gives elasticity and flexibility.

Hold the handle with one hand and beat a selected part of the body at about 80 beats per minute. The therapist may hold one club in each hand and beat them alternately. Be attentive to the patient's reactions.

Indications: Feeling of fullness and heaviness in the chest and diaphragm, hiccups, nausea, vomiting, pain in waist, back and limbs.

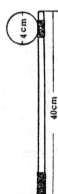

Small Ball Club

This club has a solid ball of 4 cm diameter attached to a rattan handle 40 cm long.

Hold the handle in one hand and beat a selected part of the body until you know the patient's reactions. As before, using two clubs alternately is an appropriate option.

Indications: Stiffness of the back, lumbago, numb joints, restricted joint motion.

Chopping Club

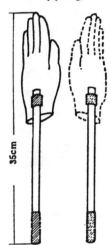

This simulates a vertical palm for techniques using the edge of the hand. It is made of rubber, 2 cm thick, with a flexible handle 35 cm long.

Chop at a selected area as if you were chopping meat. Establish a regular rhythm. Again, this may be done with two such clubs in alternation.

Indications: Spasms of the back or limbs, pain and numbness due to Wind-Cold-Dampness or trauma.

Patting Club

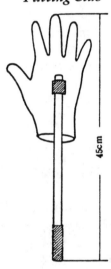

This simulates an open hand, and is made of rubber 2 cm thick. A flexible handle 45 cm long is attached at the center of the back of the hand.

Hold it in one hand and pat the patient's back with the concave palm. You may also use two such clubs, patting both sides of the spine alternately along the Urinary Bladder Meridian. The patting should be gentle and rhythmic.

Indications: Abdominal distension and heaviness due to overeating, cough, dyspnea due to retention of phlegm, shortness of breath, feeling of heaviness in the chest and diaphragm, stiffness of the back and spine.

Rubber Hammer

The head of the hammer is made of comparatively hard rubber. It is cylindrical, 5-6 cm long by 2-2.5 cm in diameter. One end is a pointed cone and the other is rounded. The handle is about 35 cm long and should be flexible. Rattan is preferable for the handle, but bamboo, plastic or other materials may be used.

This appliance was created and manufactured by Zhao Xinting and associates in Qingdao to combine Plum-blossom needle therapy with massage.

Proper execution of the beating-rebounding technique and amount of force applied are critical. The location must be accurately struck, and, in its

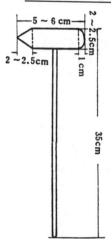

rise and fall, the hammer head should be vertical, rapid and rhythmic. The force used should be uniform and elastic. The frequency of rhythm should not be too rapid, because it is necessary for the beaten area to bounce back and transmit the force.

Beating gently along the direction of the Meridian brings about invigoration. Beating firmly against the path of the Meridian is for reduction. After beating with the hammer, it is essential to make several pushes and strokes on the area. Bruises may arise, but they will not influence the therapeutic effects, and they may later disappear spontaneously.

There are two types of rubber hammer therapy:

Routine therapy: Allow the Governor Vessel Meridian to be the central line, and draw 4 parallel lines on each side of it. Moving outward from the Governor Vessel, the distance between the lines are 0.5, 1, 2, and 4 Body Inches respectively. Beat the central line from the cervical spine to the coccyx or sacrum, then beat the parallel lines left and right alternately, progressing outward from the midline.

Local therapy: Beat the following areas—the triangular area of the upper abdomen, the triangular area of the lower abdomen, the abdomen around and around, the head, and the intercostal spaces.

The proper order when beating points of the entire body is to proceed from top to bottom (head, arms, trunk, legs) and from midline outward along the course of the Meridians.

In clinical practice, after routine hammer beating, local points or areas may be manipulated in the same way.

Rubber hammer therapy is safe, reliable and easy to perform. It is effective in preventing and treating various diseases. Patients may also beat themselves with this kind of hammer.

Porcelain Utensils

This is a traditional therapeutic method. Use the smooth thick lip of a porcelain utensil, such as a wine cup, tea cup, small plate, bowl, etc., with water, oil or juice as a lubricant, and scrape or rub a selected area along a definite direction for invigoration or reduction. This is effective in treating headache, body pains, fever, rubella, measles, poxes and other External syndromes.

Ancient Coins

Most of these are made of copper, and can be used in the same way as porcelain utensils and with the same therapeutic effects. These are also effective in tranquilizing the mind and expelling Wind.

Jade Thimble

This is about 2 cm long, with walls about 3-4 mm thick. It is usually worn on the index finger. The jade is delicate and smooth. Its properties are sweet and placid, without toxicity. This special appliance is used in the massage of children, and may promote blood circulation, expel Wind, tranquilize the mind, and nurse the skin.

Essentials of Therapeutic Massage

Diagnosis must be clear and unequivocal.

In massage, as in all areas of TCM, the data you collect through the Four Examinations (Looking, Hearing- Smelling, Asking, and Touching), should be sorted and analyzed according to the Eight Principles, Six Pernicious Influences, Yin and Yang Organs, Triple Warmers, Nutrient-Defense-Energy-Blood Systems, and Meridians and Collaterals. Modern medical diagnostic techniques may be useful to learn the exact cause and details of the disease condition. On these bases, you can form a strategy of treatment.

Let yourself be guided by the admonitions of the ancient doctors:

> *Both the root cause and its branch manifestations should be examined carefully . . . Facing an emergency, treat the urgent symptoms first. When the emergency is relieved, treat its fundamental cause.*

Remember, massage therapy is not a panacea. Avoid treating a symptom but missing the disease.

> *Treat the head when there is headache, treat the foot when the foot hurts.*

Neck and shoulder pains are frequently encountered in clinic, but their relationships should be carefully studied. Although symptoms of the shoulder may be serious, the origin of the pathology may be at the neck. Many symptoms of the leg are related to pathology in the waist. Before you begin massage, your diagnosis must be clear and definite. This is the foundation of a proper therapeutic course of treatment.

*The selection of points and areas should be correct and the location
should be accurate.*

Symptoms at a specific part of the body may indicate a disorder there, or
may merely be a reflection of disease of internal organs. Generally, traumatic injury may be massaged locally. If local massage is not proper, you
may select near or distant points according to Meridian theory.

Both the theory of Meridians and the current medical theory of neuro-
humoral transmission should be considered when selecting points or areas
for massage, because some points and areas influence internal organs
through the neural pathway reflex arc.

You may obtain synergistic therapeutic effects when you massage sensi-
tive areas such as the superclavicular fossa, the popliteal fossa, or the armpit
in conjunction with the selected points.

The proper selection of points or areas and the sequence of massage
determines the best position for your patient. Generally, when treating the
chest or abdomen, the patient is supine. When treating the head, neck,
shoulder and arms, sitting is appropriate. When treating the waist and legs,
the patient may lie prone, supine or on his/her side. The position of the
patient should ease the work of the massage therapist as long as it does not
add unnecessary pain or suffering for the patient.

The techniques should be performed correctly

This is crucial to success. Techniques should be light without being
superficial, and heavy but flowing. The force you apply should be gentle
and soft, but also deep and penetrating. The manipulation should be nimble
and skillful. The sequence should flow coherently from step to step, and
the rhythm of the movements should be regular. Different therapists will
achieve different therapeutic effects using the same techniques.

During massage, the Vital Energy you motivate and the force you apply
must be proportionately appropriate. Localized sensations of warmth,
numbness, soreness or distension, or the radiating sensations induced by
the technique can initiate the patient's convalescent mechanisms. Generally, the therapeutic effects are better when such sensations are felt. The
force you apply in massage generally should follow a curve: mild at first,
gradually increasing, and finally decreasing again.

Comparatively speaking, when treating newly diseased patients or
adults with sturdy constitutions, massage on the waist, back or limbs
should be vigorous. When treating the chronically ill, patients with feeble
constitutions, or children, massage on the chest, abdomen, head and Meridian pathways should be more subdued. When massage is employed to
improve a patient's general health, the force applied should also be gentler.

The speed of the manipulation is determined by the state of the Vital Energy you motivate, the amount of force applied, and the requirements of the disease condition.

The methods of Invigoration and Reduction should be properly done: generally, soft, slow, long-lasting and inwardly-moving manipulation belongs to Invigoration; heavy, fast, transient and outwardly-moving manipulation is part of Reduction. In clinical practice, the principle of "Invigorate the Deficiency, reduce the Excess" should guide the entire course of massage.

Although you may encounter differing viewpoints, we caution that "Treating the same disease with different methods and treating different diseases with the same method — one manipulation for all," is not a good choice. Special techniques should be adopted and developed to improve therapeutic effects and shorten the period of treatment.

Duration and frequency in therapeutic massage

Generally, this depends on the patient's condition. Acute traumatic illness should be massaged one or more times a day for about 20 minutes. Chronic illnesses should be massaged every other day at most. In these, and in self-massage for hygiene, the treatments are generally longer than 30 minutes.

Standards of environment and demeanor

Comfortable environment

The room should be at a temperature of about 28 degrees Centigrade (82.4 F), clean and dry and well lighted, with circulating fresh air. Equipment and appliances should be sturdy and convenient.

Amiable attitude

Your role is to serve your patients, and it is best to do this whole-heartedly. Clinical experience shows that the positive attitude of medical workers plays an important role in treatment.

General demeanor

You should be careful, conscientious and responsible to your patient. Be accurate and attentive, observe your patient's responses and, if you're not sure, ask what he/she is feeling.

Contraindications to Therapeutic Massage

Unknown diagnosis, overeating, excessive drinking, drunkenness, anger or rage, deep sorrow, being extremely tired or hungry.

Infectious diseases such as leprosy, plague, hepatitis, open wounds or fractures, scalds, burns, various malignant tumors, disorders with tendency to hemorrhaging, tuberculosis, psychosis. Pregnant or menstruating women should be treated later or with great caution.

Perfunctory manipulation, clumsy or harsh procedures, or making jokes are clinically inappropriate. (It is a good thing to use some levity to put a patient at ease, but a joking attitude undermines confidence and is not desirable.)

Techniques

Classification of Techniques

Classification of Techniques

The massage schools of Shandong Province divide techniques into 5 principle categories:

Simple techniques: Each is one single technique and is descriptively named. This category includes techniques done with both hands on the same area.

Compound techniques: These combine two or more simple techniques into one. These also include techniques done with both hands on the same area.

Special techniques: In this category, both hands and/or arms are used in different areas, and each performs one or more techniques simultaneously. The action of both hands should be coordinated to be harmonious, rhythmic, and sequential to shorten the time of treatment, achieve increased results, and therefore, improved therapeutic effect. Stepping Method and others are included in this category.

Passive movements: In this category, the therapist manipulates the joints and the vertebrae according to their structure, function and range of motion.

Routine techniques: These common clinical techniques are specific to the part of the anatomy where they're used.

There are also a few special techniques which are not easily classifiable, and which we will describe as they appear in prescriptions.

Simple Techniques

Pushing

Pushing involves pressing firmly on the body with the fingers, palm or fist.

Where used
Various parts of the body.

Essentials
The practitioner sits upright or stands. Pressure should be deep and penetrating. Push outward along a straight line. Coordinate each push with respiration for rhythmic intermittent motion.

Techniques

1. Pushing with the thumb

Make a fist with the thumb extended and press the thumb firmly into the area to be massaged. Contact is with the tip, pad or side of the thumb, with the other fingers held in a loose fist. Keep your wrist flexible. Push forward along a straight line. This technique is used on the head, face, neck, nape, back, and waist.

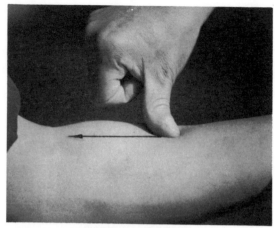

Pushing with the thumb

2. Pushing with the thenar mound

Straighten your wrist and fingers. Keep your fingers together, press the thenar mound down firmly and push out sideways. Both hands may do this simultaneously. This is commonly used to massage the chest, sides, abdomen, back, waist and limbs.

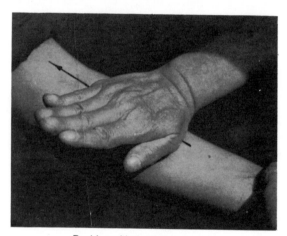

Pushing with the thenar mound

3. Pushing with the heel of the hand

Raise your hand to bend your wrist up slightly, and straighten and separate your fingers. Press with the heel of your hand. Pushing may be done with one hand, both, or with one

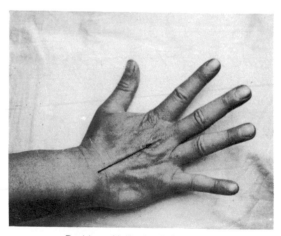

Pushing with the heel of the hand

hand on top of the other to increase pressure. This is commonly used to massage the back, waist, buttocks and lower limbs.

4. Pushing with the entire hand

Straighten your wrist with the fingers slightly separated, and press down with your entire hand. Don't lock your elbow, but keep it slightly crooked. Push forward along a straight line with one hand, both hands, or one on top of the other. All areas of the body may be massaged with this

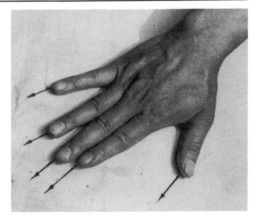

Pushing with a single hand

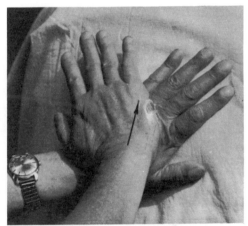

Pushing with one hand on the other

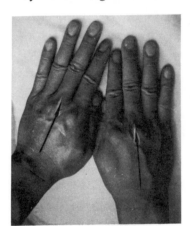

Pushing with both hands

technique except the head, face, neck and nape.

5. Pushing with the fist

Make a loose fist with the palm down. Press down with the middle segment of the four fingers, the thenar mound and the heel of the

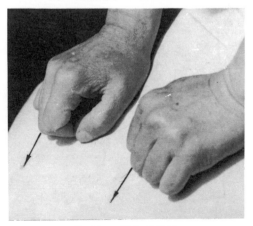

Pushing with both fists

hand. If necessary, reinforce the pressure with the other hand on top of the fist. This technique is appropriate for the back, waist and sole of the foot.

6. Intermittent pushing

In this technique, the entire hand is used, pushing forward and stopping abruptly, like a carpenter planing a board. In fact, it is also called Pushing the Plane. This technique should be coordinated with respiratory rhythm. Suitable for the chest, abdomen, back and waist.

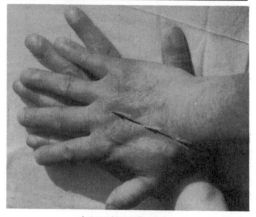

Intermittent Pushing

Indications: Headache, dizziness, stiff neck and nape, heaviness in the chest, abdominal distension, belching, hiccups, rheumatic or rheumatoid joint pain, spasms of tendons and muscles, strained waist muscles, sudden distress in the chest, trauma, bruises.

Effects: Can clear and rectify the head and eyes, ventilate the chest, help the diaphragm, improve digestion, remove food retention, warm Meridians, dredge Collaterals, activate Blood, resolve stasis, relax spasms, and relieve pain.

Grasping

This involves grasping a part of the body with the pads of the thumb and fingers, or pressing an area from both sides with the entire hand. You may use one hand on top of the other to increase force.

Where used
The head and neck, shoulder, abdomen, back, waist and limbs.

Essentials
Grasping should be done gently with appropriate force at a selected spot. Avoid nipping with the fingernails.

Techniques

1. Grasping with the fingers

Use the pad of the thumb and one or more of the fin-

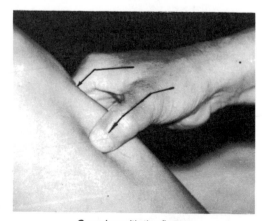

Grasping with the fingers

gers, applying force on the area of tendons, muscles, joint openings, or points. You may use all five fingers or add the fingers of the other hand as needed to reinforce the pressure.

2. Grasping with the entire hand

With the center of your palm over the selected spot, grasp with the entire hand or both hands simultaneously. Keep your wrist flexible.

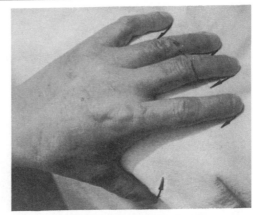

Grasping with the entire hand

Indications: Common cold, dizziness, stiff neck, shoulder neuralgia, hemiplegia, lumbago, leg pain, sprained limbs, dislocation of joints.

Effects: Open Apertures, improve eyesight, expel Wind, disperse Cold, relax Tendons, activate Blood, dredge Meridians, and relieve pain.

Pressing

Press a point with a finger, a part of the palm, or the entire palm. You may sustain the pressure while holding your breath. The force you apply should not be too strong.

Where used
Various points on the body.

Essentials
Apply force for a steady, sustained, gradually deepening and penetrating pressure. Don't be too forceful. Don't allow your hands to shift away from the point. Your respiration should be relaxed, although you may hold your breath moderately.

Techniques

1. Pressing with the fingers

Press accurately on the selected point with the thumb or another finger. Support and stabilize the pres-

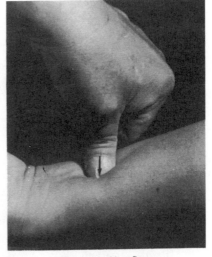

Pressing with a finger

sure with the remaining fingers. Two thumbs (or fingers) may be used simultaneously, and/or add fingers on top to increase pressure.

2. Pressing with the palms

Straighten your arm, bend your wrist, and press rhythmically with the entire palm, with the large or small thenar mound, or with the heel of the hand. Add the other hand on top to increase pressure as needed.

Indications: Headache, toothache, oppressive feeling in the chest, abdominal distension, blockage syn-

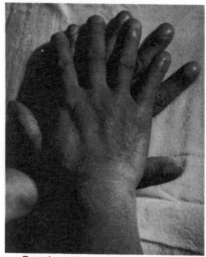

Pressing with one palm on the other

drome of the waist and back, dislocation of joints, etc.

Effects: Open and dredge obstruction, regulate Vital Energy, activate Blood, relieve pain, correct dislocation, arrange bones, rectify joints.

Round-rubbing

This involves smooth, circular, facile sliding and rubbing at a selected area or point with the fingers or parts of the palm.

Where used
Various parts of the body.

Essentials
Apply uniform force. The round-rubbing should be smooth and sequential with moderate speed. Your fingers, palm and wrist should be flexible and coordinated. Herbal preparations should be used with these techniques.

Techniques

1. Round-rubbing with the fingers

Press the pad(s) of your straightened finger or fingers to a selected spot, while rubbing in a circle. Allow your other fingers to curl naturally.

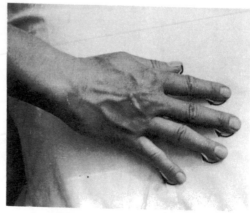

Round-rubbing with the fingers

Use one or more fingers, as indicated.

2. Round-rubbing with the palm

Stretch your fingers upward to avoid contact. Press your hand or hands to the skin and rub in a circular motion. Use the large or small thenar mounds, or the heel of the hand. When you enfold your hands with each other in using this technique on the abdomen, it is called Taiji round-rubbing of the abdomen. (Taiji is an ancient cosmological principle represented by a Yin fish with Yang eyes and a Yang fish with Yin eyes encircling each other in an embrace.)

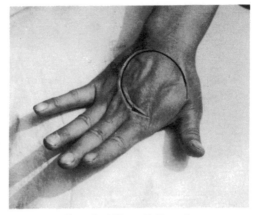

Round-rubbing with the palm

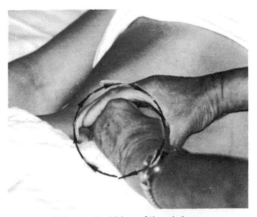

Taiji round-rubbing of the abdomen

3. Round-rubbing with the entire hand

This combines the two previous techniques. It is also called "stroke and caress."

Indications: Headache, insomnia, heaviness in the chest and rib cage, mental agitation, abdominal pain, diarrhea, bruises from falling or beating, collapse, shock.

Effects: Regulate and harmonize Ying and Wei systems, expel Wind, disperse Cold, rectify Vital Energy, reduce the Middle Warmer, resolve stasis, reduce swelling.

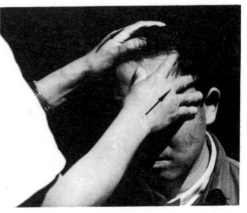

Stroke and caress

Kneading

Press one or more fingers or your entire hand on a selected spot. Move the fingers or hand in a circular or back-and-forth motion.

Where used
Various parts of the body.

Essentials
The underlying muscles should be kneaded. This differs from round-rubbing in that the fingers or hands do not slide or shift from the selected spot. Take care to avoid scratching the skin. The force applied should be deep and penetrating but still gentle and soft.

Techniques

1. Kneading with the fingers

Press the pad or side of the thumb to the selected place, and knead the spot in a circular motion. Keep your wrist relaxed. This may also be done with up to all five of the fingers. In that situation, move the wrist to do the kneading.

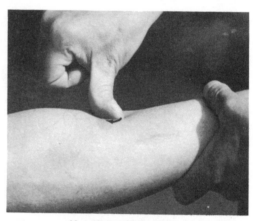

Kneading with the thumb

2. Kneading with the hand

Bend your elbow, and with your wrist raised and fingers together, press your hand to the area. Move your hand in a circular motion or in a spiral from place to place. You may apply force with the large or small thenar mound, the heel of the hand, or with the other hand on top to reinforce the kneading.

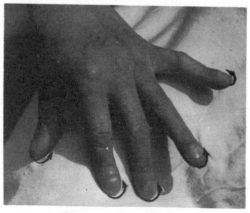

Kneading with the fingers

Indications: Pain in various parts of the body, numbness, spasm or contraction, stiffness, painful or difficult urination, bruising trauma, etc.

Effects: Relax muscles, activate Blood, ease spasms, open obstructions, resolve stasis, reduce swelling, dredge Meridians, and relieve pain.

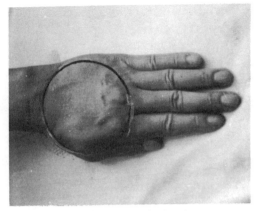

Kneading with the hand

Revolving

Press your forearm or the elbow to an area and use a revolving motion over a relatively wide area and with moderate speed.

Where used
The shoulder, chest, abdomen, back waist, buttocks and limbs.

Essentials
The motion should be circular, with enough pressure to involve the underlying muscles. It is important to stay in the selected area. The force should be deep and penetrating, but still soft and gentle. Don't scratch the skin. Choose a direction in accordance with the principle of Meet-Follow Invigorate-Reduce. Revolving surpasses kneading in the size of the area treated and the depth of treatment.

Techniques

1. Forearm revolving

Bend your elbow, and with a bare forearm, press the ulnar side of your arm, where the muscles are full and round, to the selected spot. Use appropriate force. Proceed until the

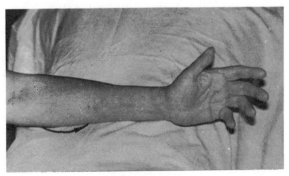

Forearm revolving

patient feels a warm sensation. Your speed should be fast enough to produce this effect.

2. Elbow revolving

Bend your forearm up, and press the bare tip of your elbow to the selected spot. Proceed until you achieve the desired effect — the patient feels warmth and distension at the area. This technique is suitable for Huantiao (GB 30), Chengfu (UB 36), Yinmen (UB 37) and other points where the muscles are full and round.

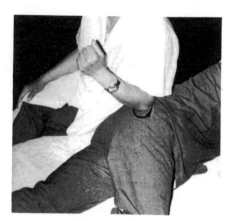

Elbow revolving

Indications: Common ailments of the head, neck, chest, abdomen, back, waist and limbs; excessive Liver Yang, depression of Liver Energy, flaming up of Liver Fire, Stomach syndrome due to attack of Liver, hemiplegia, neuralgia of the hip, flaccid paralysis of the legs, and common diseases of the Liver and Gall Bladder Meridian.

Effects: Guide and depress Vital Energy and Blood, quell the Liver, dispel Wind, reduce the Liver, clear Heat, clear excess Fire of the Upper Warmer, moderate Stomach, and lead Fire back to its origin.

Dotting (Tapping)

Grip your middle finger firmly with thumb and forefinger for support. Using the tip of the middle finger, tap the point or area firmly.

Where used
Points, apertures and openings of joints.

Essentials
Hold your breath and motivate Vital Energy to flow through your middle finger. The dotting location should be accurate, with appropriate force applied. Avoid injuries of the skin from poking.

Technique
Raise your forearm with the elbow slightly bent and the wrist bent down. Concentrate your mind to bring strength to your middle finger, and tap the point or area.

Indications: Hemiplegia, numbness, flaccid paralysis, muscle wasting and atrophy, difficult joint motion, joint pain due to Wind-Cold-Dampness, common convulsions, dementia, the five kinds of flaccidity in infants, infantile paralysis, etc.

Effects: Relax tendons and muscles, activate Vital Energy and Blood, disperse Cold, expel Wind and Dampness,

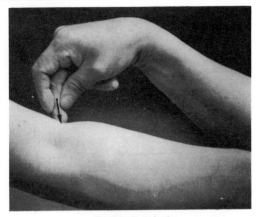

Dotting (tapping)

dredge Meridians and Collaterals, relieve pain, ease joints, promote tissue regeneration, open closed Apertures, relieve spasm, harmonize Yin and Yang, and regulate the functions of internal organs.

Rubbing

Press your palm and fingers to the skin and rub back and forth briskly and swiftly.

Where used
Various parts of the body.

Essentials
Control your breath, motivate Vital Energy to flow through your hand and fingers, and rub briskly and swiftly to induce a warm surface sensation. The underlying muscles are not involved. Herbal preparations may be used as adjuncts.

Techniques

1. Rubbing with joined hands

Interlace the fingers of your hands to form an arc. Press the arc against a protruding part of the patient's body (the head, nape, shoulder, knee). Open and shut the arc quickly and repeatedly, with your hands sliding and rubbing with each motion, until a warm sensation is induced. Without

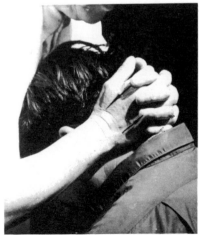

Rubbing with joined hands

the warm sensation, there will
be no effects.

2. Rubbing with the fingers

Press your thumb and fin-
gers against the skin and rub
back and forth. If you desire,
use both hands simul-
taneously.

3. Rubbing with the palm

Support the patient with
one hand. Raise your fingers
slightly, press the palm of the
other hand to the area and
rub vigorously. The rubbing
involves the entire base of the
hand — the large and small
thenar mounds and the heel
of the palm. When appro-
priate, use both hands simultaneously.

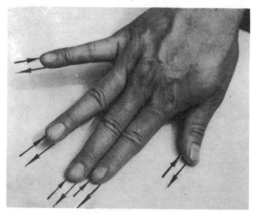

Rubbing with the fingers

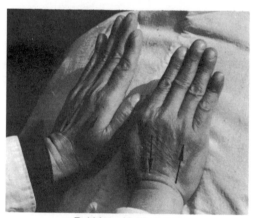

Rubbing with the palm

Indications: Common
cold, headache, stiff neck, ailments of the neck and nape,
misalignment of the eye and
mouth, acute blurring of vision, abdominal pain, diarrhea, joint pain due
to Cold-Wind-Dampness, numbness and excessive menstrual bleeding.

Effects: Warm and dredge Meridians and Collaterals, expel Wind, disperse Cold, open Apertures, improve eyesight, cultivate and invigorate
Primordial Yang.

Rolling

Move various parts of the hand freely, briskly and repeatedly with a
rolling motion over a selected area.

Where used
The shoulder, back, waist, buttocks and limbs.

Essentials
Drop your shoulders, relax your elbow and flex the wrist. Roll the back
of your hand on the selected area along or against the trend of the

meridian. The rolling action may stay in the original site or shift away along a select course. Avoid scratching or rubbing.

Techniques

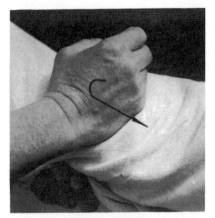

Rolling with the palm

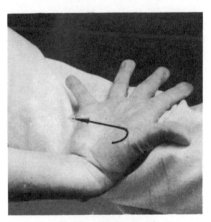

Rolling with the hand

1. Rolling with the hand

Relax your hand with fingers curved, bend the wrist, and place the ulnar side of the hand on the area or pathway of a particular meridian. Roll your hand out across the area onto its back, while gradually stretching out the fingers. When the palm faces up, your fingers should be completely outstretched. Then roll the hand in, allowing the fingers to curl again as it moves until it returns to the original position. You may use both hands in this manner, either alternating or in concert, symmetrically.

2. Rolling with the small thenar mound

Make a loose fist. Apply force through the small thenar mound. Using the forearm and the wrist, roll your fist along the selected area. Stretch out your fingers while the fist rolls out. Curl your fingers in while

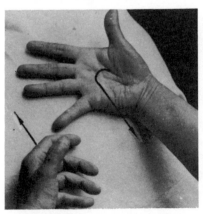

Rolling with two hands alternating

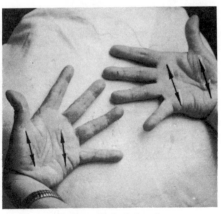

Rolling with both hands

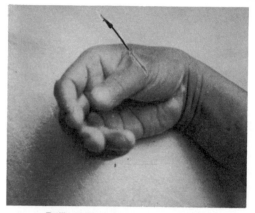

Rolling with the small thenar mound

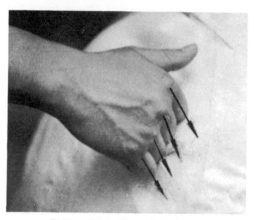

Rolling with the back of the fingers

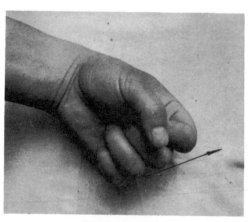

Rolling with the fist

the fist rolls in. Repeat quickly. Don't scratch, rub, clap or beat the particular area.

3. Rolling with the back of the fingers

Stretch out your elbow and flex your wrist. Clench your fingers with the thumb held out. Press the area with the backs of the fingers, applying force. Sway your forearm and wrist back and forth rapidly, to roll your fingers up and down on the area.

4. Rolling with the fist

Clench your fist. Press the small thenar mound to the selected area. Reinforce the pressure with your other hand by pressing down on your fist or by holding your wrist. Apply force with the back of the fist or the joints of the fingers and roll your fist back and forth repeatedly.

Indications: Blockage syndrome of the back and waist, numbness of limbs, hemiplegia, spasm or contractions of tendons and muscles, feeling of distension and fullness in the abdomen, abdominal pain, swelling due to Blood stasis, soft tissue trauma.

Effects: Warm and dredge Meridians and Collaterals, regulate and harmonize Vital Energy and Blood, resolve stasis, reduce swelling, relax muscular spasm and relieve pain.

Pinching

Squeeze the appropriate part of the patient's body between the thumb and any one or all of the fingers. Keep the palm high, away from contact with the skin. Pinch and loosen the area repeatedly and nimbly.

Where used
Various parts of the body.

Essentials
The action of the wrist and fingers should be nimble and well coordinated, never still or remaining in one place. The force applied should be deep and penetrating, but also soft and gentle.

Techniques

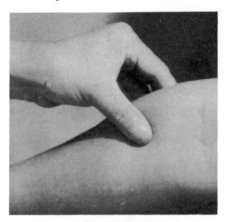

Soft pinching

1. Soft pinching

Allow your mind to become quiet, and your spirit peaceful. Press your fingers to the skin on both sides and squeeze it gently and superficially. You may use an addition circular motion of the fingers, as if nipping a Buddhist rosary. For this reason, this is also called Nipping Beads method.

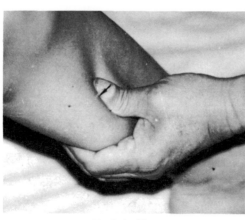

Hard pinching

2. Hard pinching

Concentrate your attention and control your breath. Apply deep and penetrating pressure. The squeezing and relaxing of muscles and tendons in this technique should be done slowly with one or both hands. Take care not to injure the skin or flesh.

Indications: Dizziness, common cold, stiff neck,

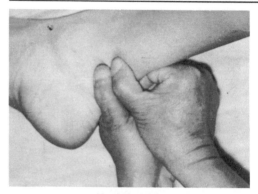

Hard pinching

nausea, vomiting, abdominal pain, diarrhea, cold limbs, difficulty in activity, traumatic bruising, injuries to tendons and dislocated joints.

Effects: Expel Wind, relieve the External, reduce Fire, clear Heat, disperse Cold, relieve pain, dredge Meridians and Collaterals, activate Blood, resolve stasis, relax Tendons, and ease joints.

Nipping

Nipping is done on a selected point using the fingernails.

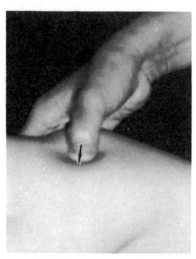

Nipping with a single finger

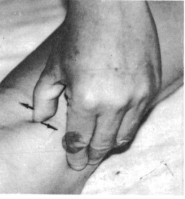

Finger Plucking Method

Where used
Points at various parts of the body.

Essentials
The force comes from the wrist, through the fingers to their tips. The nipping location should be accurate and the depth of the nipping should be appropriate. Take care not to injure the skin or flesh.

Technique
Nip a selected point with the thumbnail and/or the nail of the index or middle finger. Nipping with the thumbnail alone is called a single finger method. You may use thumbnails and/or fingernails of both hands simultaneously. Moving the nail back and forth during nipping is called Finger Plucking Method.

Indications: Sunstroke, fainting, coma, listlessness, collapse, edema of the face, epilepsy, lockjaw, tetanic spasm, contraction of limbs.

Effects: First aid, resuscitation, sober the mind, open Apertures, divide Tendons, pluck Collaterals.

Rectifying

The process of this technique is to hold, compress and stroke limbs or digits with your fingers, moving along Meridian pathways.

Where used
Arms, legs, fingers, toes.

Essentials
Bend your fingers into an arch. The degree of this depends on whether you are rectifying digits or limbs. The movement of your hand should be brisk, quick, facile and flexible. Apply uniform, symmetrical force.

Techniques

1. Rectifying the fingers and toes

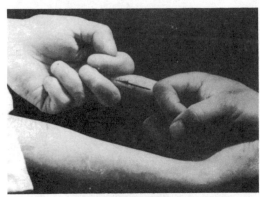

Rectifying the fingers

Grasp the sides of one digit of the patient between the knuckles of your bent index and middle fingers. Hold, compress and stroke, applying force while pulling from the root to the tip. Manipulate each finger or toe in order by the same method. You may also hold, compress and stroke the digits along their top and bottom in order.

2. Rectifying the arms and legs

Hold the patient's hand with one hand. With your other, rectify the arm along the Three Yin Meridians of the Hand. Change hands and rectify the Three Yang Meridians of the Hand. You

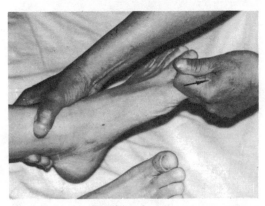

Rectifying the toes

may use both hands simul-
taneously. Rectify the Six
Meridians of the Foot by the
same method.

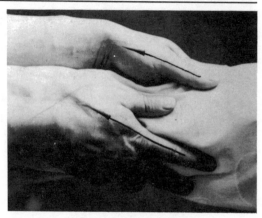

Indications: Fullness of
the head, dizziness, headache due to congestion, listlessness, weakness of the
digits, hands or feet, acute
swelling and pain in the
breast, pain and numbness
of limbs, difficult physical
activity, weakness of legs.

Rectifying the arms and legs

Effects: Dredge Meridians, activate Collaterals, expel Wind, disperse
Cold, relax spasm.

Deep-pressing

On a selected area, press and hold down the forearm or elbow, applying
considerable force to the deep tissues.

Where used
The shoulder, back, waist, buttocks and limbs.

Essentials
Drop your elbow and control your breath, and apply force to the chosen
area with the forearm or elbow. The deep-pressing force should be
increased gradually from light to heavy. The location should be accurate. Don't allow your elbow or forearm to slide or shift from the spot.
Be careful to avoid injury to bones or joints.

Techniques

1. Deep-pressing with the forearm

Press a selected area with
the full, round muscles of
the forearm (i.e., ulnar
side). The action should be
continuing and forceful accompanied by rocking and
intermittent pauses. You
may hold your forearm

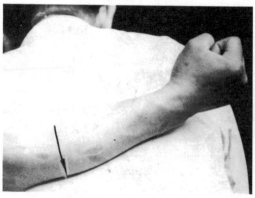

Deep-pressing with the forearm

with the other hand to reinforce the pressure.

2. Deep-pressing with the elbow

Make a fist and bend your arm so your knuckles face your chest. Press the tip of your elbow to the selected spot. The force applied should start light and gradually become heavy. In this technique, the deep-pressing action may be continuing or intermittent. This method is commonly used to massage the buttocks or parts of the legs where the muscles are full and thick.

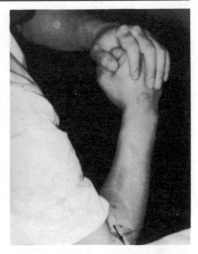

Deep-pressing with the elbow

Indications: Excessive uprising of Liver Yang, dizziness, disharmony between Liver and Stomach, neuralgia of the hip, soreness and distension of the back and waist, joint pain due to Wind-Cold-Dampness, contraction of the limbs.

Effects: Activate Vital Energy and Blood, open the obstructed, disperse Cold, expel Wind, relax spasms, relieve convulsions, dredge Meridians, alleviate pain.

Pulling

Hold the selected part of the body firmly with one or both hands, or two parts of the body with your hands on either side of or astride a joint. Rotate or pull the joint or joints along one or more directions.

Where used
The neck, shoulder, back, waist, and limbs.

Essentials
Control your breath. Your hands must be coordinated. The direction of pulling must be precise and correct. The angle of bending (of the joint) and the speed of the pulling should be appropriate to the location. The signal of successful therapy is an audible crack. This type of technique is not suitable for swollen or rigid parts of the body.

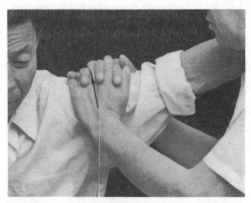
Straight pulling

Techniques

1. Straight pulling

Hold the specific part of the body firmly with both hands and apply force to pull in a straight line. This may also be done with one hand on either side of the joint, or with the fingers interlaced.

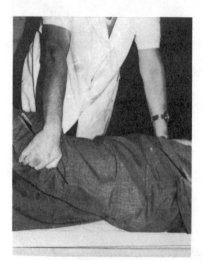
Oblique pulling

2. Oblique pulling

Hold the part of the body in place with one hand. With the other, take hold of the part across the joint and pull obliquely.

3. Circular pulling (Twisting)

Hold the part of the patient's body to be worked on firmly with your both hands on either side (for example, the head). Apply force to perform a circular clockwise or counter-clockwise pulling motion. The extent of the circular pull should be appropriate.

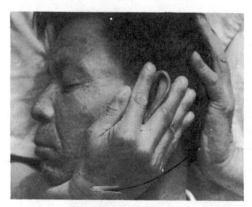
Circular pulling (Twisting)

Indications: Stiff neck, cervical spondylosis and numbness of extremities due to this, shoulder neuralgia, dislocated shoulder, stiffness of the back or spine, acute or chronic sprained waist, protruding intervertebral disc, traumatic bruising.

Effects: Divide and rectify Tendons, lubricate and ease joints, activate Blood, resolve stasis, dredge Meridians and Collaterals, set and reposition bones, relax spasms, relieve pain.

Rotating (Twisting)

Hold the affected part with both hands. Twist it in alternating directions against its own resistance. Force should be applied in both directions.

Where used
Flanks and extremities

Essentials
The interactions of the therapist's fingers, palms and wrists should be well coordinated and nimble. The patient's underlying muscles should be involved in the motions. The speed of the rotating should be appropriate to the location and condition. The procedure should be continued until the patient feels a warm sensation at the spot.

Techniques

1. Rotating the hand

Have the patient raise his/her hand with the elbow bent and the back of the hand facing you. Hold the thumb and index finger with one hand, and the ring and little fingers with the other. Twist the patient's hand right and left alternately, quickly and deftly. This method is also used on the foot.

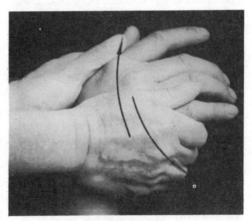

Rotating the hand

2. Clasping-rotating

Clasp an area with both hands. Apply force to twist it repeatedly from top to bottom. The twisting may be done with each of the thenar mounds, the heel of the hand and the entire hand at once.

Indications: Numbness of fingers (toes) and hands (feet), difficulty bending and stretching digits, weakness of grip, cold and aching limbs, cracking fingers, writer's cramp, depression of Liver Energy, heaviness and distension in the chest and rib cage, joint pain due to Cold-Wind-Dampness, spasm and contraction of tendons and muscles.

Effects: Relax Tendons, activate Blood, disperse and regulate Liver Energy, dredge Meridians and Collaterals, relieve spasm, alleviate pain.

Knocking

Knock a specific area rhythmically with the finger tips, or with the large thenar mound, small thenar mound and heel of the hand in sequence.

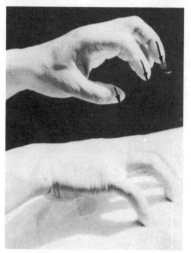

Where used
The head, chest, abdomen, back, waist, and limbs.

Essentials
Bring the fingertips together. Your wrist should be relaxed and flexible. Quiet your mind and calm your spirit. The knocking should be brisk and bouncing.

Knocking with the fingertips

Techniques

1. Knocking with the fingertips
Drop your shoulders, spread your elbows out and relax your wrist. Bend your fingers, bring them together and allow force to flow through your fingertips. This technique may be done as three, four, and five fingers knocking. In the last one, the fingertips should form the shape of a plum blossom.

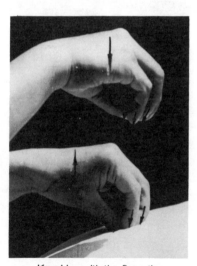

Knocking with the fingertips

2. Knocking with a cupped palm
Flex your elbow naturally and bring all five fingers together, slightly bent. This raises the center of the palm away from contact. Knock up and down rhythmically and repeatedly so that air rushes on each knock. This may be done with both hands.

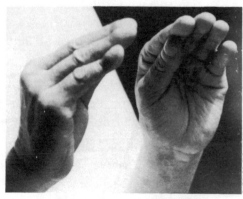

Knocking with a cupped palm

3. Knocking with the back of the hand

Bend your fingers so that your palm faces up. Knock with the back of one hand, both hands simultaneously or alternately. The knocking should be rhythmic and regular. You may also do this technique with both hands joined by interlacing your fingers. Best results come with a loud knocking sound and rushing air.

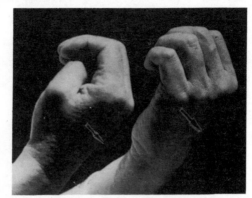

Knocking with the back of the hand

Indications: Headache, dizziness, tinnitus, insomnia, heaviness and distension in the chest and abdomen, hiccups, labored breathing due to Phlegm, joint pain due to Wind-Cold-Dampness, difficult movement of joints, restricted physical motion.

Effects: Improve hearing and eyesight, tranquilize the mind, relieve the chest, eliminate Phlegm, disperse Cold, expel Wind, dredge Apertures, ease joints.

Vibrating

Allow Vital Energy to flow to your finger or hand. Apply force by quickly vibrating the finger or hand on the point or area. While doing this, draw Vital Energy from the patient, or lead Vital Energy into the patient, as desired.

Where used
All points of the body.

Essentials
Concentrate your mind, motivate Vital Energy to your hand, and allow force to flow from your finger or hand. Do not press with force. Use the principle of Meet-Follow Invigorate-Reduce and shift the finger or hand with or against the trend of the Meridian as appropriate.

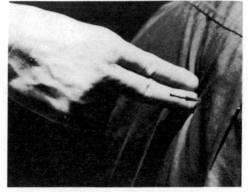

Vibrating with sword-like fingers

Techniques

1. Vibrating with the finger

Extend the index and middle fingers, pressed together as a sword, or into the position for dotting. Straighten your arm and elbow, touch the selected point with your fingertips, and motivate Vital Energy to begin the vibration. This may also be done by pressing the touching finger with another of the same hand to produce the vibration.

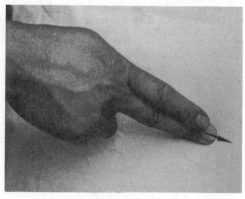

Vibrating with dotting fingers

2. Vibrating with the palm

Drop your shoulders, extend your elbow and straighten your wrist. Press the center of your palm, Laogong (Per 8), precisely on the selected spot and vibrate quickly. You may also do this with the large and small thenar mounds or the heel of the hand.

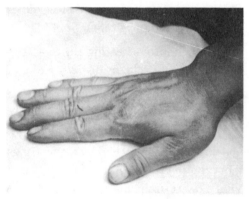

Vibrating with the palm

Indications: Headache, vertigo, sunstroke, nausea, cold limbs, abdominal and diaphragmatic pain, severe palpitations, palpitations due to fright, insomnia and amnesia.

Effects: Dredge Meridians and Collaterals, regulate Vital Energy and Blood, clear the head and eyes, ease the chest and diaphragm, calm fright, tranquilize the mind.

Scratching

Send Vital Energy through all five fingers and hold your hand as if an eagle's talons. Press the pads of the fingers closely to the patient's back and waist, and scratch straight and forcefully from top to bottom. This is also called Manipulation with the Eagle's Talons.

Where used
The back and waist.

Essentials
Motivate Vital Energy through your arm and wrist, and initiate force from your fingers. The speed of scratching should be fast. The patients should feel a burning hot sensation. Be careful not to injure the skin.

Technique

Bend your elbow and straighten your wrist. Spread out your hand, straighten and separate the fingers with only the last joint flexed. Press the middle finger to Dazhui (GV 14), with the other fingers in order. Scratch forcefully in a straight line from top to bottom. Scratch the middle first, then the left side, then the right.

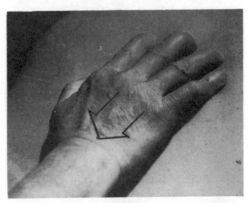

Scratching

Indications: Soreness of back and waist, lassitude, weakness, chills, aversion to Cold, Meridians attacked by Dampness, impeded Blood circulation, loss of appetite, difficulty in urination and defecation.

Effects: Relieve muscles, expel pathogens from the exterior, open the obstructed, dredge and rectify Vital Energy and Blood, warm the Middle Warmer, disperse Cold, strengthen Spleen, eliminate Dampness, reinforce body resistance, expel pathogens, invigorate True Yang significantly.

Chopping

Chop a selected area with the outside of your hand, both hands alternately, or joined hands, as if mincing meat. This is also called cutting-beating.

Where used
The chest, abdomen, back, waist and limbs.

Essentials
Your elbow and wrist should be nimble and flexible. Apply brisk force. The chopping should be rhythmic, moving gradually from slow to fast.

Techniques

1. Chopping with one hand

Bend your elbow in toward your body and hold your hand perpendicular to the selected spot. Chop with the side of your hand.

2. Chopping with two hands

Hold your hands the same way as above. Your two hands may chop simultaneously or alternately.

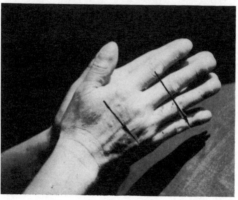
Chopping with joined hands

3. Chopping with joined hands

Press your hands and fingers together with fingers outstretched and separated. Chop up and down with a loud sound of chopping and rushing air. You may also do this with your fingers interlaced and palms against each other.

Indications: Cough, labored breathing due to Phlegm, abdominal distension and flatulence from overeating, stiffness of the back, sprain in the waist, sudden chest distress, pain in the extremities, general weakness.

Effects: Relieve the chest, ease the diaphragm, eliminate Phlegm, rectify Vital Energy, relax Tendons, activate Blood, dredge Meridians, alleviate pain.

Pounding

Clench your fist loosely with the thumb inside. Pound the area briskly, rhythmically and nimbly.

Where used

The head, shoulders, back, waist, limbs and various joints.

Essentials

Keep your fist loose, with your wrist flexible and relaxed. The force you apply should not be too heavy. Be quiet in mind and peaceful in spirit. Avoid violent beating, stiff wrist or solid fist.

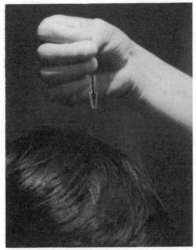

Pounding with an open fist

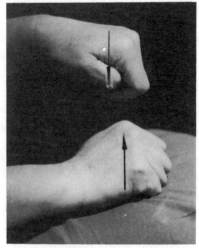

Pounding with a prone fist

Techniques

1. Pounding with an open fist

This is also called the lateral fist. Bend your wrist slightly in, with the thumb up. Do not hurry the rising and falling of the fist. The selected area should be pounded softly. It is appropriate to hear the sound *kwa, kwa* during the pounding. A single fist is adequate for the head and shoulders. Both fists may be used in other areas, alternating.

2. Pounding with a prone fist

Straighten your wrist and turn your fist so that the fingers are down. Pound with one or two fists.

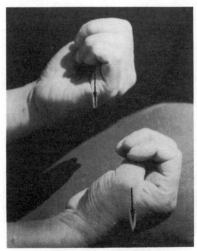

Pounding with a supine fist

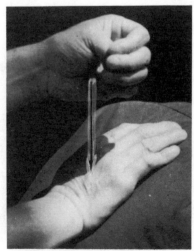

Padded pounding

3. Pounding with a supine fist

Stretch out your fist with the fingers facing up. Pound a selected area with the back of the fist. Use one or two fists.

4. Padded pounding

Place one cupped palm with its center above the afflicted spot as if you were knocking with an open hand. Pound the back of this hand with the clenched fist of the other. There will be a sound of rushing air with each pounding. The area can be shifted around.

Indications: Headache, dizziness, listlessness, cough, labored breathing due to Phlegm, nausea, vomiting, pain of shoulder, back, waist and legs, tendon spasms, Blood stasis.

Effects: Relax Tendons, activate Blood, clear Heat, depress Fire, stop cough, eliminate labored breathing, tranquilize the mind, ease spasm, alleviate pain, dredge Meridians and Collaterals.

Compound Techniques

Pinching-grasping

In this, as in most of the grasping techiques, both are done simultaneously as one, each as part of the other, rather than separately or successively. This has a synergistic effect and brings much more dynamic results than the sum or either technique done separately.

Where used
Various muscles.

Essentials
The force you use should be soft and gentle, gradually deepening and penetrating. This technique should be repeated nimbly in successive steps until the patient feels sensations of soreness, distension and numbness at the area being treated.

Technique
Take and hold a handful of soft tissue with one or two hands. Pinch and grasp it, then loosen your grip. Repeat successively at the same spot or along or against the

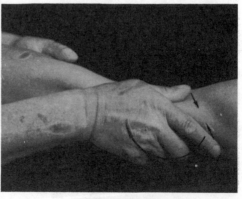

Pinching-grasping

trend of the Meridian. This is often used to treat disorders of all the Meridians of the Hand and Foot.

Indications: Palpitations, panic, epigastric pain, cough and labored breathing due to Phlegm, distress in chest and rib cage, asthma, hiccups, abdominal distension and flatulence due to overeating, abdominal pain and Stomach ache, common disorders of any of the Meridians of the Hand or Foot.

Effects: Clear and ventilate Lung Energy, stop cough, resolve Phlegm, promote digestion, remove stagnation, activate Blood, alleviate pain, relax spasm, tranquilize the mind.

Holding-grasping

Where used
Muscles of the back, waist and limbs.

Essentials
This is a gentler version of the previous technique. Using your fingers and palm to apply force, hold and grasp an area, lift it and loosen your grip. Pause and repeat successively. Maintain a moderate speed.

Technique
Press the palm and fingers of one or both hands to the selected area. Hold and grasp a handful of soft tissue quickly, then loosen. Pause and repeat using moderate force and speed in a fixed spot or shifting along the muscles.

Holding-grasping

Indications: Common cold, headache, dizziness, muscle spasms, soreness of back or waist, cold limbs, difficulty in walking.

Effects: Expel Wind, disperse Cold, warm Meridians, dredge Collaterals, resolve stasis, relax spasm, activate Blood, alleviate pain.

Grabbing-grasping

Where used
The head, neck, nape, back, abdomen and limbs.

Essentials

Control your breath, motivate Vital Energy through your fingers and form "Eagle's Talons" with your hand. Grasp and lift, applying force through the fingers with your palm raised. Take care not to injure the skin or underlying muscles.

Technique

Stretch out your fingers. Grab-grasp the area quickly and loosen it. Repeat rhythmically. When you use this technique on the abdomen, have the patient synchronize breathing with the rhythm of the procedure.

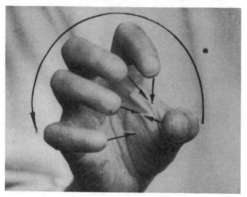

Grabbing-grasping

Indications: Headache, stiff neck, cervical spondylosis, stiff back muscles, abdominal pain, diarrhea, spasms or contractions of limbs.

Effects: Activate Blood, expel Wind, warm Meridians, disperse Cold, eliminate Dampness, promote urination, relax spasm, relieve pain.

Nipping-grasping

Where used

The neck, nape, shoulder, and various limb joints (fissures, apertures, fossae, points, etc.).

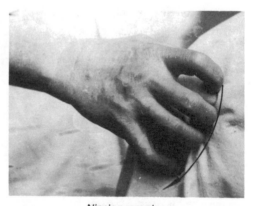

Nipping-grasping

Essentials

Both techniques are done as one and should be skillfully coordinated. Apply energetic force, without penetrating too quickly. The patient should feel soreness, numbness and distension.

Technique

Bend the fingers of one or both hands into hooks. Probe the fissures, fossae and points around the joints. Nip and grasp nimbly and intermittently, pressing and relaxing in turn.

Indications: Pain or stiffness of joints, difficult flexion and extension in joints, severe and migratory joint pain, trauma and common disorders of the bones.

Effects: Disperse Cold, expel Wind, dredge Meridians and Collaterals, relax Tendons, activate Blood, lubricate and ease joints.

Plucking-grasping

Where used
The neck, nape, shoulder, back and limbs.

Essentials
Apply force through your fingertips, palpating the soft tissues to find the selected tendon. Grasp the tendon and pluck it repeatedly. Proceed slowly and intermittently. Avoid nipping with fingernails or rubbing the skin with the fingertips.

Technique
Probe for the tendon with the tip of your thumb, index and middle finger. Grasp it firmly, lift it, then pluck it gently as if playing a guitar.

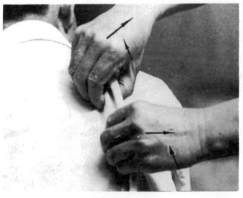

Indications: Stiff neck and nape, joint pain due to Wind-Cold- Dampness, numbness, stiff back and waist, tendon and muscle spasms.

Plucking-grasping

Effects: Dredge Meridians and Collaterals, relax and rectify the Tendons, resolve stasis, activate Blood, eliminate spasms, relieve pain.

Lifting-grasping

Where used
Muscles of the back and abdomen.

Essentials
Grasp, lift and rotate with both hands acting symmetrically. Keep the speed moderate. Continue until the patient feels warmth. Do not grasp internal organs.

Technique

Grasp and lift the muscles of the abdomen or along the ribs with both hands, or hold them with the thenar mounds. Rotate them back and forth symmetrically several times. Repeat successively.

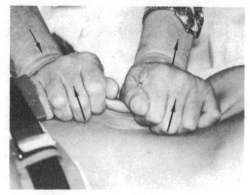

Lifting-grasping

Indications: Acute pain in abdomen and back, heaviness and distension in the chest and rib cage, hiccups, belching, disharmony between Liver and Stomach.

Effects: Relax spasms, relieve pain, dredge and clear obstructions, disperse and rectify Liver Energy, regulate and harmonize Spleen and Stomach.

Pulling-grasping

Where used
The neck, shoulder, back, waist and limbs.

Essentials
Combine these two techniques skillfully and nimbly. You may use them as one movement, or sequentially with either one first. The position, extent and angle of pulling should be accurate and the speed appropriate to the condition. Avoid being rough or grasping persistently.

Technique
Let the patient rest in a comfortable position (sitting, lying prone, supine or on his/her side). Pull on the selected part of the body to ease the movement of the joint, and grasp the area or point with the other hand. Both hands should work in coordination. You may work with both hands at once by supporting the patient with your leg or chest for stability. For further applications, see Passive movements.

Indications: Restricted motion of the neck, cervical spondylosis, dislocation of cervical vertebra, scapular pain, inflammation around the shoulder joint, stiffness of back and spine, acute or chronic sprain of the waist or leg, strained lumbar muscles, protruding lumbar disc, trauma due to falling, beating, pulling, wrenching, etc.

Effects: Relax and rectify Tendons and muscles, relieve spasm, set and reposition bones, lubricate and ease joints, activate Blood, reduce swelling, dissipate stasis, alleviate pain.

Kneading-grasping

Where used
Various muscles.

Essentials
Both procedures are done as one, with each aspect in harmony, grasping and kneading selected muscles. The progression is circular and may be shifted along the body. Apply soft, penetrating force through the palm and fingers.

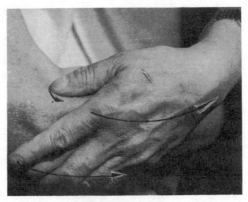
Kneading-grasping

Technique
Press the palm and fingers of one or both hands to the area and grasp it. Revolve the hand from the wrist and elbow in a circular motion, kneading and grasping at moderate speed.

Indications: Common cold, headache, rigidity of the back and nape of neck, stiff neck, shoulder neuralgia, joint pain in the back and waist due to Wind-Cold-Dampness, aching and distension of muscles, numbness of limbs, difficult joint motion, cramping in the calf, swelling and Blood stasis due to trauma.

Effects: Expel Wind, eliminate Dampness, disperse Cold, relax muscles and Tendons, activate Blood, dredge Meridians and Collaterals, relieve pain.

Kneading-pinching

Where used
Various parts of the body.

Essentials
The two procedures are done as one. The force should be soft but penetrating, and the rolling movement of the fingers uniformly nimble. Keep your palm raised.

Technique
Grasp the skin and superficial fascia between the thumb and any or all of the other fingers. Knead and pinch the area lightly and nimbly, moving the tissues back and forth. You may use both hands at once.

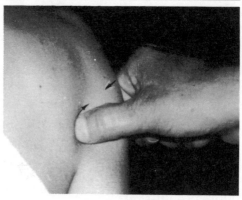
Kneading-pinching

Indications: Dizziness, nausea, vomiting, listlessness, weakness, cervical spondylosis, stiff neck, joint pain in the back or waist caused by Wind-Cold-Dampness, swelling due to Blood stasis, numbness, aching of various parts of the body.

Effects: Regulate and invigorate Vital Energy and Blood, sober the mind, open Apertures, resolve stasis, reduce swelling, warm Meridians, relieve pain.

Kneading-nipping

Where used
Various points.

Essentials
Both procedures are blended harmoniously into one. Locate the point to be treated precisely and apply appropriate force. Start slowly and gradually increase the speed. Effects are best when the patient feels strong sensations. Take care not to injure the skin or muscles.

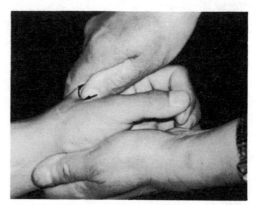
Kneading-nipping

Technique
Apply force to the selected point with the tip of the thumb and any or all of the fingers. Knead and nip repeatedly in a circular motion, until the patient feels soreness, numbness and distension. You may use both hands at once.

Indications: For common diseases of Heart, Lung, Triple Warmer, Large Intestine and Small Intestine, knead and nip the primary points of the Yin and Yang Meridians of the Hand. To treat common diseases of the Liver, Kidney, Stomach and Gall Bladder, knead and nip the Yin and Yang Meridians of the Foot.

Effects: Dredge Meridians and Collaterals, balance Yin and Yang, promote the flow of Vital Energy and Blood. This technique will strengthen the body's resistance if done regularly.

Kneading-vibrating

Where used
Various parts or points of the body.

Essentials
Hold your strength in your forearm, and apply force from the hand or finger. These two techniques are done as one. Apply soft, brisk force which gradually becomes deep and penetrating.

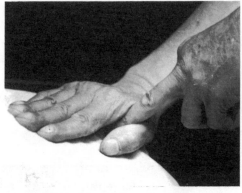

Techniques

1. Kneading-vibrating with a finger

Press your hand lightly on the area with the fingers closed and palm raised. Grip the

Kneading-vibrating with a finger

middle finger of your other hand between the thumb and index finger. Curl the other fingers up and press your middle finger to the selected spot. Dot with your middle fingertip, then knead with the cupped palm while you vibrate the middle finger by rotating and quivering your wrist. The vibrating may also be done with the thumb or the index and middle finger in sword-style.

2. Kneading-vibrating with the palm

Extend your hand and straighten your wrist. Press the thenar mounds, the heel of the hand, or the entire hand to the area. Knead softly in a circular motion while vibrat-

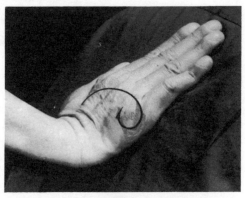

Kneading-vibrating with the palm

ing quickly. You may move the hand along from one area to another.

Indications: Rigidity of the neck and nape, stiff neck, wryneck, swelling and pain of the throat, heaviness in the chest, flatulence, abdominal masses, aching of the back and waist, swelling of limbs and joints due to Blood stasis, difficulty in movement, dysmenorrhea and other menstrual irregularities.

Effects: Rectify Vital Energy, eliminate retention, soften hardnesses, dissipate the stagnant, warm and dredge Meridians and Collaterals, activate Blood, resolve stasis.

Pressing-pushing

Where used
Subclavicular fossa, armpit, popliteal fossa.

Essentials
Allow your mind to become quiet and your spirit calm. Press and push steadily at a specific place, "helping the strong with the flexible, and the flexible with the strong." The Vital Energy you bring up and the force you apply should be appropriate. Your action should be quick and nimble. The best effects are seen when the patient has a strong response.

Technique
Let the patient relax comfortably. Concentrate your mind, breathe naturally, and bring Vital Energy to your hand, particularly the middle finger. Crook your fingers slightly and probe the fossa. Press in and push up and down, forward and back, right and left. Gradually increase the speed from slow to fast. This is also called, "Pressing-pushing the three fossae."

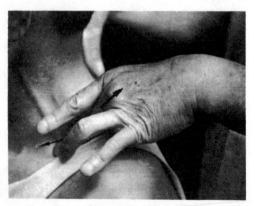

Pressing-pushing

Indications: Epigastric pain, heaviness and feeling of suffocation in the chest, cough, labored breathing due to Phlegm, hiccups, belching, nausea, vomiting, oppression and distension in the rib cage, abdominal distension, stomach ache, strained waist, sudden discomfort of the chest, leg pain, restricted or difficult knee motion, urticaria.

Effects: Ventilate Lung Energy, depress adverse uprising, stop vomiting, eliminate heaviness and distension, regulate and harmonize Vital Energy and Blood, dredge Meridians, activate Collaterals, relax spasms, relieve pain.

Whisking-sweeping

Where used
The back and waist.

Essentials
Concentrate your mind and breathe naturally. Relax your shoulders, elbows, wrists and hands. The motion of your hands should be like whisking or sweeping, rising and falling gracefully.

Technique
Have the patient sit in a stable posture with the back straight. Sit behind and stretch your arms out naturally. Apply force with both hands, moving them outward from either side of the spine. Increase speed from slow to fast.

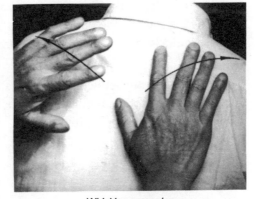
Whisking-sweeping

Indications: Lassitude, weakness, scapular pain, hiccups, belching, congested chest and diaphragm, cough and labored breathing due to Phlegm, disorders of the back and waist due to Wind-Cold-Dampness.

Effects: Resolve Phlegm, ventilate Lung Energy, relieve the chest, ease the diaphragm, expel Wind, disperse Cold, warm Meridians, alleviate pain.

Whirling with the thumb

Where used
Pain in fissures or gaps around joints, tenderness or pain in muscles.

Essentials
Bring Vital Energy to the tip of your thumb and hold your breath. Whirl your thumb energetically at the painful spot.

Technique
Let the patient lie in a prone position. Clench your fist with the thumb
extended as if hitch-hiking. Press the most painful spot with the tip of
the thumb. Hold your breath and apply force to whirl the thumb. The
underlying muscles should be pushed along in a single direction.

Indications: Severe deep pain in the gaps of joints, spasm and cramping
of muscles.

Effects: Relax spasms, relieve pain. The effect is immediate.

Jerking-dragging

Where used
The waist and legs.

Essentials
The patient's leg should be relaxed. Use energetic force.

Technique
The patient lies in a supine position with arms down. Stand below the
feet. Hold the leg of the diseased side above the ankle with both hands.
Push the leg toward the patient's chest, then yank it back toward you
sharply, quickly and energetically. Repeat the procedure on the other
leg.

Indications: Acute and chronic injuries to the soft tissues of the waist,
protruding lumbar disc, trauma of tendons of the legs, difficult flexion and
extension, neuralgia of the hip.

Effects: Promote the flow of Vital Energy and Blood, resolve stasis,
dissipate stagnation, stretch and rectify Tendons and muscles.

Special techniques

Hand rolling with forearm revolving

Where used
The back, the waist, the abdomen and the limbs.

Essentials
These two techniques should be coordinated harmoniously, with each
done appropriately. Movements should be gentle, circular and nimble.
The force applied should gradually deepen and penetrate.

Techniques

1. The back, the waist and the legs

Sit beside the patient, who is prone. Your forearm revolves on the back or waist while your hand rolls on the leg (usually

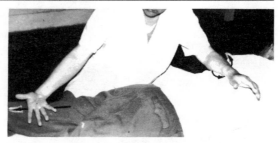

Hand rolling with forearm revolving

along the Urinary Bladder Meridian). When completed, shift to the other side and repeat.

2. The abdomen and the legs

Sit beside the patient, who is supine with his/her toes extended and pointed in. Your forearm revolves on the abdomen while your hand rolls on the leg (usually along the Stomach Meridian). Repeat on the patient's other side.

3. The arms and the legs

Sit beside the patient, who is either prone or supine. Roll your hand on the Three Yin or Yang Meridians of the Hand, while revolving your forearm on either the front or back of the leg (usually along the pathway of a Meridian). Repeat on the other side.

Indications: Pain of the back, waist and legs due to Wind-Cold-Dampness; Kidney deficiency or trauma, acute and chronic stomach ache, chronic appendicitis, flaccid paralysis and weakness of limbs, irregular menstruation, leukorrhea.

Effects: Activate Blood, resolve stasis, strengthen Spleen, eliminate Dampness, promote urination and defecation, soften Tendons, enrich muscles, warm Meridians, dredge Collaterals, relieve pain.

Forearm revolving with pinching-grasping

Where used
The back, the waist, the abdomen and the limbs

Essentials
The revolving should be circular, involving the underlying muscles. The pinching and grasping should be soft, gradually deepening and penetrating. Your arms should be coordinated in actions and sequence.

Techniques

1. With the patient supine

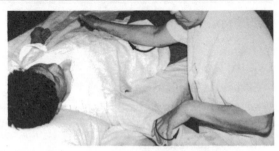

Sit beside the patient. Revolve your forearm on the abdomen, and pinch and grasp the arm along a Yin Meridian with your

Forearm revolving with pinching-grasping

hand. Then revolve your other forearm on the abdomen and pinch and grasp the leg along a Yin or Yang Meridian. Continue in sequence until completed, then shift to the other side and repeat.

2. With the patient prone

Sit beside the patient. Revolve your forearm on the back and waist, and pinch and grasp along a Yang Meridian on the arm. Then revolve your other forearm on the back and waist, and pinch and grasp along a Yang Meridian on the leg. Continue in sequence and then do the other side.

Indications: Pain of the chest and back, cough and labored breathing due to excessive Phlegm, severe palpitation, palpitation due to fright, disharmony between Liver and Stomach, aching or soreness of the waist and legs, numbness of limbs, flaccid paralysis and weakness, irregular or excessive menstruation, amenorrhea.

Effects: Ventilate and rectify Lung Energy, disperse Liver Energy, harmonize Stomach, relax spasms, relieve convulsions, strengthen the waist and Kidney, regulate menses, activate Blood, resolve stasis, relieve pain.

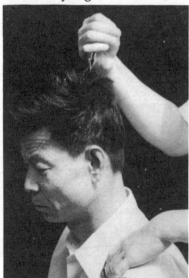

Open-fist pounding with pinching-grasping

Open-fist pounding with pinching-grasping

Where used

The head, the shoulder and the limbs.

Essentials

These two movements should be coordinated in harmony, matching the number of poundings to the number of pinching-graspings. The procedure should be brisk and nimble.

Techniques

1. The head and the shoulder

The patient sits in a stable position, while you stand behind. Pound the top of the patient's head with the open fist and pinch and grasp the shoulder with the other hand. The actions of the two hands should be balanced, without one or the other dominating.

2. The arms and the legs

A. The Three Yang Meridians of the Hand and Foot. The patient lies on his/her side with straightened arms and legs. Sit beside the patient and pound with the open fist and pinch-grasp with the other hand, along the Yang Meridians. Your two hands may work either simultaneously or alternately.

B. The Three Yin Meridians of the Hand and Foot. The patient lies on his/her side, but facing upward a bit, with the lower arm outstretched, palm up, and the lower leg slightly bent. Sit beside the patient and work on the Yin Meridians of the Hand and Foot. Shift to the other side if both arms and legs require this procedure.

Indications: Migraine, headache, deviation of the eye and mouth, hemiplegia or hemiplegia accompanied by numbness and pain.

Effects: Normalize Yin and Yang, dredge Meridians and Collaterals, relax Tendons, activate Blood, disperse Cold, relieve pain.

Elbow revolving with dotting

Where used
The back, the buttocks, the legs and their points.

Essentials
The two different procedures are done simultaneously. Areas and points should be accurately chosen. The force should increase gradually. Maintain a moderate pace — don't allow yourself to hurry.

Techniques

1. The back and the buttocks

Sit beside the patient, who is prone. Revolve the buttock with the elbow while dotting selected points on the patient's back.

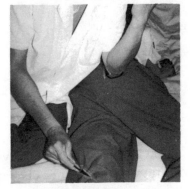

Elbow revolving with dotting

2. *The buttocks and the legs*

Sit beside your patient who is prone. Revolve your elbow on the buttock, primarily Huantiao (GB 30), and dot selected points on the patient's leg.

Indications: Rheumatic and rheumatoid joint pain, blockage syndrome of the back and waist, flaccid paralysis of the legs, hemiplegia, traumatic pain of the waist and legs, after-effects of bone trauma, difficult movement of the leg joints.

Effects: Relax and rectify Tendons, resolve stasis, activate Blood, open and dredge the obstructed, disperse Liver Energy, regulate the flow of Vital Energy, expel Wind, eliminate Cold, dredge Meridians, relieve pain.

Hand-rolling with clapping-knocking

Where used
The back, the waist and the legs.

Essentials
The rolling hand should be nimble. When clapping, your hand should have a raised palm, with your fingers together and straight. When knocking, your hand should be open with fingers curved. Coordinate the movements of your hands.

Techniques

1. *The back*

The patient is prone. Clap and knock the points of the Urinary Bladder Meridian along one side of the spine, and roll your hand along the points

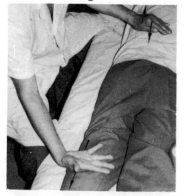

of the same Meridian on the other side. The actions of the two hands may be reversed.

2. *The waist and the legs*

Sit beside the prone patient. Clap and knock a selected area of the waist with one hand and roll your other hand on the leg. You may shift your sitting position to change hands, or perform this technique on both sides of your patient.

Hand-rolling with clapping-knocking

Indications: Cough, labored breathing due to Phlegm, wheezing, heaviness in the chest, hiccups, vomiting, pain in the waist and legs due to trauma or Wind-Cold-Dampness, neuralgia of the hip.

Effects: Relax the chest, ease the diaphragm, promote digestion, resolve Phlegm, depress adverse uprising, stop vomiting, activate Blood, expel Wind, warm and dredge Meridians and Collaterals, relieve spasms and pain.

Pounding-chopping with round-rubbing

Where used
The back, the lumbosacral area and the limbs.

Essentials
Let your mind become quiet and your spirit calm. Focus your attention. The pounding and chopping should be rhythmic, and the round-rubbing agile. Coordinate the two techniques systematically.

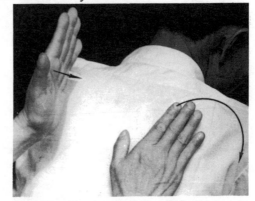

Pounding-chopping with round-rubbing

Techniques

1. *The back and the arms*

Sit behind and slightly to one side of the patient, who should sit in a stable posture. Pound and chop the selected area of the patient's back while round-rubbing the shoulder, elbow and wrist sequentially along a straight line. Shift to the other side and repeat.

2. *The lumbosacral area and the legs*

Sit beside the prone patient. Pound and chop the waist or lumbosacral area with one hand, and with the other, round-rub the leg from Chengfu (UB 36) down to the ankle in a straight line. Depending on the patient's condition, you might choose to whirl and round-rub the lumbosacral area while pounding and chopping the leg, or shift your seat and change hands, or work on both sides.

Indications: Distension and heaviness due to overeating, cough and labored breathing due to Phlegm, pain and coldness of the limbs, strained waist, sudden distress in the chest, stiffness of the knee, irregular menstruation. ·

Effects: Relax the chest, ease the diaphragm, eliminate the stagnated, resolve Phlegm, relax and rectify Tendons and muscles, regulate and harmonize Vital Energy and Blood.

Whisking-sweeping and pounding-chopping

Where used
The back and the legs.

Essentials
Become quiet in mind and calm in spirit. Pound with an open fist, chop with the edge of the palm. The whisking and sweeping should be agile. The force applied should be nimble and brisk.

Techniques

1. The back
Sit behind the patient, who is sitting in a stable posture. Whisk and sweep one side of the back from the spine outward while pounding and chopping alternately on the other side. Change hands as desired.

2. The legs
Sit beside your patient who is supine with toes outstretched and pointing in. Pound and chop a selected area on the front of the thigh with one hand while whisking and sweeping the side of the lower leg with the other. Change hands as needed.

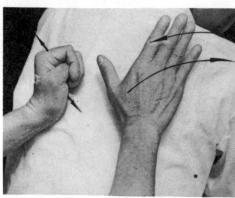

Whisking-sweeping and pounding-chopping

Indications: Heaviness in chest and distension of the rib cage, backache, soreness of the waist, pain and numbness in the leg, stiff joints, etc.

Effects: Smooth the flow of Vital Energy, eliminate heaviness and distension, activate Blood, expel Wind, relax spasms, relieve pain, warm Meridians, dredge Collaterals.

Knocking-clapping-pounding-chopping-hitting

Where used
The back, the lumbosacral area and the limbs.

Essentials
Be quiet in mind and calm in spirit. Relax your hands. Knock with the fingertips, clap with a raised palm, pound with an open fist, chop with the

edge of the hand, and hit softly with the heel of the hand. Change techniques in sequence during this set of procedures. Your hands should work nimbly, swiftly and regularly. The beating sounds should be rhythmic.

Techniques

1. The shoulder and the back

You and the patient are both sitting, with you behind. Work along both sides of the Urinary Bladder Meridian with noth hands from the shoulder down to the back repeatedly.

2. The lumbosacral area and the legs

Sit beside the patient, who is prone. Work at a part of the lumbosacral area with one hand, and along the Urinary Bladder Meridian of the leg with the other. Repeat on the opposite side.

3. The arms and the legs

Sit beside the patient, who is supine with both arms stretched out. Work along the Three Yin or Yang Meridians of the Hand with one hand, and along the front of the leg with the other. Do the patient's other side the same way.

Indications: Cough with much spitting, slow heart beat, disharmony between Liver and Stomach, feeling of distension and heaviness due to overeating, lumbago and leg pain, stiff joints, numbness in the limbs, flaccid paralysis, weakness, irregular menstruation, amenorrhea, dysmenorrhea, etc.

Effects: Stop cough, quell asthma, eliminate distension and heaviness, activate Blood, resolve stasis, lubricate and ease joints, warm and invigorate the waist and Kidney, enrich muscles.

Stepping

Where used
The back, the waist, the spine and the back of the leg.

Essentials
Inhale and hold your breath momentarily and lighten your body. Step gently and steadily, applying force appropriately, from light to heavy. The speed of this procedure should not be too fast. This technique should be coordinated with the patient's breathing. Take extreme precautions against injuring the patient with overly forceful steps.

Technique
Hang rings or a suspended wooden frame from the ceiling. You may want to use sturdy canes or a stable structure for climbing. The patient

lies in a prone position. Cushions may be indicated, according to the patient's condition. Hold the ring (frame, cane, structure) with one or both hands. Inhale and hold your breath momentarily, lighten your body and control the force of your step according to what is needed. Step on a selected area at the spine, waist, buttocks, or leg with your toes, your heel, the entire foot, or both feet. You may want to vibrate your foot slightly while pressing it to a fixed location, or stretch the pressure along a Meridian pathway, shifting the location with agility. Have your patient exhale while you are stepping down and inhale as you lift your foot. Keep the patient calm and relaxed. Breath naturally.

Indications: Sudden sprain of the waist, sudden distress in the chest, tendon spasm, stiff joints, blockage syndrome of the back and waist due to Wind-Cold-Dampness, rickets.

Effects: Dredge and rectify Vital Energy, expel Wind, disperse Cold, relax Tendons, activate Collaterals, relieve pain, open the obstructed, reposition joints.

Scraping

This is a simple and easy therapeutic technique which has been passed along from generation to generation. It is also called "Scraping therapy."

Where used
The neck and nape, both sides of the spine, the chest and rib cage, the abdomen, the cubital fossa, the popliteal fossa.

Essentials
Scraping should be brisk and easy. The force should be appropriate,

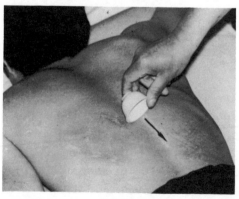
Scraping

gradually deepening and penetrating. The edge of the utensils used should be smooth. Don't injure the skin. Watch the change of skin color continually.

Technique
The patient is either prone or supine. Place one hand on the area to hold the skin in place, and hold an appropriate utensil with the other hand. This could be a wine cup, a spoon, a comb, etc. Apply a suitable medium to the area. Scrape the skin with the utensil along straight lines from top to bottom or outward from the

center, until the area becomes darker, red or purple. The middle joint of the index finger or the back of the thumb-nail may be used instead of a utensil. This technique is often used to treat the elderly, weak patients or children.

Indications: Fever due to common cold, sunstroke, infantile convulsions, heaviness in the chest, nausea, vomiting, diarrhea, epidemic diseases, febrile diseases, numbness of limbs, etc.

Effects: Clear Heat, cool Blood, depress adverse uprising, stop vomiting, eliminate retention, remove the stagnated, activate Blood, resolve masses.

Passive Movements

Passive movements of the neck and nape

Where used
The neck and nape.

Essentials
The patient's neck should be relaxed. Pull, twist, drag (see below) and stretch the neck with both hands. Use an appropriate speed, with the extent of pulling and the angle of bending accurately controlled. Avoid any harsh actions.

Techniques

1. Rotate the neck

Let the patient sit in a stable position with the neck relaxed. Hold the back of the head firmly with one hand and support the jaw with the other. To begin, twist the head gently several times the the end of its range of motion, then turn it quickly and deftly in the chosen direction to reach the proper angle. After you hear the crack, immediately begin to pinch and grasp until the patient feels a warm sensation.

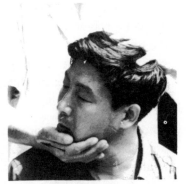
Rotate the neck

2. Twist the neck
This is commonly practiced as a circular twisting-pulling-grasping technique, which may be done in two different styles.

A. The patient lies prone, with arms crossed under the chin. Stand behind and to one side. Press the healthy side of the cervical vertebra with the thumb of one hand. Support and hold the chin with the other. Pull, twist and stretch the head toward the diseased side with appropriate angle and extent of rotation. Once this is done, begin pinching and grasping, or push and press on the occiput to twist the head toward the healthy side.

B. The patient sits in a stable posture with the occiput pressed against your chest. Pull and twist the neck with both hands according to the method described above. (Refer to Circular pulling)

3. Drag the neck (Traction)

This is a straight pulling and grasping technique to drag and stretch the neck. It also has two variations.

A. The patient sits in a stable posture. Put your forearm on the left shoulder to support and hold the chin. With the tip of the thumb and index finger of the other hand, deep-press on both Fengchi (GB 20), or on both sides of a cervical vertebra. Pull, rock, drag and stretch upwards with both hands.

B. The patient is prone. Sit in front of the patient's head with knees bent, legs apart, and feet propped against his/her shoulders. Hold the jaw with the fingers of both hands. Slowly press the shoulders away from you with your feet and drag to stretch the neck, or gently turn the head from side to side, or rock it while dragging and stretching.

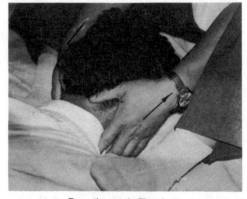

Drag the neck (Traction)

Indications: Injuries of neck tendons, dislocation of cervical vertebrae, pain and stiffness of the neck and nape, cramp in the neck involving the shoulder, wryneck, difficult physical movements, cervical spondylosis, protruding cervical disc, pathological changes of cervical vertebrae due to falling, beating, wrenching, etc.

Effects: Set bones and reposition joints, relax Tendons, ease joints, open the obstructed, resolve stasis, relieve spasm, alleviate pain.

Passive movements of the arms

Where used
The shoulder, the elbow, the wrist, the hand, the fingers.

Essentials
Both hands work together as a coordinated unit. Be very accurate about the part of the arm you are working on. Strictly control the extent of the stretching, dragging, twisting, rocking, jerking, deep pressing, rectifying and arranging. Use appropriate force. The technique should be done skillfully and nimbly, without sharp or harsh motions. Take care not to dislocate any joints.

Techniques

1. Arrange the shoulder

This may be divided into four approaches.

A. Support the elbow and twist the shoulder joint. The patient sits in a stable position. Hold the diseased shoulder. Nip or grasp selected points with one hand, support the elbow of the affected side with the other, and deep-press Quchi (LI 11) with the thumb. Then, turn the arm inward, outwards, and lift the arm up; or support the arm to twist it clockwise and counterclockwise, thereby activating the shoulder joint.

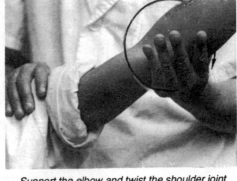

Support the elbow and twist the shoulder joint

B. Hold the arm, stretch the shoulder. The patient is sitting and stable. Stand behind the affected side. Deep-press the diseased shoulder (front, upper or back part) with one hand; hold the forearm near the wrist at the ulna with one hand and drag and stretch it upwards laterally or obliquely. Results are improved

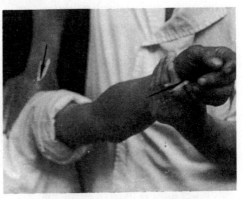

Hold the arm, stretch the shoulder

when you incorporate this technique with a swaying motion.

C. Pull the arm to spread the shoulder. The patient is supine with the affected arm alongside and slightly away from the body. With one hand, pinch and grasp Zhongfu (Lu 1), Yunmen (Lu 2) or the front and underside of the armpit. Hold the arm with the other hand and pull it up and out to the side to spread the shoulder. This may also be done by pulling the arm upwards along a curving line.

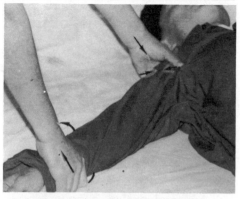

Pull the arm to spread the shoulder.

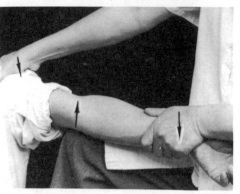

Pull the arm to spread the shoulder.

In another approach to this technique, the patient sits in a stable position. Straighten the diseased arm, resting the forearm on your shoulder. Deep-press the shoulder with both hands. At the same time you may also rock your body right and left or up and down to drag, stretch and spread the shoulder. (Refer to Straight Pulling) You may also support the patient's forearm on your knee, deep-press the shoulder with one or both hands, or pinch and grasp Jianjing (GB 21), or whirl Jianyu (LI 15) with your thumb.

D. Twist the arm with rocking and jerking. Hold the wrist of the diseased side with one or both hands and rock the arm in a large circle, drag and stretch it, or straighten and jerk it rapidly. This may also be done by supporting the elbow from below while holding the wrist and pressing it downwards with one hand and jerking it. In this way, the shoulder joint is twisted, stretched and spread.

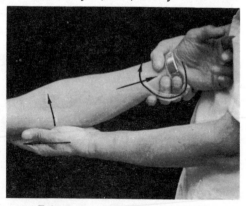

Twist the arm with rocking and jerking

2. Reposition the elbow

This consists of three techniques: dragging to stretch, twisting and rocking, and flexing.

A. Drag to stretch the elbow. Have the patient sit in a stable position and raise the affected arm. Hold and support the forearm near the elbow with one hand, hold the wrist with the other, and drag to stretch it out.

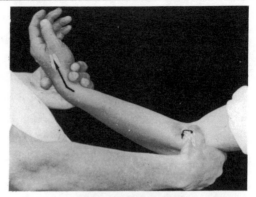

Drag to stretch the elbow

B. Twist and rock the elbow. Support and hold the elbow with one hand, while nipping Quchi (LI 11) with the thumb and Shaohai (H 3) with the middle finger. With the other hand, hold the wrist from below and rock it clockwise and counterclockwise.

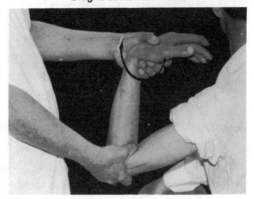

Twist and rock the elbow

C. Hold, grasp and flex the elbow. Hold the elbow joint with one hand keeping the forearm vertical, palm toward the shoulder. Hold the wrist with your other hand and press it down gradually, forcing the elbow joint to flex. This method is commonly used in treating dislocation of the elbow.

3. Rectify the wrist

Nip or pinch selected points around the wrist with the fingers of one hand. Hold the patient's four fingers with the other hand to stretch, drag, tug or pull to flex and extend them up and down, right and left. This may also be done by rotating the fingers in both directions accompanied by rocking and jerking. It is important to also incorporate hand twisting and finger rectifying into this technique.

Indications: Injuries to tendons, numbness, difficult

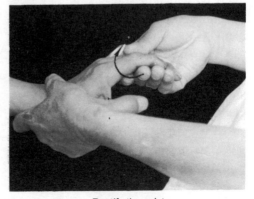

Rectify the wrist

physical activity, dislocation of the shoulder, neuralgia of the shoulder, scapular pain, trauma to the shoulder, arthritic and periarthritic shoulder joint, dislocation of the elbow, pain in the elbow, difficult flexion and extension, arthritic elbow, wrist pain, difficult flexion and extension of the hand and fingers, writer's cramp, snapping fingers, injuries due to falling, beating, wrenching, tugging, etc.

Effects: Divide Tendons, rectify joints, set bones, reposition joints, regulate and harmonize Vital Energy and Blood, resolve stasis, open the obstructed, lubricate and ease joints, relax spasms, relieve pain.

Passive movements of the back, the waist, and the spine

Where used
The spine, the back, the waist, the sacroiliac, and the legs.

Essentials
Let the patient rest comfortably, completely relaxed, and, when you begin, synchronize his/her breathing to your actions. Select the techniques carefully according to your patient's condition. The force you use should be energetic but flexible. Avoid injuries or dislocations. Carefully control the extent of motion and the degree of flexing. Avoid any harsh or careless moves.

Techniques

1. Jerk and drag to relax the waist
Have the patient lie supine and completely relaxed, with arms down along the sides of the body. First, hold the leg of the affected side above the ankle with both hands and jerk it several times. Flex and press the patient's knee toward the chest, then immediately drag the leg down with sharp force. Repeat the procedure on the healthy side. This approach is also the most suitable for jerking and dragging both legs simultaneously.

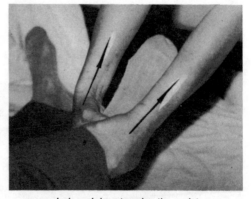

Jerk and drag to relax the waist

2. Deep-press bent legs to tug at the waist

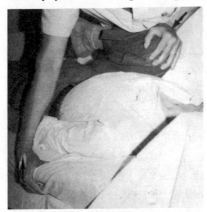

Deep-press bent legs to tug at the waist

A. The patient is supine, with the leg of the healthy side straight, the leg of the diseased side bent. Don't let the patient's body tilt to one side or the other during this procedure. Hold the diseased knee with one hand, and grasp the side of the table (for leverage) with the other. Increase the force gradually, have the patient breathe deeply, and press the bent knee down as far as it will go toward the chest. Repeat the procedure on the healthy side.

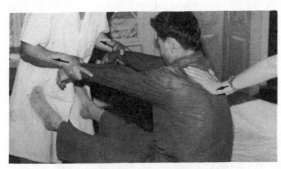

Drag the arms to tug at the waist

B. The patient is supine with both legs straight, feet propped on your thighs. Grasp the patient's wrists firmly and pull them strongly toward you until the patient is sitting upright. Continue pulling until the patient's upper body is facing down. You may have an assistant push on the patient's back to complete this last portion of waist motion.

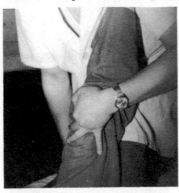

Bend the hip to tug at the waist.

C. The patient is supine with knees up. Squat on the table (or sick-bed) with your feet propped against the patient's buttocks. Place one of the patient's heels on your shoulder. Take the other knee and (1) hold and deep- press with both hands, or (2) stroke the knee with one hand and deep-press with the other. As the procedure progresses, gradually stand up, lifting the foot and leg on your shoulder to bend the hip and tug at the waist. Alternate legs. After this procedure is done, hold the ankle and jerk each leg separately.

D. The patient is prone. Deep-press the selected area on the back, waist or spine with one hand or one knee. Hold the ankle of one or both legs with

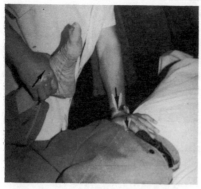

Deep-press bent legs to tug at the waist

the other hand and lift up or pull toward the back to tug at the waist. You may also do this procedure by having the patient bend the knees in order to have the heels touch to the buttocks, or hold the ankle with both hands and lift and tug it back.

3. Rectify the waist back-to-back

Stand steadily back-to-back with your patient. Put your arms back through the patient's bent elbows. Pull the patient onto your back and bend forward slightly. The patient's body will be facing up, with the occiput nestled against the nape of your neck, and the waist against your sacroiliac. Continue bending over, lifting the patient's feet off the floor and tugging farther at the waist. Repeat several times until you can hear a crack from the patient's waist. Have the patient exhale to help relaxation. Safety is very important in this procedure.

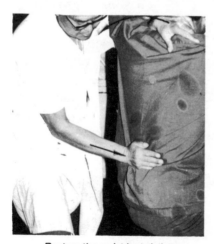

Restore the waist by twisting

4. Restore the waist by twisting

The patient sits in a stable posture, feet on the floor, buttocks firmly in place. The buttocks should not move during this procedure. If you're starting on the left, stand to the left and behind the patient and move in a forward lunge. Pass your left arm below the patient's left armpit and over the body to hold the back of the right shoulder with your left hand. Have the patient hold your left elbow steadily with his/her right hand. With your right hand, deep-press the diseased area of the waist. Have the patient rotate his/her waist from right to left as far as possible. At the end of his/her range of motion, add force by twisting the shoulders, pushing and pressing with your right hand until you hear a crack. To do the other side, reverse your posture, position and hands, and repeat.

5. Straight and oblique pulling of the waist

A. Stand behind your sitting patient with one foot up on a stool or other support. Push your knee against the appropriate part of the patient's back

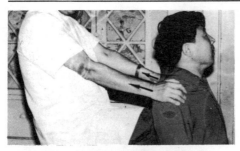

Straight and oblique pulling of the waist

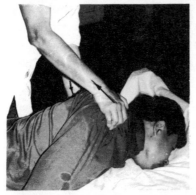

Straight and oblique pulling of the waist

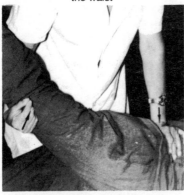

Straight and oblique pulling of the waist

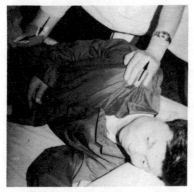

Straight and oblique pulling of the waist

to stabilize it. Hold both shoulders with your hands and pull back moderately to expand the chest and stretch the back.

B. The patient is prone with both arms loose and at his/her sides. Stand alongside. Apply deep pressure to Mingmen (GV 4) or other points on the back with one hand, and pull the opposite shoulder with the other hand. Apply force with both hands to twist the spine and stretch the shoulder back as far as possible. The hand applying the deep pressure may be shifted up along the spine.

The same results may be achieved by applying deep pressure to the waist with one hand, and lifting and holding the opposite thigh with the other. Pull, lift and twist, rock, stretch and drag the thigh. Repeat on the other side.

C. The patient is on his/her side with the lower leg straight and the top leg bent, while you stand in front. Push and press the diseased area of the waist with one hand and hold the front of the thigh and push it backwards with considerable force. Repeat on the healthy side.

Other approaches: Stand behind the patient and press the shoulder with one hand, pushing it back, while you deep-press the hip with the elbow of the other arm and push it forwards; or deep-press the shoulder and hip with both elbows; or press and push the hip forward with one hand and pull the shoulder back with the other. Apply force with both hands simultaneously in opposing directions. When you have twisted the waist to its natural extent, increase the

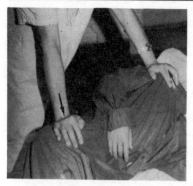

Straight and oblique pulling of the waist

force quickly with both hands or elbows to over-stretch it past that limit. Take care to avoid injury to the patient. Reverse and repeat on the opposite side.

Indications: Injuries to the psoas major, sacrospinalis, supraspinal ligaments, interspinal ligaments, anterior and posterior longitudinal ligaments, and the lumbosacral area; protruding lumbar disc, cryptogenic sacral hiatus, dislocation of lumbar vertebrae and other bone injuries due to trauma; blockage syndrome due to Wind-Cold-Dampness, disorders of the waist and legs due to Kidney Deficiency.

Effects: Relax Tendons and muscles, activate Blood, dredge Meridians and Collaterals, relieve pain, expel Wind, eliminate Dampness, disperse Cold, set bones and reposition joints, invigorate and benefit Kidney.

Passive movements of the legs

Where used
The hip, the knee, the ankle and the foot.

Essentials
The patient should be relaxed and at ease. Select appropriate techniques and areas. Be skillful in performing techniques. Twisting and rocking should begin in the center and move outward. Gradually increase the range of motion from small to large. Use appropriate force and degree of joint flexion.

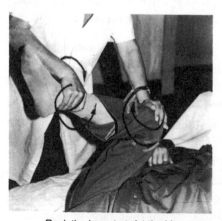

Rock the knee to twist the hip

Techniques

1. Rock the knee to twist the hip
The patient is supine with one leg bent and the other straight. Hold the bent leg with one hand at the knee and the other just above the ankle. Lift the ankle, pressing the knee partially in towards the chest, rock and rotate the knee repeatedly to twist the hip.

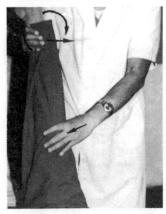

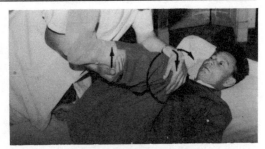

Rock the knee to twist the hip

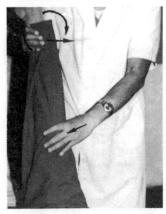

Rock the knee to twist the hip

After rocking and twisting a few times, press the knee and tug up on the ankle to straighten the leg. Flex the knee and rock and rotate it again.

Motivate Vital Energy into Dantian (the Elixir Field). Press the bent knee to straighten it with one hand and lift the leg, holding it just above the Achilles tendon. Pull it out from the body, then bend and press it in, and

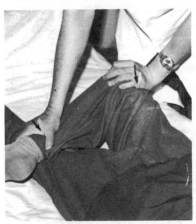

rock the knee to twist the hip, increasing the dragging force to the hip joint.

All of these techniques may be used on alternate sides. Also, you may incorporate such techniques as Lifting up the Straight Leg, 4-Shaped Technique, and Pulling the Straight Leg Outward.

2. *Weighty Floodgate bending method*

The patient stands steadily, relaxed, arms hanging naturally, toes pointing out. Have the patient bend the knees gradually to a semi-squatting position. Stand behind and press both Jianjing (GB 21) points, hold your breath, motivate Vital Energy to both arms and push down on the shoulders quickly and forcefully as if a weighty floodgate falls suddenly, forcing the patient to squat. Do this three times. This technique is appropriate for patients whose knees are stiff, and who cannot squat or stand up freely. Do not use if the patient's knees are swollen.

Rock the knee to twist the hip

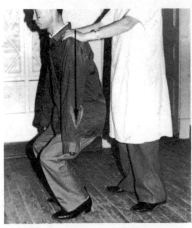

Weighty Floodgate bending method

3. Pad the popliteal fossa and bend the knee

The patient is prone or supine with one leg straight and the diseased leg bent. Stand by the diseased side and pad the popliteal fossa with your hand, fist or forearm. Hold the ankle with your other hand and bend the leg down to tug and

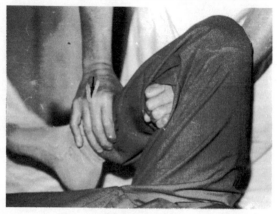

Pad the popliteal fossa and bend the knee

stretch the knee joint. You may go so far as to touch the heel to the buttock.

4. Drag and rock the ankle

Sit beside the patient, who should be supine with both legs straight. Support the heel of the affected foot with one hand and grasp its toes with the other. Drag the ankle, rotate it in and out, or rotate and rock it.

Therapeutic effects will be best if they are combined with revolving Huantiao (GB 30), grasping Weizhong (UB 40), pressing Chengshan (UB 57), pinching Kunlun (UB 60), and rubbing Yongquan (K 1).

Indications: Injury to the hip, difficulty in raising the leg, restricted motion squatting or standing up, stiff knee, spasms and contractions of tendons, flaccidity and paralysis of the legs, cramped calf muscles, traumatic pathological changes of the lower limbs.

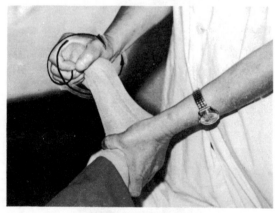

Drag and rock the ankle

Effects: Set bones and reposition joints, lubricate and ease joints, stretch and rectify Tendons, resolve stasis, activate Blood, dredge Meridians and Collaterals, relax spasms, relieve pain.

Routine Techniques

The head and face

Where used
The head and face.

Essentials
The techniques should be soft and gentle but deeply penetrating, and not superficial. The principle of Meet-Follow Invigorate-Reduce should be followed. Manipulation should be systematic and flowing, going from front to rear, middle to outside, and from dot to area.

The massage proceeds in three stages. (1) The adaptive stage begins with soft and slow motions. (2) The analgesic stage, in which force and speed increase. (3) Dissipating/propagating stage, when the manipulations become gentle and nimble and the force and speed gradually decrease.

Techniques

1. Stroke and caress the head to benefit the brain

The patient sits comfortably with you in front. Hold the patient's head in place with one hand. Bring Vital Energy through the other hand and fingers. Stroke the head front to back from hairline to hairline. Stroking increases from slow to fast, rubbing the scalp repeatedly. For patients with long hair, wrap it with a piece of cloth and manipulate

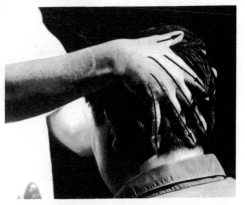

Stroke and caress the head to benefit the brain

through the cloth. Rub the left side of the scalp first, the right side second and the middle last until your patient feels a scorching hot sensation. Then interlace your fingers and rub both Fengchi points (GB 20) with the small thenar mounds joined together. Finally, clutch and grasp large handfuls of hair with both hands. Pounding Baihu (GV 20) and its surrounding area with open fists may be added.

2. Open Passes and dredge Apertures

This involves many single manipulations. In clinical practice, they may be selected according to the disease condition. There is no need to use all of them. The general order of operation is as follows:

The patient sits comfortably or is supine. Divide his/her forehead rubbing outward with both thumbs from Yintang (Ex-HN 2) to the lateral hairlines. This is called The Method of Dividing the Forehead.

Pinch the space between the eyebrows nimbly and skillfully with the thumb and index finger of both hands, and continue pinching along the eyebrows from inner to outer ends several times. This is called the Method of Pinching Eyebrows.

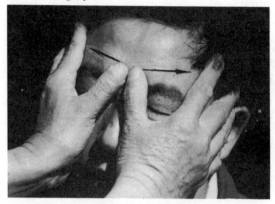

Dividing the forehead

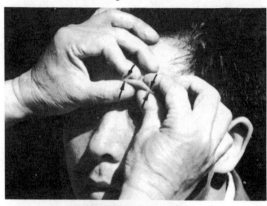

Pinching the eyebrows

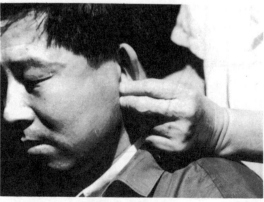

Beat Heaven's Drum

Nip Yintang (Ex-HN 2) and Renzhong (GV 26) with your thumb nail, pinch Duidan (GV 27), nip Chengjiang (CV 24), nip both Jingming (UB 1) with your thumb nails, knead both Yingxiang (LI 20); nip and knead Dicang (St 4), Xiaguan (St 7) and Jiache (St 6) with your thumb, index finger and middle finger; then nip and knead Taiyang (Ex-HN 4), Tinggong (SI 19), and Yifeng (TW 17) the same way. Ideally, your patient will feel sensations of numbness, soreness, distension and pain when these points are manipulated. Finally, lift and pull both ears from behind and rock them moderately. This is called Beat Heaven's Drum.

During these procedures, the patient should have closed eyes, be calm, and breathe evenly. Select points and areas with accuracy. The force should not be too strong. The procedure should be nimble, flexible and skillful.

Indications: Common cold, headache, migraine, dizziness, collapse, fainting, unconsciousness, listlessness, insomnia, amnesia, neurasthenia, dreaminess, blurred vision, facial paralysis, sunstroke, epilepsy, twitching of lips, lockjaw, nasal obstruction, facial edema, glossy pale complexion, pain around the eyes, toothache, tinnitus, acute deafness.

Effects: First aid, resuscitation, raise and promote the restoration of Yang, sober the mind, open Passes, dredge Apertures, improve eyesight, relax spasms, tranquilize, quell convulsions, relieve pain, relieve the External, expel Wind.

N.B. According to the holistic principles of Traditional Chinese Medicine and clinical experiences, manipulations of the head and face should be combined with treatment of remote points, such as Quchi (LI 11), Shousanli (LI 10), Neiguan (Per 6), Shenmen (H 7), Hegu (LI 4) and others of the arms; and Huantiao (GB 30), Weizhong (UB 40), Zusanli (St 36), Sanyinjiao (Sp 6), Yongquan (K 1) and others of the legs.

The neck and nape

Where used
The neck and the nape.

Essentials
The patient should be comfortable. Choose the appropriate operative direction according to the principle of Meet-Follow Invigorate-Reduce. Pay close attention to the angles of rotation and the extent of motion. These techniques should be gentle and nimble, slow without stopping, swift and calm. The force should be moderate but deeply penetrating.

Techniques

1. Push, pull and knead the neck

The patient sits in a stable position. Begin to pull and rotate the neck in the chosen direction. Then push, knead, pinch and grasp points along the nape, such as Yamen (GV 15), Fengfu (GV 16), Dazhui (GV 14), and

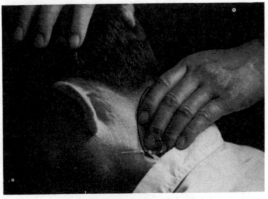

Push, pull and knead the neck

Fengchi (GB 20); or along the large tendons of the nape, such as Jianwaishu (SI 14), Jianzhongshu (SI 15), Jianjing (GB 21). Keep repeating until the patient feels a warm sensation. Depending on the patient's condition, you may add revolving with the forearm, in which case the patient should lie prone or on his/her side.

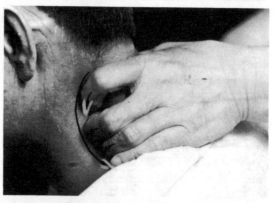

Push, pull and knead the neck

2. Pluck, vibrate and knock the neck

Stand beside your patient, who is sitting comfortably. Choose points or areas relevant to the disease, and pluck, nip, knead, vibrate and knock repeatedly. You may also use rolling.

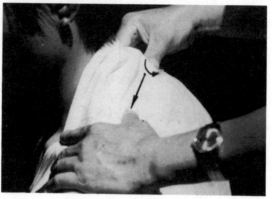

Push, pull and knead the neck

3. Knead and grasp to relax the throat

Stand beside the patient, who may either sit or be supine. Hold the occiput with one hand. Knead and grasp the throat with the thumb and index finger of the other at Renying (St 9), Futu (LI 18), Tianding (LI 17), Shuitu (St 10) and other points. These

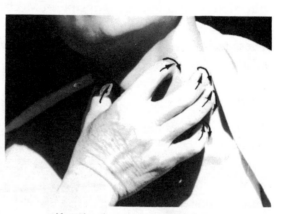

Knead and grasp to relax the throat

manipulations should be soft, nimble and precise. Push the neck and shift it right and left. Continue repeatedly.

4. Rock and deep-press to initiate vocalization

The patient may be either sitting or supine. Hold the forehead with one hand to keep the head in place. Deep-press, knead, grasp, and rock from Renying (St 9) to Qishe (St 11), and from Lianquan (CV 23) to Tiantu (CV 22) with your thumb and index or middle finger as those fingers push along the sides and midline of the larynx. During the procedure, either have the patient try to pronounce the syllable, "Ye," (Yuh) to strengthen the opening and closing ability of the glottis; or swallow repeatedly to shift the larynx, synchronizing this with the manipulations. Continue repeatedly.

Indications: Restricted neck motion, stiff neck, cervical spondylosis and numbness in the limbs from this condition, hoarseness, swollen and painful throat, sudden loss of voice, aphasia due to apoplexy, stiff tongue, difficulty in swallowing, flaccid tongue, slobbering.

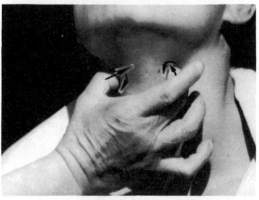

Rock and deep-press to initiate vocalization

Effects: Divide Tendons, pluck their Collaterals, reposition cervical vertebrae, dredge Meridians and Collaterals, resolve stasis, activate Blood, clear the pharynx and ease the larynx, rectify Vital Energy, initiate vocalization.

Rock and deep-press to initiate vocalization

N. B. Although diseases of the neck and nape are comparatively simple, they are situated in a critical section of the body through which many Meridians pass. For this reason, diagnosis must be correct and unequivocal. For example, patients suffering from cervical spondylosis should be examined by X-ray or MRI. Avoid violent pulling, hard grasping, and harsh operations. In order to improve therapeutic effects, points of the arms, such as Quchi (LI 11), Hegu (LI 4), Neiguan (Per 6), and points of the legs, such as Waiqu (GB 36), Xuanzhong (GB 39), and Yongquan (K 1) may also be treated.

Back and waist

Where used
The spine, the back, the waist and the sacral area.

Essentials
The position of the patient and the techniques selected must be appropriate. Work on the back should begin gently, becoming deep and penetrating. Work on the spine should be heavy but flowing. Work on the waist and sacral area should be moderate. Energetic dragging and deep-pressing must be kept safe and pulling and twisting must stay within definite limits. Knocking should be regular and rhythmic. Pushing, revolving, scratching and rubbing should continue until the patient feels a warm sensation.

Techniques

1. Push the back with pinching and grasping

The patient is prone. Push the back along the Governor Vessel Meridian and Urinary Bladder Meridian with one or both hands from Dazhui (GV 14) to Eight Liao (UB 31 - 34). Continue by pinching and grasping repeatedly along these Meridians. The back pinching is also called the method of Pinching the Back.

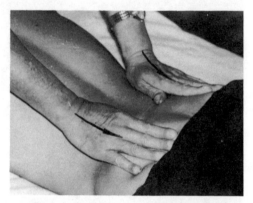

Push the back with pinching and grasping

2. Deep-press the spine with kneading and revolving

Stand beside your patient, who is prone. Press, deep-press, knead and revolve the diseased area on both sides of the spine along the Meridians

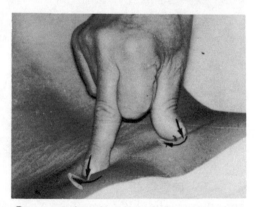

Deep-press the spine with kneading and revolving

from top to bottom with fingers, palms, forearm and/or your elbow. The direction you choose may be along or against the trend of the Meridian according to the guiding principle.

3. Pull the waist with jerking and dragging

Refer to "Straight and oblique pulling of the waist," and "Jerk and drag to relax the waist," in Passive movements. Choose one or both according to the situation.

4. Strengthen the waist by rolling and rubbing

The patient is prone. Revolve one or both forearms on the waist, then rub it or roll it with your hands. Best results will accompany a warm sensation.

5. Pluck Collaterals with knocking and scratching

The patient is prone. Using one or both thumbs, divide Tendons and pluck their Collaterals to the sides along the Meridians and Tendinomuscular Meridians of the back, from top to bottom. Then immediately knock the

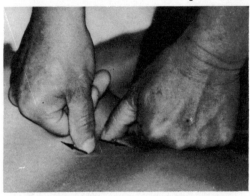

Pluck Collaterals with knocking and scratching

area with open fists. This is called the method of Knocking the Back. To finish, scratch downwards or outwards from Dazhui (GV 14).

Indications: Common spine disease caused by trauma, Wind-Cold-Dampness, or Deficiency of Kidney.

Effects: Relax Tendons, activate Blood, dredge Meridians, relieve pain, expel Wind, disperse Cold, set and reposition bones.

Note: Clinical experience shows therapeutic effects may be improved by simultaneously treating points of the leg, such as Weizhing (UB 40), Chengshan (UB 57), Xuanzhong (GB 39), Kunlun (UB 60), Taixi (K 3).

Chest and rib cage

Where used
The chest and rib cage.

Essentials
Select points along the Meridians. Avoid harsh movements. With female patients, avoid touching their breasts except for treating diseases of the mammary glands.

Techniques

1. Relieve the chest by dotting and vibrating

The patient is supine. Dot and vibrate the points of the Conception Vessel Meridian from Tiantu (CV 22) to Tanzhong (CV 17), bypassing Yutang (CV 18). Continue with points of the Kidney Meridian from Shufu (K 27) to Shenfeng (K 23), bypassing Shencang (K 25). Dot the Stomach Meridian from Kufang (St 14) to Rugen (St 18), bypassing Yingchuang (St 16). Finish with Lung Meridian points Zhongfu (Lu 1) and Yunmen (Lu 2).

2. Relax the chest by pressing and kneading

The patient is supine. Press the chest with your hands and knead it with your fingers along the same four Meridians, from top to bottom. Repeat many times.

3. Push and wipe to divide the ribs

Standing above the supine patient's head, place your hands symmetrically on the chest, fingers pointing out and down. Begin at the upper intercostal spaces, and apply force to both sides, pushing and wiping the ribs from the midline outward. Continue to the eighth intercostal space. This may also be done by rubbing the two sides separately.

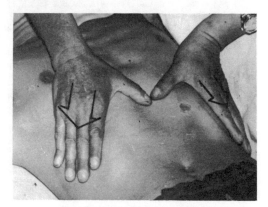

Push and wipe to divide the ribs

Indications: Distension and pain in the chest and rib cage, cough, adverse uprising of Vital Energy, swelling and pain in the throat, nausea, vomiting, dysphagia, loss of appetite, acute mastitis, deficient milk secretion, depression of Liver Energy, disharmony between Liver and Stomach, injuries of the chest and flanks due to overexertion while holding breath.

Effects: Ventilate the chest, benefit the diaphragm, eliminate phlegm, promote expectoration, depress adverse uprising, stop vomiting, disperse and rectify Liver Energy.

N.B. When manipulating the chest, add Xiabai (Lu 4), Shaohai (H 3), and Neiguan (Per 6). When manipulating the flanks, select Huantiao (GB 30), Sanyinjiao (Sp 6), Xingjian (Liv 2) and Taichong (Liv 3). You will have better results when you work the points of both sides.

Abdomen

Where used
The abdomen.

Essentials
Procedures should be coordinated with the patient's breathing, and done along Meridian pathways. Don't be too quick with deep-pressing and kneading. Be gentle when knocking and vibrating. Lifting and jerking should be brisk. All actions should be light and gentle to avoid injuries to internal organs.

Techniques

1. Push the abdomen with round-rubbing and revolving

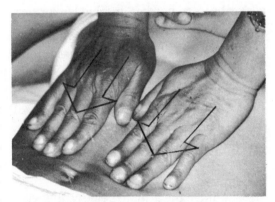

Push the abdomen with round-rubbing and revolving

Let the patient relax in a supine position. Push the abdomen with one or both hands along Meridian pathways according to the principle of Meet-Follow Invigorate-Reduce. Continue with round-rubbing and revolving. Alternately, you may begin with round-rubbing and revolving and go on to the pushing.

2. Press the abdomen with deep-pressing and kneading

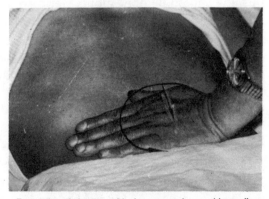

Press the abdomen with deep-pressing and kneading

The patient is supine. Press and deep-press selected points one by one with your fingers or palms, then knead and rotate them along Meridian pathways.

3. Grasp the abdomen with lifting and jerking

The patient is supine. Hold and firmly grasp a part of the abdominal wall along Meridian pathways. Lift it and jerk it right or left, or twist it while shifting back and forth.

4. Roll the abdomen with knocking and vibrating

The patient is supine. Roll one or both hands on the abdomen along Meridian pathways, then knock selected areas with empty fists, or vibrate them using motivated Vital Energy.

Indications: Fullness and distension in the abdomen, abdominal pain, abdominal mass due to stagnation of Vital Energy, malnutrition due to parasites, stomach distress, loss of appetite, loose stools with undigested grains, diarrhea, borborygmus, intestinal colic, constipation, fecaloma, abdominal mass in females, collapse of Spleen-Stomach Energy, abdominal ptosis, painful or difficult urination, impotence, premature ejaculation, nocturnal emissions, involuntary emission, irregular menstruation, dysmenorrhea, amenorrhea, morbid leukorrhea, prolapsed uterus.

N.B. Abdominal manipulations should be coordinated with the patient's breathing and combined with the selection of the following points: Quchi (LI 11), Neiguan (Per 6), Hegu (LI 4), Yanglingquan (GB 34), Xuehai (Sp 10), Zusanli (St 36), Sanyinjiao (Sp 6), Yinbai (Sp 1), Taibai (Sp 3), Gongsun (Sp 4), Neiting (St 44), Taixi (K 3), Yongquan (K 1).

Arms and shoulders

Where used
The shoulder, the arm, the elbow, the wrist, the hand.

Essentials
Pinching, nipping and grasping are especially suitable for points around the shoulder, the elbow, and the wrist. Kneading, rolling and pushing should be done along Meridian pathways. Pulling, twisting, rocking and jerking and generally used to dredge the entire limb. Rotating and rectifying are done on the arm and hand. Techniques should be done sequentially. The force used should be within reasonable limits. Avoid harsh dragging and unyielding pulling.

Techniques

1. Pinch the arm with nipping and kneading

Have the patient sit or lie supine with arms straight. Hold his/her elbow to support the arm with one hand, and pinch points along the pathway of the Three Yin or Yang Meridians of the Hand, or at fossae and apertures around the shoulder, elbow and wrist, as well as the hand. Continue with nipping, then kneading.

2. Roll the arm with pushing and grasping

Again, the patient is either sitting or lying supine with arms straight. Roll on his/her arm along or against the trend of the Meridian. The rolling may also be done in a selected spot. Follow this with pushing and grasping. Repeat several times.

3. Pull the arm with rotating and rectifying

Pull the patient's shoulder and rotate the arm and hand and rectify the fingers from top to bottom.

4. Twist the arm with rocking and jerking.

This is used to energize the arm. For specific technique, refer to this entry under Passive movements of the arms.

Indications: Disorders caused by trauma, Wind-Cold-Dampness, cervical spondylosis.

Effects: Divide Tendons, rectify and ease joints, clear Apertures, warm Meridians, dredge Collaterals, activate Blood, relieve pain.

N.B. Disorders of the arms are often caused by cervical spondylosis. For this reason, diagnosis must be correctly identified and relevant treatment prescribed. (Refer to Simple Techniques, Compound Techniques, and Passive Movements.)

Legs and hips

Where used
The hip, buttock, knee, ankle and foot.

Essentials
Dragging should be performed with great force in the correct direction, and with the patient in the proper position. The sites for plucking and grasping should be accurately selected. Pulling and tugging should be done within reasonable limits. Knocking and vibrating should be regular and rhythmic. Rolling, revolving, pinching and grasping should follow the pathways of the Meridian or Tendinomuscular Meridian. Rotating and round-rubbing should produce a warm sensation. Various techniques may be selected and deftly incorporated according to the situation.

Techniques

1. Drag the leg with plucking and grasping

The patient may be either prone or supine, with you either by the side or at the feet. Drag the leg, then pluck the points along the Three Yin or Yang Meridians of the Foot, then grasp them.

2. Pull the leg with knocking and vibrating

Stand beside the patient, who may be prone, supine or on his/her side. After pulling and twisting the leg, knock and vibrate selected areas in rhythmic succession.

3. Roll the leg with revolving and pinching

Your position and the patient's are the same as above. Roll successive points along selected Meridians of the Foot, revolve the leg with your elbow or forearm according to the situation, then pinch selected points of areas. In clinical practice, the pinching is usually done along the midline and both sides of the calf with a distance of one Body Inch between pinches. In other words, the pinching begins at the popliteal fossa and goes to Kunlun (UB 60) and Taixi (K 3) This is also called the method of Calf Pinching.

4. Knead the calf with rotating and round-rubbing

Same positions as above. Depending on the situation, do various types of kneading, then follow with rotating and round-rubbing.

Indications: Common disorders of lumbosacral area and legs due to trauma or Wind-Cold-Dampness.

Effects: Relax Tendons, ease joints, set and reposition bones, expel Wind, disperse Cold, activate Blood, resolve stasis, dredge Meridians, relieve pain.

N.B. Disorders of the legs are often related to disease in the lumbosacral area. Incorporate appropriate techniques. The waist and the leg are often treated together.

Applications

Treatment of Diseases

Internal Medicine

Catching cold

Cold is a common disease. Its chief signs and symptoms are stuffy nose, nasal discharge, headache, cough, fever, and aversion to cold.

Etiology: Caused by Wind evil, especially during sudden changes of weather or abnormal variations of environmental temperature. Wind is the first and foremost pathogenic factor among Six Exogenous Evils, but it is often accompanied by other factors such as seasonal or epidemic pathogens. Wind evil invades the body through the nose and skin and attacks the Lung first. The Lung then fails to control Vital Energy and the External Defense System is impaired. Deficiency of Healthy Energy and attenuated Defense mechanism due to irregular habits, over-tiredness or weak physical constitution are internal causes. Wind (often combined with Cold) and other evils are external causes. Since there is so much variety in seasonal change, climate, physical constitution and pathogenic factors, aspects of Cold and the degree of seriousness are many. People Deficient in Yang are susceptible to Wind-Cold; those Deficient in Yin to Dryness-Heat; those with an Excess of Phlegm to Wetness.

Diagnosis & Treatment

1. Wind-Cold

Signs & Symptoms: Aversion to cold, fever without perspiration, headache, aching of limbs, stuffy nose, nasal discharge, itching larynx, twangy voice, cough, expectoration of white phlegm, no thirst. *Tongue:* thin white fur. *Pulse:* superficial, tense.

Therapeutic Principle: Expel Wind, relieve External, ventilate Lung Energy, disperse Cold.

Principal Measure: Stroke and caress the head to benefit the brain, pluck and grasp the neck and nape, rectify all four limbs, scratch the back along Urinary Bladder Meridians.

Subordinate Measure: Nip Lieque (Lu 7), Hegu (LI 4); knead Dazhui (GV 14), grasp Jianjing (GB 21).

2. Wind-Heat

Signs & Symptoms: Fever, perspiration, aversion to Wind, sore throat, headache, feeling of distension in the head, cough, expectoration of yellow phlegm, thirst, aching of whole body. *Tongue:* white/yellowish fur. *Pulse:* superficial, rapid.

Therapeutic Principle: Expel Wind, relieve External, ventilate Lung Energy, diffuse Heat.

Principal Measure: Pinch eyebrows, rub the forehead with joined hands, stroke and caress the head, pluck and grasp the neck and nape.

Subordinate Measure: Knead Taiyang (Ex-HN 4) and Dazhui (GV 14), nip Quchi (LI 11), Waiguan (TW 5), Fenglong (St 40) and Shaoshang (Lu 11).

3. Wind-Cold with Dampness

Signs & Symptoms: Recessive fever, aversion to cold, feeling of distension in the head, joint pain, epigastric heaviness, loss of appetite, vomiting. *Tongue:* yellow, greasy fur. *Pulse:* superficial and rapid.

Therapeutic Principle: Clear Heat, eliminate Dampness, relieve External, harmonize the Middle Warmer.

Principal Measure: Round-rub the head with the entire hand, pinch and grasp the neck, drag, vibrate and knock the neck. Grasp Fengchi (GB 20), revolve the middle abdomen with the forearm, knead Pishu (UB 20) and Weishu (UB 21) with the fingers, chop the legs with joined hands.

Subordinate Measure: Nip Lieque (Lu 7), Hegu (LI 4), Neiguan (Per 6) and Zusanli (St 36); knead Zhongwan (CV 12).

4. Summer-Heat with Dampness

Signs & Symptoms: Fever with perspiration, thirst, short temper, headache, feeling of heaviness in arms and legs, epigastric fullness and distension, diminished and dark urination. *Tongue:* yellow, greasy fur. *Pulse:* soft, floating, rapid.

Therapeutic Principle: Relieve External, clear Summer Heat, relax the chest, resolve turbidity.

Principal Measure: Stroke and caress the head, lift and grasp both ears, pluck and grasp the neck and nape, relieve the chest by dotting and vibrating, divide the ribs by pushing and wiping, revolve the lower abdomen (chiefly Guanyuan [CV 4]) with the forearm.

Subordinate Measure: Push Xinshu (UB 15 - reducing), Dazhui (GV 14), Quchi (LI 11); nip Sanyangjiao (on the opposite side of Sanyinjiao [Sp 6]), and Zusanli (St 36).

Sunstroke

Sunstroke is an acute disease caused by intense heat in summer. It happens particularly to those who are exposed to the direct sun, or those who work in an environment of high temperature. It varies in degree of seriousness and in manifestations of signs and symptoms. Generally, it may be classified as Attack of Summer-Heat, Summer-Heat Syncope, Summer-Heat Spasm, Summer Atrophy, or Summer Infection.

Etiology: Summer-Heat or Summer-Heat with Dampness and/or Turbidity takes advantage of a weak constitution or a Deficient state. Summer-Heat is a Fire-evil which clogs the Exterior of the body and impedes free perspiration. The accumulated Heat cannot be expelled from the body, and invades the Pericardium and obscures the Heart Aperture, resulting in high fever, coma, cold and clammy limbs. When the intense Heat stirs Internal Wind, there are spasms or convulsions. Patients often drip with perspiration during the high fever, and both their Vital Energy and body fluids are depleted, resulting in collapse.

Diagnosis & Treatment

1. Attack of Summer-Heat

Signs & Symptoms: Dizziness, headache, heaviness in the chest, labored breathing, thirst, nausea, insufficient perspiration, fever, short temper, weakness and exhaustion. *Pulse:* superficial and feeble.

Therapeutic Principle: Clear away heat, open Apertures.

Principal Measure: Nip Renzhong (GV 26), pinch Duiduan (GV 27), stroke and caress the head, pluck and grasp the neck and nape, pinch and grasp both Jianjing (GB 21).

Subordinate Measure: Nip Shixuan (Ex-UE 9), Hegu (LI 4), Quchi (LI 11); knead Guanyuan (CV 4), Weizhing (UB 40), Chengshan (UB 57) and Yongquan (K 1).

2. Summer-Heat Syncope

Signs & Symptoms: Sudden fainting, fever, slight perspiration, cold clammy limbs, labored breathing, unresponsiveness, reddened complexion, lockjaw. *Tongue:* Thick, yellow fur. *Pulse:* Full, rapid.

Therapeutic Principle: Clear Heart, open Apertures.

Principal Measure: Open Passes, dredge Apertures, stroke and caress the head, grasp Fengchi (UB 20), pluck and grasp the neck and nape, relieve the chest with dotting and vibrating.

Subordinate Measure: Grasp Kunlun (UB 60), nip Weizhong (UB 40), nip and knead Quze (Per 3) and Hegu (LI 4), nip Shixuan (Ex-UE 9).

3. Summer-Heat Spasm

Signs & Symptoms: Sudden fainting, spasm, twitching, sallow complexion. *Tongue:* red with yellow fur. *Pulse:* superficial, rapid.

Therapeutic Principle: Clear Heat, calm Wind.

Principal Measure: Open Passes and dredge Apertures; pluck, vibrate and knock the neck; grab and grasp the neck and nape, push the back with pinching and grasping; push the legs along the Six Meridians, pinch the calf.

Subordinate Measure: Nip Yanglingquan (GB 34), Chengshan (UB 57) and Weizhong (UB 40); nip and knead Quchi (LI 11), Neiguan (Per 6) and Hegu (LI 4); nip Zhongchong (Per 9).

4. Summer Atrophy

Signs & Symptoms: Oppressive fever, thirst, dizziness, cough, labored breathing, bloody sputum, perspiration, cold limbs. *Tongue:* white, greasy fur. *Pulse:* superficial, full and feeble.

Therapeutic Principle: Clear Heat, protect Lung.

Principal Measure: Stroke and caress the head, push and grasp the neck and nape, relieve the chest with dotting and vibrating, relax the chest by pressing and kneading, push and grasp both shoulders, chop the legs with joined hands.

Subordinate Measure: Knead Feishu (UB 13), nip and grasp Weizhong (UB 40), nip Fenglong (St 40).

5. Summer Infection

Signs & Symptoms: Dizziness, nausea, vomiting, profuse perspiration, abdominal distension and heaviness, abdominal pain, diarrhea, foul and filthy stool. *Tongue:* greasy fur. *Pulse:* full.

Therapeutic Principle: Clear Dampness, resolve Turbidity, regulate and harmonize Spleen-Stomach.

Principal Measure: Pinch Duiduan (GV 27), stroke and caress the head, grab and grasp the neck and nape, relieve the chest with dotting and vibrating, revolve the middle abdomen with the forearm, push the abdomen with round- rubbing and revolving.

Subordinate Measure: Nip Renzhong (GV 26), Chengjiang (CV 24), Weizhong (UB 40) and Zusanli (St 36); grasp Kunlun (UB 60).

Headache

Headache is a subjective symptom involved in a variety of acute and chronic diseases. Generally, it is classified in two categories: the externally attacked and the internally damaged.

Etiology: The head is a meeting place for Yang. All the essences in Blood from the Five Yin Organs and Vital Energy from the Six Yang Organs converge in the head. When a person is attacked by exogenous evils or impaired by internal damage, there is pain due to the stagnation of Vital Energy and the stasis of Blood, the dysfunction of Meridians and Vessels, or the failure of clear Yang to disperse. Various types of headaches occur at different areas of the head. Taiyang headache is at the occiput, involving the neck and nape; Yangming headache is at the forehead and eyebrows; Shaoyang headache is at the side of the head, involving the ear; Jueyin is at the crown of the head and involves the eyes.

Headache due to attack of exogenous evils: If a person is not attentive to health, Wind-Cold may attack the upper part of the body, obstruct Collaterals and induce headache. Wind-Heat may attack clear Apertures, harass the circulation of Vital Energy and Blood and bring headache. Wind-Dampness may attack the body, soak and cover up clear Yang, stopping the rise of clear Yang and the descent of Turbid Yin and cause headache.

Headache from Internal damage: This is usually due to disorders of Liver, Kidney and Spleen. This can happen in various ways. Internal Wind from the Liver may harass Clear Apertures during a period of emotional excitement; during a period of disharmony between sentiment and aspiration, depressed Liver Energy may become Fire and disturb the Clear Apertures; there may be an excessive uprising of Liver Yang when Fire damages Yin or when Kidney Yin is Deficient; Clear Yang may fail to nourish the brain when the reservoir of marrow is depleted of Vital Energy and Blood, or when Kidney Yang declines; malnutrition of the brain, spinal cord and Meridians due to Deficiency of Spleen; retention of Dampness or Phlegm can disturb the reservoir of marrow due to Deficiency of Spleen.

Diagnosis & Treatment

1. Headache caused by Wind-Cold

Signs & Symptoms: Headache, stiff nape, fever, aversion to cold, headache aggravated by Wind or Cold, aching joints, stuffy nose, nasal discharge, no thirst. *Tongue:* thin white fur. *Pulse:* superficial and tense.

Therapeutic Principle: Expel Wind, disperse Cold.

Principal Measure: Stroke and caress the head, nip and knead Fengfu (GV 16), pluck and grasp the neck and nape, pinch and grasp both Jianjing (GB 21), scratch the back, rectify the fingers.

Subordinate Measure: Nip Quchi (LI 11), Waiguan (TW 5) and Hegu (LI 4); knead Dazhui (GV 14).

2. Headache caused by Wind-Heat

Signs & Symptoms: Intermittent splitting pain and distension of the head and eyes, fever, aversion to Wind, thirst, swollen and painful throat, reddened complexion, conjunctivitis. *Tongue:* red tip with yellow fur. *Pulse:* superficial and rapid.

Therapeutic Principle: Expel Wind, clear Heat.

Principal Measure: Pinch and grasp the neck and nape, stroke and caress the head, grasp Fengchi (GV 20), knead Taiyang (Ex-HN 4); pluck, vibrate and knock the neck, and rectify limbs.

Subordinate Measure: Knead Dazhui (GV 14) and Fengchi (GB 20), nip Lieque (Lu 7), Shaoshang (Lu 11), Weizhong (UB 40) and Xingjian (Liv 2).

3. Headache caused by Wind-Dampness

Signs & Symptoms: The head aches as if wrapped, heavy sensation in body and limbs, heaviness in the chest, lack of appetite. *Tongue:* white, greasy fur. *Pulse:* soft, floating.

Therapeutic Principle: Expel Wind, dry Dampness.

Principal Measure: Open Passes and dredge Apertures, rub Fengchi (GB 20) with joined hands, pound the crown of the head with an open fist, push and grasp the neck and nape, pluck and grasp both Jianjing (GB 21), rectify limbs.

Subordinate Measure: Nip Yanglingquan (GB 34) and Neiting (St 44); dot Shangxing (GV 23), Baihu (GV 20) and Touwei (St 8).

4. Headache caused by excessive uprising of Liver Yang

Signs & Symptoms: Headache, dizziness, rash behavior, short temper, tinnitus, insomnia, pain and distension in chest and rib cage, reddened complexion, dry mouth, bitter taste. *Tongue:* red with thin yellow fur. *Pulse:* stringy, energetic.

Therapeutic Principle: Quell Liver, retrieve Yang.

Principal Measure: Stroke and caress the head, drag and lift both ears, pinch and grasp the neck and the nape; pull, push and knead the neck.

Subordinate Measure: Nip and knead Quchi (LI 11), rub Yongquan (K 1), nip Taichong (Liv 3).

5. Headache caused by Deficient Kidney

Signs & Symptoms: Headache with feeling of weightlessness, dizziness, tinnitus, insomnia, amnesia, tiredness, feebleness, soreness of the waist and weariness of legs, seminal emission, morbid leukorrhea. *Tongue:* red with minimal fur. *Pulse:* deep, thready and feeble.

Therapeutic Principle: Nourish Yin, invigorate Kidney.

Principal Measure: Knead the back, revolve Shenshu (UB 23) and Zhishi (UB 52) with the forearm, rotate and rub to strengthen the waist, revolve lower abdomen with the forearm, roll the abdomen with knocking and vibrating.

Subordinate Measure: Nip Yintang (Ex-HN 2), knead Taiyang (Ex-HN 4); nip Lieque (Lu 7), Zusanli (St 36), Sanyinjiao (Sp 6) and Taixi (K 3).

6. Headache causes by Deficient Vital Energy

Signs & Symptoms: Continuous headache with feeling of dizziness and weightlessness, symptoms aggravated by overwork, weariness, feebleness, severe palpitations, remoteness, poor appetite. *Tongue:* pale, swollen with thin fur. *Pulse:* weak and feeble.

Therapeutic Principle: Invigorate Vital Energy, raise Yang.

Principal Measure: Pound the top of the head with open fists, pinch the eyebrows, rock the rim of the ear, pluck and grasp both Jianjing (GB 21), nip Zanzhu (UB 2), pinch and grasp the neck and nape (all of these to invigorate).

Subordinate Measure: Knead Dazhui (GV 14); nip Shenmen (H 7), Neiguan (Per 6), Zusanli (St 36) and Chongyang (St 42).

7. Headache caused by Deficient Blood

Signs & Symptoms: Headache, dizziness, dry eyes, pale lips and complexion, palpitation from fright, severe palpitations, insomnia. *Tongue:* pale. *Pulse:* deep, thready, feeble.

Principal Measure: Open Passes and dredge Apertures, pound the top of the head with open fists, stroke and caress the head, roll the abdomen with knocking and vibrating, relax the chest with pressing and kneading, Taiji round-rub the abdomen.

Subordinate Measure: Revolve Jueyinshu (UB 14), Xinshu (UB 15), Pishu (UB 20), Ganshu (UB 18) and Shenshu (UB 23); nip Xuehai (Sp 10) and Sanyinjiao (Sp 6).

8. Headache caused by Phlegm and Turbidity

Signs & Symptoms: Headache with muddled feeling, dizziness, short temper, confusion, fullness and heaviness in chest and epigastrium, vomiting and spitting of sputum and saliva. *Tongue:* white, greasy fur. *Pulse:* stringy, slippery.

Therapeutic Principle: Eliminate Phlegm, subdue the adverse uprising of Vital Energy.

Principal Measure: Stroke and caress the head, relieve the chest with dotting and vibrating, relax the chest with pressing and kneading, rub Fengchi (GB 20) with joined hands, revolve the middle abdomen with the forearm, press the abdomen with deep-pressing and kneading, revolve the lower abdomen with the forearm.

Subordinate Measure: Knead Tiantu (CV 22), nip Neiguan (Per 6), grasp Fenglong (St 40) and Kunlun (UB 60).

Vertigo

Vertigo is a common symptom — a feeling of giddiness or confusion in which your patient feels as if he/she or the surroundings seem to be spinning.

Etiology: Deficiency of Vital Energy and Blood due to weak constitution or extended illness; uprising of Liver Wind due to a constitutional Excess of Yang with emotional depression accompanied by depletion of Liver Yin; excessive uprising of Liver Yang due to a Deficiency of Kidney Yin; obstruction of the Middle Warmer by Dampness or Phlegm due to Deficient Spleen.

Diagnosis & Treatment

1. Deficiency of Vital Energy and Blood

Signs & Symptoms: Dizziness, pale complexion, palpitation, insomnia, desire to stay in bed, remoteness, shortness of breath, feebleness, tiredness, poor appetite. *Tongue:* pale with pale lips. *Pulse:* thready, weak.

Therapeutic Principle: Benefit Vital Energy, nourish Blood.

Principal Measure: Pound the head with both open fists; stroke and caress the head; nip Renzhong (GV 26), vibrate both Jianjing (GB 21) with your palms; revolve Pishu (UB 20), Weishu (UB 21), the back and waist, and Dantian (all invigorating).

Subordinate Measure: Revolve Jueyinshu (UB 14), Xinshu (UB 15), Ganshu (UB 18) and Shenshu (UB 23) with your forearm; nip and knead Zusanli (Sp 36) — all invigorating.

2. Excessive uprising of Liver Yang

Signs & Symptoms: Dizziness, feeling of distension in the head, fretfulness, short-temper, reddened complexion, dreaminess, hot palms and soles, dry mouth, dryness and discomfort of the eye. *Tongue:* red with small amount of fur. *Pulse:* thready, stringy.

Therapeutic Principle: Quell Liver, conceal Yang.

Principal Measure: Lift and grasp Fengchi (GB 20), nip and knead Chize (Lu 5), pinch and grasp the elbow tendon, nip Quze (Per 3), push the back with pinching and grasping.

Subordinate Measure: Dot Quchi (LI 11) and Hegu (LI 4), revolve Huantiao (GB 30) with your elbow, nip and grasp Weizhing (UB 40), nip Xingjian (Liv 2), push Yongquan (K 1).

3. Deficiency of Kidney Yin

Signs & Symptoms: Dizziness, tinnitus, listlessness, insomnia, amnesia, blurred vision, soreness and pain in waist and knees, lassitude, feebleness, involuntary discharge of semen, emotional irritation, hot palms and soles. *Tongue:* reddened. *Pulse:* thready, stringy.

Therapeutic Principle: Invigorate Kidney, benefit the brain.

Principal Measure: Vibrate both Jianjing (GB 21) with your hands, knead the back, round-rub the abdomen with joined hands, revolve Dantian with your forearm, nip Zanzhu (UB 2), pull and lift both ears.

Subordinate Measure: Revolve Eight Liao (UB 31-34, both sides) with your forearm, revolve Huantiao (GB 30) with your elbow, nip Yongquan (K 1), nip and knead Rangu (K 2) and Kunlun (UB 60).

4. Obstruction of Middle Warmer by Phlegm and Turbidity

Signs & Symptoms: Dizziness with heaviness and weighted sensation, feeling of heaviness in the chest, nausea, attempts to vomit, heaviness of the body and limbs, poor appetite, somnolence. *Tongue:* white greasy fur. *Pulse:* soft, floating, slippery.

Therapeutic Principle: Dry Dampness, eliminate Phlegm.

Principal Measure: Stroke and caress the head, relieve the chest by dotting and vibrating, vibrate both Jianjing (GB 21) with palms, relax the chest by pressing and kneading, revolve lower and mid-abdomen with your forearm.

Subordinate Measure: Revolve Feishu (UB 13), Jueyinshu (UB 14),Xinshu (UB 15), Pishu (UB 20) and Dachangshu (UB 25) with your forearm; nip Chize (Lu 5), Zhigou (TW 6), Neiguan (Per 6) [all three on both sides], Fenglong (St 40), Kunlun (UB 60) and Lieque (Lu 7).

Insomnia

Insomnia has several varieties — lying awake at night is the best known, but it also includes difficulty in falling asleep and easiness of being awakened.

Etiology: Damage of Heart and Spleen due to overwork or overthinking; Deficiency of Blood from illness or loss of blood during childbirth; Deficiency of Heart and timidity of Gall Bladder from fright; disharmony between Spleen and Stomach from overeating; depletion of Kidney Yin from over-indulgence in sexual intercourse; breakdown of the normal physiological co-ordination between Heart and Kidney.

Diagnosis & Treatment

1. Depletion of Blood in Heart and Spleen

Signs & Symptoms: Dreaminess, easily awakened, palpitation, amnesia, dizziness, lassitude, weariness, loss of appetite, pale complexion. *Tongue:* pale with thin fur. *Pulse:* thready, weak.

Therapeutic Principle: Invigorate Spleen, nourish Heart.

Principal Measure: Stroke and caress the head, nip Zanzhu (GB 2), vibrate Baihu (GV 20) with a finger, push the back with pinching and grasping, revolve the waist with your forearm (all invigorating).

Subordinate Measure: Nip Shenmen (H 7), Tongli (H 5), Yinxi (H 6), Neiguan (Per 6) and Sanyinjiao (Sp 6).

2. Hyperactivity of Fire due to Deficiency of Yin

Signs & Symptoms: Fretfulness, insomnia, dizziness, tinnitus, dry mouth, vexation with hot palms and soles, soreness and lassitude of the waist and knees, seminal emission. *Tongue:* reddened. *Pulse:* thready, rapid.

Therapeutic Principle: Nourish Yin, clear Heat.

Principal Measure: Stroke and caress the head, pinch and grasp the neck and nape, pull and lift both ears, rub the waist, scratch the back.

Subordinate Measure: Nip Shenmen (H 7) and Lingdao (H 4), knead Laogong (Per 8) and Sanyinjiao (Sp 6), push Yongquan (K 1) (all invigorating).

3. Deficiency of Heart and Timidity of Gall Bladder

Signs & Symptoms: Palpitation, timidity, dreaminess, easily frightened, distracted mind, shortness of breath, feebleness, clear and long-passing urine. *Tongue:* pale. *Pulse:* stringy, thready.

Therapeutic Principle: Benefit Vital Energy, calm fright.

Principal Measure: Pound the top of the head with open fists, stroke and caress the head, revolve the chest with your forearm, vibrate both Jianjing (GB 21) with your palms, scratch the back, revolve the waist with your forearm (all invigorating).

4. Disharmony between Spleen and Stomach

Signs & Symptoms: Insomnia, feeling of epigastric heaviness, belching, loss of appetite, abdominal distension after eating, stomach distress, constipation. *Tongue:* greasy fur. *Pulse:* slippery.

Therapeutic Principle: Promote digestion, remove stasis, harmonize the Stomach.

Principal Measure: Vibrate the chest with your fingers, relax the chest by pressing and kneading, divide the ribs with pushing and wiping, round-rub Zhongwan (CV 12) with a finger, roll the abdomen with knocking and vibrating, vibrate Pishu (UB 20) and Weishu (UB 21) with your palms, knock the back (all reducing).

Subordinate Measure: Nip and knead Quchi (LI 11), Yinbai (Sp 1), Lidui (St 45) and Zusanli (St 36).

Epigastric pain

This occurs near the area of the heart.

Etiology: Stomach attacked by transversely hyperactive Liver Energy from emotional depression or resentment; Stasis of Blood and obstruction of Collaterals from Stagnation of Vital Energy; Retention of food from overeating, which damages Spleen and Stomach; depressed Liver Heat transforms into Fire, scorching the Stomach; Deficiency and Cold of Spleen and Stomach leading to food retention; depletion of Yin by depressed Heat, which impedes the flow of Vital Energy and Blood in Vessels and Collaterals.

Diagnosis & Treatment

1. Stagnation of Vital Energy

Signs & Symptoms: Fullness and distension in the epigastrium and rib cage, belching, heartburn, feeling of heaviness and obstruction in the chest, tendency to sigh deeply, feeling of relief when epigastrium is pressed, aggravation of condition when angry, poor appetite. *Tongue:* white, thin fur. *Pulse:* stringy.

Therapeutic Principle: Disperse and rectify Liver Energy.

Principal Measure: Revolve middle abdomen with your forearm, chop all four limbs with joined hands, pound and chop the back, push the abdomen with round-rubbing and revolving, roll the abdomen with knocking and vibrating, revolve Huantiao (GB 30) with your elbow, chop the legs with both palms.

Subordinate Measure: Knead Neiguan (Per 6); nip Taichong (Liv 3), Xingjian (Liv 2) and Zusanli (St 36).

2. Blood stasis

Signs & Symptoms: Fixed stabbing pain and tenderness at the epigastrium, resistance to pressing, pain is aggravated after eating. *Tongue:* dim purple. *Pulse:* uneven.

Therapeutic Principle: Resolve Blood stasis, rectify Vital Energy.

Principal Measure: Grasp the abdomen with lifting and jerking, round-rub the abdomen with joined hands, knock and clap the back, divide the ribs with pushing and wiping.

Subordinate Measure: Nip Neiguan (Per 6), Zusanli (St 36), Shangjuxu (St 37) and Gongsun (Sp 4).

3. Retention of food

Signs & Symptoms: Distension, fullness and pain in the epigastrium, resistance to pressing, belching with foul odor, heartburn, aversion to the smell of food, nausea, vomiting, relief after vomiting, constipation. *Tongue:* thick, greasy fur. *Pulse:* slippery.

Therapeutic Principle: Promote digestion, remove stasis.

Principal Measure: Clap and beat the back, chop the back with both hands, push the abdomen with round-rubbing and revolving, roll the abdomen with knocking and vibrating, grasp the abdomen with lifting and jerking, pinch the spine, chop the legs with both hands (all reducing).

Subordinate Measure: Nip Liangqiu (St 34), Zusanli (St 36), Tiaokou (St 38), Neiting (St 44).

4. Depressed Heat in Liver and Stomach

Signs & Symptoms: Urgent scorching epigastric pain, heartburn, Stomach distress, belching with foul odor, thirst, desire for cold water, bitter taste in mouth, constipation. *Tongue:* thin yellow fur. *Pulse:* rapid.

Therapeutic Principle: Clear Stomach, discharge Heat.

Principal Measure: Pound the back with open fists, grasp the abdomen with lifting and jerking, press the abdomen with deep-pressing and kneading, revolve both Huantiao (GB 30) with your elbow, chop the legs (all reducing).

Subordinate Measure: Nip Zusanli (St 36), Gongsun (Sp 4) and Neiting (St 44).

5. Deficiency-Cold of Spleen and Stomach

Signs & Symptoms: Continuous abdominal pain, nausea, vomiting clear water, poor appetite, abdominal distension, desire for being warmed and pressed, lassitude, feebleness, cold limbs, loose stool. *Tongue:* pale, tender with thin white slippery fur. *Pulse:* soft, floating, weak.

Therapeutic Principle: Warm the Middle Warmer, benefit Spleen.

Principal Measure: Revolve Pishu (UB 20) and Weishu (UB 21) with your forearm, scratch the back, pinch the spine, push the abdomen with round-rubbing and revolving, round-rub the abdomen with joined hands, press the abdomen with deep-pressing and kneading, revolve the lower abdomen with your forearm, rotate the arms, pinch the Six Meridians of the leg.

Subordinate Measure: Nip and knead Zusanli (St 36), Yanglingquan (GB 34) and Tiaokou (St 38).

6. Deficiency of Yin

Signs & Symptoms: Vague pain in the stomach, dry mouth and cracked lips, loss of appetite, retching, hiccups, constipation. *Tongue:* reddened with insufficient saliva and sparse fur. *Pulse:* thready, rapid.

Therapeutic Principle: Nourish Yin, benefit Stomach.

Principal Measure: Revolve middle abdomen with your forearm, roll the abdomen with knocking and vibrating, grasp the abdomen with lifting and jerking, Taiji round-rub the abdomen, vibrate Shenque (CV 8) with a finger, chop the legs with joined hands.

Subordinate Measure: Nip and knead Zhigou (TW 6), Hegu (LI 4), Sanyinjiao (Sp 6), Jiexi (St 41), Neiting (St 44) and Dadun (Liv 1).

Abdominal pain

This is pain beneath the epigastrium, around to the navel.

Etiology: Overeating of raw and cold meals, or the abdomen attacked by exogenous cold; Deficiency of Kidney Yang impairs Spleen Yang — "Fire cannot generate Earth;" accumulation and stagnation of Cold and Dampness due to Deficiency of Spleen and Kidney; damage of Spleen and Stomach from too much greasy and pungent food. At first, depression of Vital Energy and retention of food occurs in the Stomach, then the Large Intestine.

Diagnosis & Treatment

1. Cold accumulated in the Interior

Signs & Symptoms: Acute, serious sustained pain — aggravated when the abdomen is cooled, relieved when the abdomen is warmed; stomach rumblings, diarrhea, cold limbs. *Tongue:* pale with white, wet fur. *Pulse:* deep, tense.

Therapeutic Principle: Warm the Middle Warmer, disperse Cold.

Principal Measure: Knead the back, whisk the back with pounding and chopping, push the abdomen with round-rubbing and revolving, grasp the abdomen with lifting and jerking, press the abdomen with deep-pressing and kneading, revolve Dantian with your forearm, pinch Diji (Sp 8).

Subordinate Measure: Nip Zusanli (St 36), Gongsun (Sp 4).

2. Despondent Spleen Yang

Signs & Symptoms: Continuous varying abdominal pain, desire to be pressed, lassitude, tiredness, shortness of breath, aversion to cold, loose stool. *Tongue:* pale with thin white fur. *Pulse:* deep, thready.

Therapeutic Principle: Warm Yang, invigorate Spleen.

Principal Measure: Scratch the back, push the back with pinching and grasping, roll the abdomen with knocking and vibrating, grasp the abdomen with lifting and jerking, round-rub the abdomen with joined hands, revolve the middle abdomen with your forearm, roll the legs with your hands.

Subordinate Measure: Nip Zusanli (St 36) and Gongsun (Sp 4), knead Baihu (GV 20).

3. Retention of food

Signs & Symptoms: Fullness, distension and pain in the abdomen, resistance to pressing, loss of appetite, foul-smelling belches, heartburn, loose bowels, sour/foul stool mixed with undigested grains, abdominal pain relieved by defecation, aggravated by constipation. *Tongue:* greasy fur. *Pulse:* slippery, replete.

Therapeutic Principle: Promote digestion, remove stasis.

Principal Measure: Vibrate Pishu (UB 20) and Weishu (UB 21) with your palms, push and wipe to divide the ribs, vibrate middle abdomen with hands, push the back with pinching and grasping, chop the legs with both hands.

Subordinate Measure: Nip Zusanli (St 36) and Jiexi (St 41).

4. Vital Energy stagnation and Blood stasis

Signs & Symptoms: Fullness and distension in the abdomen, belching, vomiting, heartburn, indignation aggravates the pain, which always occurs at the same place; loss of appetite. *Tongue:* dim purple fur. *Pulse:* deep, stringy, uneven.

Therapeutic Principle: Promote the flow of Vital Energy, dissipate stasis.

Principal Measure: Revolve the middle abdomen with your forearm, grasp the abdomen with lifting and jerking, round-rub the abdomen with joined hands, press the abdomen with deep-pressing and kneading, push and wipe to divide the ribs, push the back with pinching and grasping, pinch Diji (Sp 8), chop the legs with both hands.

Subordinate Measure: Nip Neiguan (Per 6); nip and knead Sanyinjiao (Sp 6), Zusanli (St 36) and Taichong (Liv 3).

Hiccups

This is the result of the involuntary adverse uprising of Vital Energy from the chest, diaphragm and Stomach.

Etiology: Weakness and Deficiency of Healthy Energy due to careless eating, drinking or emotional depression; Cold accumulated in Stomach due to overeating of raw and cold food, or Stomach attacked by Cold evil; Heat accumulated in Stomach due to overeating of fatty and pungent food; abnormal uprising of Liver energy with Phlegm, tugging at the diaphragm; depletion of Stomach Yin due to serious or extended disease.

Diagnosis & Treatment

Hiccups may be classified as either Deficiency or Excess. Those caused by Cold, Fire or depression of Vital Energy are often Excess; those caused by weakness of the Middle Warmer or Deficiency of Stomach Yin are often Deficiency.

1. Cold hiccups

Signs & Symptoms: Deep, slow and energetic sound, feeling of coldness, heaviness and pain in the Stomach; symptoms are relieved when epigastric region is warmed and aggravated when it is cooled. *Tongue:* white moist fur. *Pulse:* slow, moderate.

Therapeutic Principle: Warm Middle Warmer, depress adverse uprising of Vital Energy.

Principal Measure: Stroke and caress the head, push and wipe to divide the ribs, push the abdomen with round-rubbing and revolving, revolve Dantian with your forearm.

Subordinate Measure: Knead Tiantu (CV 22) with a finger; nip Neiguan (Per 6) and Zusanli (St 36), grasp Weizhong (UB 40).

2. Heat hiccups

Signs & Symptoms: The sound is sonorous and sudden, halitosis, excessive thirst, desire for cold water, diminished urination with deep color. *Tongue:* yellow dry fur. *Pulse:* slippery, rapid.

Therapeutic Principle: Clear Heat, depress the adverse uprising of Vital Energy.

Principal Measure: Push the chest with your thenar mounds, revolve the middle abdomen with your forearm, revolve Huantiao (GB 30) with your elbow, push the abdomen with round-rubbing and revolving, deep-press the back with kneading and revolving, rectify the fingers, chop the legs with joined hands.

Subordinate Measure: Knead Tiantu (CV 22) and Neiguan (Per 6), nip Hegu (LI 4), Jianshi (Per 5) and Jiexi (St 41).

3. Food retention

Signs & Symptoms: The sound is energetic; fullness and distension in the epigastrium and stomach, sour fetid breath, belching, heartburn, vomiting undigested food, impeded diarrhea. *Tongue:* dirty, greasy fur. *Pulse:* deep, uneven.

Therapeutic Principle: Remove stasis, depress the adverse uprising of Vital Energy.

Principal Measure: Revolve middle and lower abdomen with the forearm, grasp the abdomen with lifting and jerking, press the abdomen with deep-pressing and kneading, rectify the fingers, revolve Huantiao (GB 30) with the elbow.

Subordinate Measure: Knead Tiantu (CV 22), nip Neiguan (Per 6) and Zusanli (St 36), grasp Weizhong (UB 40).

4. Deficiency of Stomach Yin

Signs & Symptoms: The sound is hurried and intermittent; vexation, restlessness, dry mouth and throat. *Tongue:* red or crimson. *Pulse:* thready, rapid.

Therapeutic Principle: Benefit Stomach, quell the adverse uprising of Vital Energy.

Principal Measure: Relieve the chest by dotting and vibrating, relax the chest by pressing and kneading, push and wipe to divide the ribs, push the abdomen with round-rubbing and revolving, grasp the abdomen with lifting and jerking, Taiji round-rub the abdomen.

Subordinate Measure: Revolve Pishu (UB 20), Weishu (UB 21) and Geshu (UB 17) with your forearm; nip Neiguan (Per 6) and Zusanli (St 36).

5. Despondent Spleen Yang

Signs & Symptoms: The sound is low and timid, shortness of breath, pale complexion, cold limbs, poor appetite, lassitude. *Tongue:* pale with white fur. *Pulse:* thready, feeble.

Therapeutic Principle: Strengthen Spleen, quell the adverse uprising of Vital Energy.

Principal Measure: Stroke and caress the head, push the chest with the thenar mounds, relieve the chest by dotting and vibrating, relax the chest by pressing and kneading, push and wipe to divide the ribs, push the abdomen with round-rubbing and revolving, roll the abdomen with knocking and vibrating, scratch the back and the waist.

Subordinate Measure: Knead Baihu (GV 20), nip Taichong (Liv 3), knead Ganshu (UB 18) and Geshu (UB 17).

Vomiting

The Stomach is concerned with the reception and digestion of food. It cooperates with the Spleen to send the clear elements of food upwards and to propel the turbid elements downwards. Vomiting is usually caused by the failure of the Stomach to harmonize and descend, resulting in adverse uprising of Vital Energy. Vomiting may occur with or without sound.

Etiology: Stomach attacked by exogenous evils; retention of Phlegm and Dampness in Spleen-Stomach; overeating of raw, cold or fatty foods; the Liver attacks the Stomach during emotional depression.

Diagnosis & Treatment

1. Attack of exogenous evils

Signs & Symptoms: Sudden onset of vomiting with fever, aversion to cold, feeling of fullness and heaviness in the chest and epigastrium, belching, loss of appetite. *Tongue:* white, greasy fur. *Pulse:* superficial.

Therapeutic Principle: Expel evils, relieve the external, rectify Middle Warmer, depress the adverse uprising.

Principal Measure: Relax the chest by pressing and kneading, revolve the middle abdomen with your forearm, push the abdomen by round-rubbing and revolving, press the abdomen with deep-pressing and kneading, push and wipe to divide the ribs, push the back by pinching and grasping, scratch the back, chop the legs with joined hands.

Subordinate Measure: Nip Lieque (Lu 7), Waiguan (TW 5), Neiguan (Per 6) and Neiting (St 44); rub Yongquan (K 1).

2. Retention of Phlegm and fluids

Signs & Symptoms: Vomiting clear water, saliva or sputum; loss of appetite, heaviness in the epigastric region, dizziness, palpitations. *Tongue:* greasy fur. *Pulse:* slippery.

Therapeutic Principle: Warm and resolve Phlegm and fluids, harmonize Stomach, depress the adverse uprising.

Principal Measure: Push the chest with your hands, relieve the chest by dotting and vibrating, relax the chest by pressing and kneading, grasp the abdomen with lifting and jerking, deep-press the spine with kneading and revolving, push the back with pinching and grasping, revolve Huantiao (GB 30) with your elbow, chop the legs with joined hands.

Subordinate Measure: Nip Neiguan (Per 6), Chize (Lu 5), Fenglong (St 40) and Lidui (St 45).

3. Stomach impaired by overeating

Signs & Symptoms: Sour, fetid vomit, fullness and distension in epigastrium and abdomen, aversion to the smell of food, belching, loss of appetite, symptoms aggravated after a meal and relieved after vomiting. *Tongue:* thick, greasy fur. *Pulse:* slippery, replete.

Therapeutic Principle: Promote digestion, remove stasis, harmonize Stomach, depress the adverse uprising.

Principal Measure: Revolve middle and lower abdomen with your forearm, push the abdomen with round-rubbing and revolving, roll the abdomen with knocking and vibrating, pinch the spine, chop the legs with joined hands.

Subordinate Measure: Nip and knead Zusanli (St 36) and Neiguan (Per 6).

4. Stomach attacked by Liver Energy

Signs & Symptoms: Nausea, belching, intermittent vomiting with little substance, fullness and heaviness in the chest and epigastrium, pain in the chest and rib cage, regurgitation (after eating), symptoms are especially aggravated during emotional depression, bitter taste in mouth. *Tongue:* yellow fur. *Pulse:* stringy.

Therapeutic Principle: Disperse and rectify Liver Energy, harmonize Stomach, depress the adverse uprising.

Principal Measure: Push the chest with both hands, relieve the chest by dotting and vibrating, push and wipe to divide the ribs, revolve the middle abdomen with your forearm, press the abdomen with deep-pressing and kneading, grasp the abdomen with lifting and jerking, revolve both Huantiao (GB 30) with your elbow.

Subordinate Measure: Revolve Ganshu (UB 18), Pishu (UB 20), Geshu (UB 17) and Weishu (UB 21); nip Taichong (Liv 3) and Zulinqi (GB 41).

5. Deficiency-Cold of Spleen and Stomach

Signs & Symptoms: Vomiting triggered by slight overeating, aggravated when cooled — relieved when warmed, tiredness, feebleness, dizziness, dry mouth but no desire to drink. *Tongue:* pale. *Pulse:* soft, floating, weak.

Therapeutic Principle: Warm Middle Warmer, strengthen Spleen, harmonize Stomach, depress the adverse uprising.

Principal Measure: Push the abdomen with round-rubbing and revolving, roll the abdomen with knocking and vibrating, round-rub the abdomen with joined hands, revolve middle abdomen with your forearm, grasp the abdomen with lifting and jerking, pinch the spine.

Subordinate Measure: Knead Baihu (GV 20), nip Neiguan (Per 6) and Zusanli (St 36).

Diarrhea

Diarrhea is described as frequent intestinal evacuations with loose or liquid stool, but without pus or blood. It may be encountered throughout the year, but seems to occur more frequently in summer and autumn.

Etiology: Generally speaking, Spleen, Stomach, and Large and Small Intestines are involved in diarrhea, which is caused by such factors as exogenous evils, impairment from overeating, or emotional depression. Although Cold, Heat, and Summer-Heat may be pathogenic factors of diarrhea, Dampness is the primary cause. It blocks Spleen Yang and impairs the normal transportation occurring within the gastrointestinal tract. Spleen and Stomach may be directly harmed by raw, cold, fatty or contaminated foods, or their overeating. Stomach may be attacked by hyperactive Liver Energy during periods of emotional depression or resentment. Spleen and Stomach may also be weakened by overwork or extended illness. Also, Deficiency of Kidney Yang may be a cause.

Diagnosis & Treatment

1. Diarrhea caused by Cold-Dampness

Signs & Symptoms: Dilute, loose stool mixed with undigested grains, feeling of fullness and distension in the stomach, abdominal pain, rumblings, poor or lost appetite, desire to be warmed and pressed, heaviness of body and limbs, tiredness, feebleness, possible chills and fever, headache, clear urine. *Tongue:* white, greasy fur. *Pulse:* soft, floating, moderate.

Therapeutic Principle: Warm Middle Warmer, eliminate Dampness.

Principal Measure: Push the abdomen with round-rubbing and revolving, press the abdomen with deep-pressing and kneading, revolve the middle abdomen with your forearm, round-rub the abdomen with joined hands, scratch the back, strengthen the waist by rolling and rubbing.

Subordinate Measure: Knead Zusanli (St 36) and Gongsun (Sp 4), push Chengshan (UB 57) and Waiguan (TW 5), knead Baihui (GV 20).

2. Diarrhea caused by Dampness-Heat

Signs & Symptoms: Hot, loose stool with a foul smell, stomach rumblings, abdominal pain, short temper, thirst, heaviness and obstruction in the chest and epigastrium, chills and fever, diminished urination with deep colored urine. *Tongue:* red with thick, yellow greasy fur. *Pulse:* slippery, rapid.

Therapeutic Principle: Clear Heat, promote the elimination of Dampness.

Principal Measure: Push the chest with both hands, knead Pishu (UB 20) and Weishu (UB 21) with your fingers, roll the abdomen with knocking and vibrating, grasp the abdomen with lifting and jerking (all clearing), vibrate Shenque (CV 8) with your fingers.

Subordinate Measure: Nip Zusanli (St 36) and Jiexi (St 41), push Chengshan (UB 57).

3. Diarrhea caused by overeating

Signs & Symptoms: Glutinous, sour, foul-smelling stool, abdominal pain, vomiting, fullness and heaviness in the epigastrium, alleviation of symptoms after defecation, foul-smelling belching, refusal to eat. *Tongue:* filthy, turbid fur. *Pulse:* stringy, slippery.

Therapeutic Principle: Promote digestion and remove stasis.

Principal Measure: Revolve the middle abdomen with your forearm, press the abdomen with deep-pressing and kneading, grasp the abdomen with lifting and jerking, roll the abdomen with knocking and vibrating, revolve the lower abdomen with your forearm, pinch the spine, chop legs with joined hands.

Subordinate Measure: Nip Yinlingquan (Sp 9) and Zusanli (St 36).

4. Disharmony between Liver and Spleen

Signs & Symptoms: Feeling of heaviness and distension in the chest and rib cage, belching, heartburn, abdominal pain and diarrhea without relief from defecation. *Tongue:* pale, red with thin white fur. *Pulse:* stringy.

Therapeutic Principle: Disperse Liver Energy, strengthen Spleen.

Principal Measure: Push the chest with the thenar mounds, push and wipe to divide the ribs, relieve the chest with dotting and vibrating, revolve the middle abdomen with your forearm, grasp the abdomen with lifting and jerking, push the abdomen with round-rubbing and revolving, knock Shenque (CV 8) with your hands.

Subordinate Measure: Knead Taichong (Liv 3) and Xingjian (Liv 2), revolve Ganshu (UB 18), Danshu (UB 19) and Pishu (UB 20).

5. Deficiency of Kidney Yang

Signs & Symptoms: Abdominal pain and diarrhea in early morning, eased after defecation; coldness in the abdomen, desire to be warmed and pressed, cold limbs, appearance of coldness, soreness and weariness of the waist and knees. *Tongue:* pale, swollen with thin white fur. *Pulse:* deep, thready, feeble.

Therapeutic Principle: Warm Kidney, strengthen Spleen.

Principal Measure: Round-rub the abdomen with joined hands, vibrate Dantian with your hands, revolve the middle abdomen with your forearm, press the abdomen with deep-pressing and kneading, roll the abdomen with knocking and vibrating, push the back with pinching and grasping (all invigorating).

Subordinate Measure: Revolve Ganshu (UB 18), Shensu (UB 23), Pishu (UB 20) and Dachangshu (UB 25) with your forearm; knead Baihui (GV 20).

Acute vomiting and diarrhea

This is a critical disorder characterized by sudden abdominal pain followed by outbursts of vomiting and diarrhea.

Etiology: Spleen-Stomach attacked by Summer-Heat, Dampness, or filthy and turbid evils in summer and autumn as part of inattentive, unhealthy living, or attraction to coldness.

Diagnosis & Treatment

1. Cold-Dampness

Signs & Symptoms: The onset is relatively quick with clear, watery vomit and foul watery stool; abdominal pain, desire to be pressed, inability to taste, thirst, cold limbs. *Tongue:* white, greasy fur. *Pulse:* soft, floating, moderate.

Therapeutic Principle: Disperse Cold, dry Dampness.

Principal Measure: Stroke and caress the head, open Passes and dredge Apertures, revolve the middle abdomen with your forearm, push the abdomen with round-rubbing and revolving, press the abdomen with deep-pressing and kneading, revolve lower abdomen with your forearm (invigorating), round-rub the abdomen with joined hands, scratch the back, roll all four limbs with your hands.

Subordinate Measure: Nip Neiguan (Per 6), Chize (Lu 5) and Chengshan (UB 57).

2. Summer-Heat and Dampness

Signs & Symptoms: Sudden onset with alternate vomiting and diarrhea; abdominal cramps; stool is yellow, foul and watery; short temper; fever and thirst with feeling of fullness and heaviness in the chest and epigastrium; reddish-yellow urine. *Tongue:* yellow, greasy fur. *Pulse:* slippery, rapid.

Therapeutic Principle: Clear Heat, eliminate Dampness.

Principal Measure: Pluck tendons of the spine, grasp tendons of the back, scratch the back, revolve lower and middle abdomen with your forearm, chop the arms with both hands, chop the legs with joined hands.

Subordinate Measure: Knead Dazhui (GV 14) and Quchi (LI 11), nip Shixuan (Ex-UE 9) and Neiguan (Per 6), knead and nip Chengshan (UB 57) and Weizhong (UB 40), grasp Achilles tendon.

Alternate Prescription

Principal Measure: Scrape the surface of the chest, neck and nape, cubital and popliteal fossae successively with the edge of a coin or a small wine cup dipped in cold water or white spirits, until you can see purple patches.

Subordinate Measure: Revolve Huantiao (GB 30) with your elbow, nip and grasp Zusanli (St 36), push Chengshan (UB 57) downwards.

Constipation

Constipation refers to painful, difficult or stopped defecation. Patients suffering from constipation have abnormally delayed bowel passage, often complicated by dry and hardened feces.

Etiology: Gastrointestinal diseases or dysfunction due to various pathogenic factors, such as accumulation of Heat from Excess of Yang, dehydration from febrile disease, disorder of Energy Mechanism from worry or anxiety, Deficiency of Spleen and Kidney Yang due to senility.

Diagnosis & Treatment

1. Accumulated Heat in Stomach and Intestines

Signs & Symptoms: Dry, hardened, unmoving feces lasting several days, feeling of distension and fullness in the abdomen, abdominal pain, resistance to pressing, reddened complexion, fever, perspiration, deep-colored urine, halitosis, lip boil. *Tongue:* yellow, thick, greasy fur. *Pulse:* slippery, replete.

Therapeutic Principle: Clear Heat, moisten Intestine.

Principal Measure: Pinch the spine, lift and grasp Shu-points on the back, push the back with both hands, roll the abdomen with knocking and vibrating.

Subordinate Measure: Nip and knead Hegu (LI 4) and Zhigou (TW 6), grasp Weizhong (UB 40) and Chengshan (UB 57), nip Dadun (Liv 1) (all on both sides).

2. Stagnation of Liver-Spleen Energy

Signs & Symptoms: Impeded movement of bowels with repeated ineffective attempts to evacuate, feeling of fullness and heaviness in the chest and epigastrium, gas under the rib cage. *Tongue:* white, greasy fur. *Pulse:* stringy.

Therapeutic Principle: Disperse stagnated Energy, remove stasis.

Principal Measure: Push the chest with the thenar mound, relax the chest by pressing and kneading, push and wipe to divide the ribs, round-rub rib cage, roll the abdomen with knocking and vibrating, revolve Huantiao (GB 30) with your elbow.

Subordinate Measure: Nip and knead Ganshu (UB 18), Pishu (UB 20), Danshu (UB 19), Dachangshu (UB 25), Quchi (LI 11), Hegu (LI 4), Zhigou (TW 6), Ligou (Liv 5) and Dadun (Liv 1) (all reducing).

3. Deficiency of Spleen-Kidney Yang

Signs & Symptoms: Coldness and pain in the abdomen, painful or difficult defecation, cyanotic complexion, cold limbs, desire to be warmed, aversion to cold, clear, lengthy urinations. *Tongue:* pale with moist fur. *Pulse:* deep, slow.

Therapeutic Principle: Warm Yang, ease bowel movements.

Principal Measure: Revolve Shu-points on the back with your forearm, scratch the back, rub the back and waist, knock the back and waist, pinch the spine, lift and grasp Shu-points on the back, round-rub the rib cage, revolve Dantian with your forearm, revolve Huantiao (GB 30) with your elbow.

Subordinate Measure: Push Eight Liao (UB 31-34, both sides) downwards; nip and knead Zhigou (TW 6), Zusanli (St 36), Sanyinjiao (Sp 6) and Dadun (Liv 1) (all on both sides).

4. Deficiency of Vital Energy

Signs & Symptoms: Dry but not hardened stool, several days duration of attempts to evacuate which are ineffective because of lack of strength, exhaustion after defecation, shortness of breath, spontaneous perspiration, glossy pale complexion. *Tongue:* pale and tender with thin white fur. *Pulse:* Deficient, feeble.

Therapeutic Principle: Benefit Vital Energy, relax bowels.

Principal Measure: Push the chest with the thenar mounds, relax the chest by pressing and kneading, push and wipe to divide the ribs, knead the abdomen, round-rub the abdomen with joined hands, revolve Dantian with your forearm, pinch the spine, grasp the abdomen with lifting and jerking.

Subordinate Measure: Nip and knead Zhigou (TW 6) and Hegu (LI 4); knead Zusanli (St 36) and Baihui (GV 20); knead Feishu (UB 13), Zhongfeng (Liv 4) and Dadun (Liv 1) 1 with your fingers (all on both sides).

5. Deficiency of Blood

Signs & Symptoms: Dry and hardened stool with ineffective attempts to evacuate, pale complexion and lips, dizziness, palpitation. *Tongue:* pale with little fur. *Pulse:* thready.

Therapeutic Principle: Nourish Blood, moisten the intestinal tract.

Principal Measure: Push the chest with your hands, relieve the chest by dotting and vibrating, round-rub rib cage, revolve Jueyinshu (UB 14), Xinshu (UB 15), Pishu (UB 20) and Weishu (UB 21) with your forearm;

round-rub the abdomen with joined hands, knead the abdomen, revolve Dantian with your forearm.

Subordinate Measure: Revolve Xinshu (UB 15), Ganshu (UB 18), Pishu (UB 20), Geshu (UB 17) and Dachangshu (UB 25) with your forearm; nip Shaohai (H 3), Quze (Per 3) and Shenmen (H 7); knead Taiyang (Ex-HN 4) and Baihui (GV 20); nip Xuehai (Sp 10) and Sanyinjiao (Sp 6) (all on both sides).

Rib cage pain

Rib cage pain may occur on one or both sides. Since Liver and Gallbladder Meridians pass through this area, this symptom is commonly associated with disorders of those organs.

Etiology: During emotional depression, Liver Energy is stagnated; during extended Liver Energy Stagnation, there will be Blood stasis; added to this, overwork or sexual overindulgence may deplete Yin and Blood, resulting in Excess of Liver Yang, bringing on rib cage pain.

Diagnosis & Treatment

Usually, rib cage pain is caused by disorders of Vital Energy and Blood. Swelling and pain around the rib cage are generally caused by stagnation of Vital Energy. Stabbing pains are generally caused by Blood stasis — vague pains are generally caused by Deficiency of Blood.

1. Stagnation of Vital Energy in Liver

Signs & Symptoms: Feeling of fullness and heaviness in the chest and abdomen, wandering distension and pain around the rib cage, symptoms are aggravated or alleviated according to emotional changes, frequent belching, poor appetite. *Tongue:* thin fur. *Pulse:* stringy.

Therapeutic Principle: Disperse and rectify Liver Energy.

Principal Measure: Push the chest with both hands, relieve the chest by dotting and vibrating, relax the chest by pressing and kneading, round-rub rib cage, push and wipe to divide the ribs, revolve Huantiao (GB 30) with your elbow, grasp the abdomen with lifting and jerking (all both sides).

Subordinate Measure: Knead Geshu (UB 17); grasp Weizhong (UB 40), Ganshu (UB 18) and Danshu (UB 19); nip Zulinqi (GB 41) and Neiguan (Per 6).

2. Blood stasis

Signs & Symptoms: Fixed stabbing pain with hardened mass in rib cage, abdominal distension, poor appetite, pain becomes especially serious at night. *Tongue:* dull, purple. *Pulse:* deep, uneven.

Therapeutic Principle: Remove stasis, dredge Collaterals.

Principal Measure: Revolve with your forearm on the back along the paths of the Urinary Bladder, rectify arms, rectify fingers; push the chest with the thenar mound, round-rub rib cage, press the abdomen with deep-pressing and kneading, push the abdomen with round-rubbing and revolving, round-rub the abdomen with joined hands, revolve Huantiao (GB 30) with your elbow.

Subordinate Measure: Knead Qimen (Liv 14); nip Zusanli (St 36), Sanyinjiao (SP 6), Zulinqi (GB 41) and Taichong (Liv 3).

3. Depletion of Liver Yin

Signs & Symptoms: Sustained vague pain in rib cage, dry mouth and throat, dizziness, vexation with feverish feeling, palpitation, dreaminess, worry, short temper. *Tongue:* red with small fur. *Pulse:* stringy, thready, rapid.

Therapeutic Principle: Nourish Yin, soothe Liver.

Principal Measure: Push and knead the eyebrow ridge, nip Zanzhu (UB 2), relax the chest by pressing and kneading, push and wipe to divide the ribs, press and push the supraclavicular fossa, pluck and grasp the arms, knead the back, revolve Huantiao (GB 30) with your elbow.

Subordinate Measure: Revolve Mingmen (GV 4), nip and grasp Yinlingquan (Sp 9), nip and knead Zusanli (St 36) and Zhongfeng (Liv 4).

Abdominal mass

Abdominal masses accompanied by feelings of distension and pain may be divided into two types. Those which are palpable with fixed form, location, and area of tenderness are called accumulated masses. These belong to disorders of Blood or Yin organs. Those which are not palpable and without fixed form and area, thereby without tenderness, are called assembled masses. These generally belong to disorders of Vital Energy or Yang organs. In most cases, accumulation of Vital Energy occurs at the first, and in others, accumulation of Blood.

Etiology: Prolonged emotional depression can lead to stagnation of Liver Energy and obstruction of Meridians; overeating impairs Spleen and Stomach resulting in accumulated Dampness, Phlegm or Turbidity; invasion of exogenous evils affecting Vital Energy and Blood.

Diagnosis & Treatment

1. Depression and stagnation of Liver Energy

Signs & Symptoms: No fixed form or location to the mass; a feeling of intermittent, wandering, swelling pain; depression, melancholy, intermittent epigastric and rib cage distress. *Tongue:* white, thin fur. *Pulse:* thready, stringy.

Therapeutic Principle: Disperse and rectify Liver Energy.

Principal Measure: Push the chest with the thenar mound, relieve the chest by dotting and vibrating, push and wipe to divide the ribs, pluck and grasp arms, roll the abdomen with knocking and vibrating, press the abdomen with deep-pressing and kneading, revolve the middle and lower abdomen with the forearm, push the back with pinching and grasping, revolve Huantiao (GB 30) with your elbow, chop the legs with joined hands.

Subordinate Measure: Nip Xingjian (Liv 2), Ququan (Liv 8) and Sanyinjiao (SP 6) (all on both sides).

2. Retention and obstruction of food and Phlegm

Signs & Symptoms: Abdominal distension and pain, constipation, loss of appetite, cord-like tender mass appears intermittently. *Tongue:* greasy fur. *Pulse:* stringy, slippery.

Therapeutic Principle: Rectify Vital Energy, promote digestion, resolve Phlegm.

Principal Measure: Revolve the middle abdomen with your forearm, press the abdomen with deep-pressing and kneading, revolve lower abdomen with the forearm, grasp the abdomen with lifting and jerking, revolve Huantiao (GB 30) with your elbow, chop the legs with joined hands, knead and press Tiantu (CV 22), relieve the chest with dotting and vibrating.

Subordinate Measure: Push Eight Liao (UB 31-34, both sides) downward, nip Weizhong (UB 40) and Zusanli (St 36).

3. Vital Energy stagnation and Blood stasis

Signs & Symptoms: Fixed, hardened and aching mass; possible chills and fever; emaciation, feebleness, poor appetite, dim complexion. *Tongue:* cyanotic. *Pulse:* stringy, slippery.

Therapeutic Principle: Promote the flow of Vital Energy, dissipate stasis.

Principal Measure: Push and wipe to divide the ribs, pluck and grasp the forearm, push the abdomen with round- rubbing and revolving, press the abdomen with deep-pressing and kneading, grasp the abdomen with lifting and jerking, knead the abdomen, push the back with pinching and grasping, revolve Huantiao (GB 30) with the elbow, pluck and grasp legs.

Stranguria

Indications of stranguria are primarily seen in the urinary tract and include abnormally frequent urination, painful or difficult urination with dripping discharge of urine, stabbing pain in the urethra, contracture and a feeling of urgency in the lower abdomen. Clinically, there are five types: Stone stranguria, Blood stranguria, Vital Energy stranguria, rice-water stranguria, and over-strain stranguria.

(*N.B.* — do not confuse this term with the Western medical term, "strangury" from which it was adapted for TCM use. Strangury refers specifically only to painful and interrupted urination. Stranguria includes a much wider range of symptoms.)

Etiology: Principally, stranguria is caused by accumulation and fermentation of Dampness-Heat in the Lower Warmer, such as may be caused by overeating pungent and rich fatty foods, or alcohol abuse. Additionally, Liver Energy may transform into Fire, depressed Energy and Fire from the Liver may then impair the function of the Urinary Bladder resulting in dysuria and dripping discharge of urine. Deficiency of Spleen and Kidney due to senility, extended illness or over-indulgence in sexual intercourse may lead to the endogenous accumulation of Dampness and Turbidity, which ferment and produce Heat.

Diagnosis & Treatment

1. Stone stranguria

Signs & Symptoms: Sand or calculi in the urine, stabbing pain during urination, interrupted urination, intolerable urgency or distress, sudden spasms of the lumbar area involving the lower abdomen, yellowish-red urine or turbid blood in the urine. *Tongue:* red with thin yellow fur. *Pulse:* stringy, rapid.

Therapeutic Principle: Clear Heat, eliminate Dampness.

Principal Measure: Push the abdomen with round-rubbing and revolving, press the abdomen with deep-pressing and kneading, grasp the abdomen with lifting and jerking, revolve Dantian, revolve the back and the waist with your forearm, chop the legs with joined hands.

Subordinate Measure: Knead Dachangshu (UB 25) and Eight Liao (UB 31-34, both sides), nip Sanyinjiao (Sp 6) and Zusanli (St 36).

Alternate Prescription: Dot Zhangmen (Liv 13) and Qimen (Liv 14), nip Weizhing (UB 40) and Yongquan (K 1) 100 times each. After massage, have your patient drink an appropriate amount of cold boiled water and rest for a while. Then have him/her jump on one leg, then the other, 100 times each, then dot and nip the above-mentioned points again, 100 times each.

2. *Vital Energy stranguria*

A. Excess syndrome

Signs & Symptoms: Fullness, distension and pain in the lower abdomen; interrupted urination, dysuria. *Tongue:* cyanotic. *Pulse:* deep, stringy.

Therapeutic Principle: Ease the flow of Vital Energy, dredge the urinary passage.

Principal Measure: Push the abdomen with round-rubbing and revolving, knead Guanyuan (CV 4) with your fingers, revolve Dantian and the waist with the forearm, roll all four limbs with your hands.

Subordinate Measure: Knead Qimen (Liv 4), nip Xingjian (Liv 2) and Taixi (K 3), push Yongquan (K 1).

B. Deficiency syndrome

Signs & Symptoms: Weighty distension and pain in the lower abdomen, abnormally frequent urination, dripping discharge of urine, glossy pale complexion. *Tongue:* pale. *Pulse:* thready.

Therapeutic Principle: Strengthen Middle Warmer, benefit Vital Energy.

Principal Measure: Roll the abdomen with kneading and vibrating, knead Guanyuan (CV 4) with your fingers, revolve Dantian with the forearm, pinch the spine, rub the back and waist, roll the arms with your hands.

Subordinate Measure: Knead Baihui (GV 20), nip Zusanli (St 36).

3. *Rice-Water stranguria*

Signs & Symptoms: The urine is turbid and milky like water in which rice has been washed, burning pain in the urethra, tiredness, feebleness, soreness of the waist and knees. *Tongue:* pale with greasy fur. *Pulse:* thready, feeble.

Therapeutic Principle: Clear Dampness-Heat.

Principal Measure: Grasp the abdomen with lifting and jerking, round-rub the abdomen, knead Shuifen (CV 9) with your fingers, revolve Dantian with the forearm, push the abdomen with round-rubbing and revolving, roll the legs with your hands.

Subordinate Measure: Knead Shenshu (UB 23), Dachangshu (UB 25) and Pangguangshu (UB 28) with the hands; rub Yongquan (K 1).

4. Over-strain stranguria

Signs & Symptoms: Protracted intermittent symptoms, becoming more serious during heavy work; dizziness, tinnitus, lassitude, soreness and weakness of the waist and legs. *Tongue:* pale, red. *Pulse:* thready, feeble.

Therapeutic Principle: Strengthen Spleen, benefit Kidney.

Principal Measure: Push the back with pinching and grasping, deep-press the spine with kneading and revolving, revolve the back and the waist with your forearm, round-rub rib cage, revolve the middle abdomen with the forearm, knead the lower abdomen with your hands, knead Guanyuan (CV 4) with your fingers, roll the legs with your hands.

Subordinate Measure: Revolve Eight Liao (UB 31-34, both sides) with the forearm, knead Weizhing (UB 40) with the fingers, nip and knead Yinlingquan (Sp 9), rub Yongquan (K 1).

Retention of urine (Uroschesis)

Uroschesis indicates difficult or painful urination (dysuria) or complete absence of urination (anuresis), resulting in the retention of urine in the bladder.

Etiology: The free discharge of urine depends on the normal functioning of the Triple Warmer — Lung, Spleen and Kidney. Excess syndrome of uroschesis is usually due to stagnation of Lung Energy or the obstruction of the water pathway. Deficiency syndrome of uroschesis is usually due to Deficiency of Spleen and Kidney Yang.

Uroschesis which originates in the Upper Warmer is often caused by Lung Heat. Uroschesis from the Middle Warmer is often caused by Damp-ness-Heat. Uroschesis from the Lower Warmer is often caused by Deficiency of Kidney Yang or depletion of Kidney Energy.

Diagnosis & Treatment

1. Dampness-Heat in the Urinary Bladder

Signs & Symptoms: Dripping discharge of urine or diminished unrination (oliguria) with deep color and scorching sensation, feeling of fullness and distension in the lower abdomen, thirst without desire for drink. *Tongue:* red with greasy yellow fur. *Pulse:* deep, rapid.

Therapeutic Principle: Clear Heat, eliminate Dampness.

Principal Measure: Press the abdomen with round-rubbing and revolving, roll the abdomen with knocking and vibrating, grasp the abdomen with lifting and jerking.

Subordinate Measure: Dot Qugu (CV 2) and Guanyuan (CV 4), nip and knead Yongquan (K 1) and Kunlun (UB 60)

2. Obstruction of water pathway by Lung Fire

Signs & Symptoms: Dysuria or anuria, shortness of breath, dry throat, excessive thirst, mild cough. *Tongue:* thin yellow fur. *Pulse:* rapid.

Therapeutic Principle: Clear Lung Heat, promote urination.

Principal Measure: Push the chest with the thenar mound, relax the chest with pressing and kneading, push and wipe to divide the ribs, revolve Dantian with the forearm, press the abdomen with deep-pressing and kneading, push the abdomen with round-rubbing and revolving.

Subordinate Measure: Dot Guanyuan (CV 4) and Zhongji (CV 3); nip and knead Hegu (LI 4), Chize (Lu 5), Neiguan (Per 6) and Yinlingquan (Sp 9).

3. Deficiency of Kidney Yang

Signs & Symptoms: Dripping discharge of urine, feeble urination, difficult bowel movement with slender and soft stool, coldness in the lower abdomen, soreness and tiredness in the waist and knees, glossy pale complexion, timid and weak facial expression. *Tongue:* pale. *Pulse:* deep, thready.

Therapeutic Principle: Warm Yang, dredge the obstructed water pathway.

Principal Measure: Revolve the back and waist with your forearm, vibrate Dantian with the fingers, push and wipe to divide the ribs, roll the abdomen with knocking and vibrating, Taiji round-rub the abdomen, scratch the back.

Subordinate Measure: Dot Qihai (CV 6), Shimen (CV 5) and Qugu (CV 2); knead Baihui (GV 20), Fuliu (K 7) and Sanyinjiao (Sp 6).

Seminal emission

This describes involuntary ejaculation of semen other than during sexual activity. It often occurs in male patients suffering from Deficiency and may be classified as spermatorrhea and nocturnal emission.

Etiology: Mental strain may deplete Heart Yin, resulting in hyperactivity of Heart Yang and failure of the Heart to consolidate and conserve Kidney; hyperactivity of Premier Fire from overindulgence in sexual intercourse;

Dampness-Heat streams down and impairs the function of the seminal Apertures.

Diagnosis & Treatment

1. Deficiency of Yin leads to hyperactivity of Fire

Signs & Symptoms: Sexual dreams, nocturnal emission, reddened complexion, palpitation, insomnia, dreaminess, dizziness, fretfulness, lassitude. *Tongue:* red with yellow fur. *Pulse:* thready, rapid.

Therapeutic Principle: Tranquilize the mind, consolidate the seminal Apertures.

Principal Measure: Stroke and caress the head; push and wipe to divide the ribs; roll the abdomen with knocking and vibrating, revolve Dantian, back and waist with the forearm.

Subordinate Measure: Nip Shenmen (H 7), Neiguan (Per 6) and Sanyinjiao (Sp 6).

2. Depletion of Kidney Yin

Signs & Symptoms: Frequent emission occurring whenever one is sexually aroused, dizziness, listlessness, soreness and weariness of the waist and knees, hotness at palms and soles of feet. *Tongue:* red. *Pulse:* thready, rapid.

Therapeutic Principle: Nourish Kidney, consolidate the seminal Apertures.

Principal Measure: Pluck Collaterals with knocking and scratching, revolve the back with the forearm, strengthen the waist by rolling and rubbing, push the abdomen with round-rubbing and revolving, Taiji round-rub the abdomen, press the abdomen with deep-pressing and kneading, vibrate Dantian with your fingers.

Subordinate Measure: Revolve Mingmen (GV 4) and Zhishi (UB 52) with the forearm; knead Baihui (GV 20); push Yongquan (K 1); nip and knead Shenmen (H 7), Sanyinjiao (Sp 6) and Taichong (Liv 3).

3. Deficiency of Kidney Yang

Signs & Symptoms: Involuntary emission of semen, listlessness, dizziness, tinnitus, soreness and weariness of waist and knees, cold dampness, shrinking scrotum, watery cold semen. *Tongue:* pale with white fur. *Pulse:* deep, thready.

Therapeutic Principle: Invigorate Kidney, consolidate seminal Apertures.

Principal Measure: Revolve the back and waist with the forearm, strengthen the waist by rolling and rubbing, push the abdomen with round-rubbing and revolving, push and wipe to divide the ribs, Taiji round-rub the abdomen, roll the abdomen with knocking and vibrating, vibrate Dantian with your palms.

Subordinate Measure: Nip and knead Baihui (GV 20), revolve Mingmen (GV 4) and Zhishi (UB 52) with the forearm, rub Eight Liao (UB 31-34, both sides), knead Zusanli (St 36) and Sanyinjiao (Sp 6).

4. Interior accumulation of Dampness-Heat

Signs & Symptoms: Frequent emission, semen in urine, hot deep-colored urine, contraction and pain in the urethra, vexation, insomnia, bitter taste in mouth, thirst. *Tongue:* yellow greasy fur. *Pulse:* soft, floating, rapid.

Therapeutic Principle: Clear Heat, consolidate seminal Apertures.

Principal Measure: Wipe to divide forehead, lift and grasp Fengchi (GB 20), Taiji round-rub the abdomen, revolve Dantian with the forearm, knead the back and waist with your hands, knock the back and waist.

Subordinate Measure: Push Shuiquan (K 5) and Yongquan (K 1).

Impotence

This describes the inability of the penis to become erect, or if able to become erect, it remains flaccid.

Etiology: Decline of Fire from the Vital Gate or depletion of Marrow Sea as a result of juvenile masturbation or overindulgence in coitus; malnutrition of the penis due to Deficiency of Vital Energy and Blood; relaxation and flaccidity of the penis due to fright or mental strain.

Diagnosis & Treatment

1. Decline of Fire from the Vital Gate

Signs & Symptoms: Impotence, dizziness, listlessness, soreness and weariness of waist and knees, feebleness, glossy pale complexion. *Tongue:* pale. *Pulse:* deep, thready.

Therapeutic Principle: Warm Kidney, foster Yang.

Principal Measure: Push the back with pinching and grasping, deep-press the spine with revolving and kneading, strengthen the waist with rolling and rubbing, press the abdomen with deep-pressing and kneading, vibrate Dantian with palms, roll the legs with your hands.

Subordinate Measure: Revolve Mingmen (GV 4) with the forearm, knead Yanglingquan (GB 34), revolve Eight Liao (UB 31-34, both sides) with the forearm, knead Chengshan (UB 57).

2. Deficiency of Spleen-Stomach Vital Energy

Signs & Symptoms: Impotence, shortness of breath, feebleness, poor appetite, listlessness, pale complexion. *Tongue:* pale, moist. *Pulse:* deep, thready.

Therapeutic Principle: Invigorate Spleen-Stomach, benefit Vital Energy.

Principal Measure: Push and wipe to divide the ribs, revolve the middle abdomen with the forearm, grasp the abdomen with lifting and jerking, press the abdomen with deep-pressing and kneading, vibrate Dantian with your palms, pinch the spine, revolve the back and waist with your forearm (all invigorating).

Subordinate Measure: Nip and knead Baihui (GV 20) and Zusanli (St 36).

3. Impairment of Kidney from fright.

Signs & Symptoms: Impotence, listlessness, timidity, paranoia, insomnia, dreaminess, involuntary emission, cold limbs. *Tongue:* thin greasy fur. *Pulse:* stringy, thready.

Therapeutic Principle: Benefit Kidney, tranquilize the mind.

Principal Measure: Drag and lift both ears, stroke and caress the head, revolve the back with the forearm, grasp tendons of the back, revolve the waist with your forearm, Taiji round-rub the abdomen, vibrate Dantian with your fingers.

Subordinate Measure: Nip Shenmen (H 7), Neiguan (Per 6), Sanyinjiao (Sp 6) and Fuliu (K 7).

Enuresis

Enuresis describes involuntary urination or nocturnal bed-wetting.

Etiology: Enuresis is associated with Lung, Spleen, Kidney and Urinary Bladder. For example: failure of Spleen and Lung to control the Apertures of the water pathway due to over-exertion; Deficiency of Kidney Yang from overindulgence in sexual intercourse or extended illness; hyperactivity of Fire due to depletion of Kidney Yin resulting in harassment of the normal function of Urinary Bladder.

Diagnosis & Treatment

1. Deficiency of Spleen-Lung Vital Energy

Signs & Symptoms: Frequent urge to urinate, incontinent dripping of urine, weighty distension of lower abdomen, shortness of breath, uncommunicative, weariness of limbs. *Tongue:* pale with small fur. *Pulse:* deficient, weak.

Therapeutic Principle: Invigorate Vital Energy, raise up Yang.

Principal Measure: Push the chest with thenar mound, push and wipe to divide the ribs, press the abdomen with deep-pressing and kneading, vibrate Dantian with your palms, push the back with pinching and grasping.

Subordinate Measure: Nip Baihui (GV 20); grasp Jianjing (GB 21), Sanyinjiao (Sp 6) and Zusanli (St 36).

2. Impairment of Kidney Yang

Signs & Symptoms: Abnormal frequency of urination, urinary incontinence, listlessness, aversion to cold, weakness, dizziness, soreness and weariness of waist and knees. *Tongue:* pale with white fur. *Pulse:* deep, thready.

Therapeutic Principle: Warm Kidney, consolidate and contract the Apertures of the water pathway.

Principal Measure: Round-rub the head with the hands, Taiji round-rub the abdomen, push the abdomen with round-rubbing and revolving, vibrate Dantian with the fingers, revolve Shenshu (UB 23) and Zhishi (UB 52) (all invigorating).

Subordinate Measure: Revolve Mingmen (GV 4) and Eight Liao (UB 31-34, both sides), knead Chengshan (UB 57) and Weizhong (UB 40), nip Xingjian (Liv 2) and Taixi (K 3) (all invigorating).

3. Hyperactivity of Fire from depletion of Kidney Yin

Signs & Symptoms: Abnormally frequent urination, diminished urination with deep color, urinary incontinence, dizziness, tinnitus, dry mouth and throat, reddened complexion and lips, insomnia, vexation, hotness of palms and soles of feet. *Tongue:* red with small fur. *Pulse:* thready, rapid.

Therapeutic Principle: Nourish Yin, depress Fire.

Principal Measure: Revolve Shu-points on the back with your forearm, push and wipe to divide the ribs, roll the abdomen with knocking and vibrating, round-rub rib cage, Taiji round-rub the abdomen, vibrate Dantian with your fingers (all clearing).

Subordinate Measure: Knead Baihui (GV 20), nip Shenmen (H 7) and Neiguan (Per 6), push Eight Liao (UB 31-34, both sides) downwards, push Yongquan (K 1).

Lumbago

A dull, aching pain in the lumbar area, which may occur at one or both sides of the waist.

Etiology: Obstruction of Meridians by Wind, Cold or Dampness; Vital Energy stagnation and Blood stasis from wrenching, straining, etc.; Deficiency of Kidney from overindulgence in sexual intercourse. Generally speaking, lumbago of internal origin is encountered more often than that of exogenous origin, and the latter is usually complicated by the former.

Diagnosis & Treatment

1. Lumbago from Wind-Dampness

Signs & Symptoms: Aversion to Wind, Cold and Dampness; fever, spontaneous perspiration; feeling of heaviness and stiffness in lumbar region; numbness and distension at the back and waist involving both legs, with aggravation of symptoms on wet days. *Pulse:* superficial, uneven.

Therapeutic Principle: Expel Wind, eliminate Dampness, dredge Meridians, activate Collaterals.

Principal Measure: Whisk the back and waist, revolve the back with the forearm, use the Stepping Method, push the waist with joined fists, jerk and drag to relax the waist, chop the legs with both hands.

Subordinate Measure: Pinch and grasp Fengchi (GB 20), knead Shenshu (UB 23) and Dachangshu (UB 25), nip Weizhong (UB 40) and Chengshan (UB 57), grasp Kunlun (UB 60) and Taixi (K 3).

2. Lumbago caused by Cold-Dampness

Signs & Symptoms: Stiffness and pain in the waist with feeling of heaviness and chilliness, cold loins, difficulty in turning around, symptoms aggravated when lying in bed or on wet days, desire to be warmed, aversion to cold. *Pulse:* deep, tense or slow, moderate.

Therapeutic Principle: Eliminate Dampness, disperse Cold, dredge Meridians, promote the flow of Vital Energy and Blood.

Principal Measure: Push the back with joined hands, push the spine with intermittent pausing, whisk the back and waist, pound and chop the back with round-rubbing, revolve the waist with the forearm, strengthen the waist by rolling and rubbing, jerk and drag to relax the waist.

Subordinate Measure: Revolve Shenshu (UB 23) and Dachangshu (UB 25), nip and grasp Weizhong (UB 40), Chengshan (UB 57), Kunlun (UB 60) and Taixi (K 3).

3. Lumbago caused by Dampness-Heat

Signs & Symptoms: Aching and pain in the sacral area with local sensation of heat, unexplained anxiety and fever, spontaneous perspiration, thirst, aversion to Dampness and Heat, desire to keep moving, reluctance to lie still, diminished urine with deep color. *Tongue:* yellow greasy fur. *Pulse:* soft, floating, rapid.

Therapeutic Principle: Eliminate Dampness, clear Heat, relax Tendons, relieve pain.

Principal Measure: Whisk and sweep the back and waist, use the Stepping Method, push Shu-points on the back with intermittent pausing, clap the back with chopping, revolve the back and waist with the forearm.

Subordinate Measure: Nip and knead Sanyinjiao (Sp 6), rub Yongquan (K 1), grasp Kunlun (UB 60).

4. Lumbago caused by Blood stasis

Signs & Symptoms: Fixed, stabbing pain varying in degree; resistance to pressing, symptoms ease during the day and increase at night, constipation, deep-colored urine. *Tongue:* dim, purple (possibly accompanied by ecchymosis). *Pulse:* deep, uneven.

Therapeutic Principle: Dredge Meridians, activate Collaterals, promote Blood flow, eliminate stasis.

Principal Measure: Push the back with joined fists; whisk and sweep the back and waist; push Shu-points on the back with intermittent pausing; knock, clap and pound the back; deep-press the bent leg to tug the waist; pluck the tendons of the spine; Taiji round-rub the abdomen; round-rub the rib cage; rectify the waist by back-to-back technique; jerk and drag to relax the waist.

Subordinate Measure: Knead Eight Liao (UB 31-34, both sides), Weizhong (UB 40), Chengshan (UB 57) and Kunlun (UB 60).

5. Lumbago caused by Deficiency of Kidney

Signs & Symptoms: Continuous lumbar pain, soreness, weakness, symptoms aggravated by exertion and alleviated by immobility, cold limbs, glossy pale complexion, loose stool, clear urine. *Tongue:* pale. *Pulse:* deep, thready.

Therapeutic Principle: Foster Yang, invigorate Kidney.

Principal Measure: Push the back with the heel of the hand, whisk and sweep the back and waist, push the back and waist with joined fists, Taiji round-rub the abdomen, push and wipe to divide the ribs, vibrate Dantian with your palms.

Subordinate Measure: Knead Mingmen (GV 4) and Yaoyangguan (GV 3) with your fingers, revolve Shenshu (UB 23) and Zhishi (UB 52) with the forearm, nip Yanglingquan (GB 34) and Fuliu (K 7).

6. Lumbago caused by Deficiency of Yin

Signs & Symptoms: Sustained lumbar pain, soreness and weakness, dry mouth, insomnia, amnesia, fevered agitation, vexation, hotness at palms and soles of feet. *Tongue:* red. *Pulse:* stringy, thready, rapid.

Therapeutic Principle: Nourish Yin, invigorate Kidney.

Principal Measure: Push the chest with the thenar mound, relieve the chest by dotting and vibrating, push the back with both hands, push the back and waist with intermittent pausing, whisk and sweep the back and waist, strengthen the waist by rolling and rubbing, pluck Collaterals with knocking and scratching, vibrate Dantian with your fingers.

Subordinate Measure: Knead Mingmen (GV 4), Shenshu (UB 23), Dachangshu (UB 25) and Eight Liao (UB 31-34, both sides); nip Sanyinjiao (Sp 6), rub Yongquan (K 1).

Chest pain

Heart and Lung reside in the chest. They participate in the rise and descent of Vital Energy and the circulation of Blood.

Etiology: Chest pain is often caused by the accumulation of Phlegm-Turbidity or the stagnation of Vital Energy. Attack of exogenous evils, impairment of internal organs, and depression may also be pathogenic factors.

Diagnosis & Treatment

1. Obstruction of Phlegm-Turbidity

Signs & Symptoms: Chest pain through the back, feeling of fullness and heaviness in the chest and diaphragm, shortness of breath, labored or rapid breathing, drooling, inability to lie flat. *Tongue:* white greasy fur. *Pulse:* slippery.

Therapeutic Principle: Remove Phlegm, benefit Vital Energy.

Principal Measure: Pinch and grasp the Three Yin Meridians of the Hand, press and push the supraclavicular fossa, relieve the chest by dotting and vibrating, relax the chest by pressing and kneading, knead the tendons of the elbows with your fingers, Taiji round-rub the abdomen, push and wipe to divide the ribs.

Subordinate Measure: Knead Tiantu (CV 22), Shaohai (H 3), Neiguan (Per 6), Taiyuan (Lu 9), Tongli (H 5), Shenmen (H 7) and Zhongchong (Per 9) with the fingers.

2. Stagnation of oppressed Vital Energy

Signs & Symptoms: Wandering distended pain in the chest involving the rib cage, symptoms aggravated by emotional depression, feeling of heaviness in the chest, shortness of breath, palpitation, insomnia. *Tongue:* white, thin fur. *Pulse:* deep, thready.

Therapeutic Principle: Relax the chest, promote the flow of Vital Energy.

Principal Measure: Press and push the supraclavicular fossa, nip and grasp the Three Yin Meridians of the Hand, whisk and sweep the back; knock, clap and pound the back, pluck the tendons of the back, relax the chest by pressing and kneading, round-rub the rib cage, revolve Huantiao (GB 30) with the elbow (all reducing).

Subordinate Measure: Nip and knead Chize (Lu 5), Quze (Per 3), Xiaohai (SI 8), Neiguan (Per 6) and Zusanli (St 36).

Apoplexy (Stroke)

According to Traditional Chinese Medicine, apoplexy is also called a stroke of Wind, since its onset is abrupt, swift and changeable. General characteristics: Sudden coma, listlessness after resuscitation, deviation of the eye and mouth, stiff tongue, inability to speak, drooling from the corner of the mouth, etc. Some patients do not lose consciousness, but facial paralysis and hemiplegia still occur.

Etiology: Apoplexy is divided into two types — the true stroke and the analogous stroke. The first is often caused by an exogenous Wind, showing pathological evidence in Six Meridians. The second is usually caused by endogenous Wind. For example, during the flaming up of Heart and Liver Fire, Fire generates Wind. Or, during Deficiency of Kidney Yin, Excess Liver Yang transforms into Wind. Or, accumulated Dampness gives rise to Phlegm due to the failure of Spleen to transport or due to the steaming action of Liver Fire, so that Phlegm obstructs Meridians and covers up clear Apertures.

Diagnosis & Treatment

1. Exogenous Wind attacks Meridians and Collaterals

Signs & Symptoms: Numb limbs, sudden deviation of the eye and mouth, drooling from the corner of the mouth, hemiplegia with or without coma. *Tongue:* white, thin fur. *Pulse:* superficial, stringy.

Therapeutic Principle: Expel Wind, dredge Meridians and Collaterals.

Principal Measure: Grasp both Fengchi (GB 20), pinch and grasp Three Yin and Yang Meridians of the Hand, nip and grasp points of Three Yin and

Yang Meridians of the Hand, open Passes and dredge Apertures, push and grasp Six Meridians of the Foot.

Subordinate Measure: Nip Hegu (LI 4) and Waiguan (TW 5), revolve Huantiao (GB 30) with the elbow, nip and knead Kunlun (UB 60), Taixi (K 3) and Yongquan (K 1).

2. Uprising and turmoil of Excess Yang and endogenous Wind due to Deficiency of Liver and Kidney Yin

Signs & Symptoms: Dizziness, tinnitus, soreness and weariness of the waist and legs, sudden deviation of the eye and mouth, stiff tongue, inability to speak, hemiplegia. *Tongue:* red with yellow fur. *Pulse:* stringy, slippery.

Principal Measure: Rock and deep-press to initiate phonation, nip and grasp both Fengchi (GB 20), open Passes and dredge Apertures, revolve Shu-points on the back with your forearm, arrange the shoulder, restore the elbow, rectify fingers; knock, clap, pound and chop the back; revolve Huantiao (GB 30) with the elbow, nip and grasp the Six Meridians of the Foot, roll legs, revolve the back and the waist with your forearm.

Subordinate Measure: Knead Taiyang (Ex-HN 4) with the fingers; nip and knead Fengfu (GV 16), Yamen (GV 15), Quchi (LI 11), Hegu (LI 4), Yanglingquan (GB 34); nip Fenglong (St 40), Sanyinjiao (Sp 6), Neiting (St 44) and Kunlun (UB 60); rub Yongquan (K 1).

3. Exogenous Wind attacks internal organs

Signs & Symptoms: Critical emergency, sudden coma. This may be classified as the blockage (Excess) syndrome or the collapse (Deficiency) syndrome. Under these circumstances, massage may be used as a means of first aid.

A. Blockage syndrome

Signs & Symptoms: Sudden coma with clenching of fists, clenching of jaw muscles, wheezing from excessive Phlegm, reddened complexion, rough breathing, halitosis, fever, restlessness, reddened lips. *Tongue:* red with yellow fur. *Pulse:* stringy, slippery, rapid. Alternately: pale complexion, dim lips, abundant phlegm and saliva, cold limbs. *Tongue:* white, greasy fur. *Pulse:* deep, slippery, moderate.

Therapeutic Principle: Open Passes, dredge Apertures.

Principal Measure: Open Passes and dredge Apertures, nip Renzhong (GV 26), relax the throat by kneading and grasping, knead Baihui (GV 20), nip and knead both Fengchi (GB 20); nip Fengfu (GV 16), Yamen (GV 15),

Quchi (LI 11), Hegu (LI 4) and Twelve Jing (Well) Points; revolve Huantiao (GB 30) with the elbow, push Yongquan (K 1) (all on both sides).

Subordinate Measure: Nip and grasp Zusanli (St 36) and Sanyinjiao (Sp 6).

B. Collapse syndrome

Signs & Symptoms: Sudden coma with opened mouth and relaxed hands, cold limbs, excessive perspiration, feeble breathing, incontinence, flaccid paralysis of the limbs and body. *Tongue:* flaccid. *Pulse:* faint, even indistinguishable.

Therapeutic Principle: Recuperate depleted Yang, rescue the patient from collapse.

Principal Measure: Open Passes and dredge Apertures, stroke and caress the head, nip Shixuan (Ex-UE 9) and Dadun (Liv 1), knead Yongquan (K 1).

Subordinate Measure: none.

Syncope (Fainting)

Syncope is a sudden loss of consciousness with cold limbs and pale complexion. Unlike apoplexy, revival is not accompanied by any sequelae such as hemiplegia, etc. Nevertheless, this can be a critical condition, and death may occur in some cases.

Etiology: Harassment and covering of Clear Apertures by adverse uprising of Vital Energy due to indignation or fright; failure of Clear Yang to ascend due to the sinking of Spleen-Stomach Energy; obstruction of Clear Apertures by the rushing up of Blood during violent anger; collapse of Vital Energy from loss of blood; Dampness-Phlegm cover Clear Apertures from overindulgence in eating and drinking; blockage of Energy Mechanism from abrupt rage.

Diagnosis & Treatment

1. Vital Energy syncope

A. Excess syndrome

Signs & Symptoms: Often brought on by emotional agitation; sudden fainting, lockjaw, clenched fists, harsh breathing, cold limbs. *Tongue:* white, thin fur. *Pulse:* deep, stringy.

Therapeutic Principle: Promote the flow of Vital Energy, dredge stagnation.

Principal Measure: First Aid — open Passes and dredge Apertures. After resuscitation, push the chest with the thenar mound, relieve the chest with dotting and vibrating, push and wipe to divide the ribs, scratch the back, rectify limbs and fingers.

Subordinate Measure: Nip Neiguan (Per 6), Lieque (Lu 7), Baixie (Ex-UE 7), Taichong (Liv 3) and Neiting (St 44).

B. Deficiency syndrome

Signs & Symptoms: Induced by overexertion or fright; sudden syncope, faint breathing, perspiration, cold limbs, pale complexion. *Tongue:* pale. *Pulse:* deep, indistinct.

Therapeutic Principle: Invigorate Vital Energy, resuscitate patient.

Principal Measure: First Aid — open Passes and dredge Apertures. After resuscitation — stroke and caress the head, scratch the back, Taiji round-rub the abdomen, vibrate Dantian with your palms, rectify the limbs and fingers.

Subordinate Measure: Nip Neiguan (Per 6), Hegu (LI 4), Zusanli (St 36) and Sanyinjiao (Sp 6); knead Yongquan (K 1).

2. Blood syncope

Signs & Symptoms: Sudden fainting, coma, cyanotic lips and complexion, lockjaw. *Tongue:* red. *Pulse:* deep, stringy.

Therapeutic Principle: Depress the adverse uprising of Blood, dredge stasis.

Principal Measure: First Aid — open Passes and dredge Apertures, nip all Twelve Jing Points. After resuscitation — rock and deep-press to initiate vocalization; knock, clap and pound the back; push the chest with your hands; rectify limbs and fingers; revolve Huantiao (GB 30) with your elbow.

Subordinate Measure: Nip Neiguan (Per 6), Chize (Lu 5), Baixie (Ex-UE 7), Zhaohai (K 6), Taixi (K 3), Neiting (St 44) and Xingjian (Liv 2).

3. Phlegm syncope

Signs & Symptoms: Sudden syncope, wheezing from excessive phlegm in the throat, vomit with frothy saliva. *Tongue:* white, greasy, thick fur. *Pulse:* deep, slippery.

Therapeutic Principle: Promote the flow of Vital Energy, eliminate Phlegm.

Principal Measure: First Aid — open Passes and dredge Apertures, dot Tiantu (CV 22). After resuscitation — stroke and caress the head, relieve the chest by dotting and vibrating, relax the chest by pressing and kneading, rub the rib cage, rectify limbs and fingers, push the back with the heel of the hand, revolve Huantiao (GB 30) with your elbow, chop the legs with joined hands.

Subordinate Measure: Nip and knead Lieque (Lu 7), Neiguan (Per 6) and Jianshi (Per 5); nip Fenglong (St 40) and Xingjian (Liv 2).

4. Food syncope

Signs & Symptoms: Sudden faint after overeating, suffocated breathing, swelling and fullness in the epigastrium. *Tongue:* greasy, thick fur. *Pulse:* slippery, replete.

Principal Measure: First Aid — open Passes and dredge Apertures. After resuscitation — stroke and caress the head; rock and deep-press to initiate vocalization; revolve the middle abdomen with your forearm; clap, chop and pound the back; rectify the fingers, pinch the spine, grasp Weizhong (UB 40), roll the legs with your hands.

Subordinate Measure: Nip Zusanli (St 36), Taichong (Liv 3) and Jiexi (St 41).

Flaccidity syndrome

Flaccidity refers to weakness, feebleness, atrophy or emaciation of the limbs.

Etiology: This syndrome is related to dysfunctions of the Liver, Lung, Kidney, etc., resulting in starvation of the Tendons, Vessels and muscles. There are various causes for flaccidity: failure of the body fluids to moisten tissues due to Lung Heat; Deficiency of Liver-Kidney Yin from sexual overindulgence or extended illness; obstruction of Tendons and Vessels from accumulation of Dampness-Heat, weakness of Spleen and Stomach.

Diagnosis & Treatment

1. Lung Heat consumes bodily fluids

Signs & Symptoms: Begins with fever. After the fever has subsided, the limbs become flaccid; short-temper, cough, dry throat, diminished urination with burning sensation in the urethra. *Tongue:* red with yellow fur. *Pulse:* rapid, thready.

Therapeutic Principle: Clear Heat, moisten Dryness, nourish Yin, foster Tendons.

Principal Measure: Pull, push and knead the neck; pluck, vibrate and knock the neck; push the back with pinching and grasping; deep-press the spine with kneading and revolving, jerk and drag to relax the waist, pluck Collaterals with knocking and scratching, roll the arms with pushing and grasping, pull the legs with knocking and vibrating, roll the legs with revolving and pinching.

Subordinate Measure: Revolve the back and the shoulder with your forearm, nip and knead Chize (Lu 5) and Shousanli (LI 10), knead Zusanli (St 36).

2. Deficiency of Liver-Kidney Yin

Signs & Symptoms: Flaccidity of legs, gradually increasing; soreness and weariness of the spine and the waist, dizziness, tinnitus, seminal emission, premature ejaculation, dripping urination and even incontinence. *Tongue:* red with little fur. *Pulse:* deep, thready.

Therapeutic Principle: Nourish Liver, invigorate Kidney, strengthen Tendons and bones.

Principal Measure: Relieve the chest by dotting and vibrating, relax the chest by pressing and kneading, push and wipe to divide the ribs, push the abdomen with round-rubbing and revolving, arrange the shoulders, restore the elbows, rock the knee to rotate the hip, flex the knee (pad the popliteal fossa), roll the legs with revolving and pinching.

Subordinate Measure: Revolve Huantiao (GB 30); nip Weizhong (UB 40), Yinlingquan (Sp 9), Sanyinjiao (Sp 6), Xuanzhong (GB 39) and Kunlun (UB 60).

3. Obstruction of Tendons and Vessels by accumulation of Dampness-Heat

Signs & Symptoms: Flaccidity of the legs with mild edema and hot sensation, feeling of heaviness in the chest and epigastrium, desire to be cooled, aversion to heat, diminished and deep colored urine. *Tongue:* yellow, greasy fur. *Pulse:* soft, floating, rapid.

Therapeutic Principle: Clear Heat, eliminate Dampness, relax Tendons, activate Collaterals.

Principal Measure: Relax the chest by pressing and kneading, push and wipe to divide the ribs, push the abdomen with round-rubbing and revolving, arrange the shoulders, restore the elbows, crook and deep-press to tug the waist, pull the legs with knocking and vibrating, knead the legs with rotating and round-rubbing, roll the legs with revolving and pinching.

Subordinate Measure: Revolve Shenshu (UB 23) and Zhishi (UB 52) with your forearm, grasp Weizhong (UB 40), nip Xuanzhong (GB 39), Zusanli (St 36) and Jiexi (St 41); grasp Kunlun (UB 60).

Arthralgia from Wind-Cold-Dampness

Arthralgia or blockage syndrome refers to pain, aching, heaviness or numbness of the joints and limbs from the obstruction of Meridians by exogenous evils.

Etiology: Constitutional weakness, Deficiency of Yang and Vital Energy with attack of Wind-Cold-Dampness. In its clinical manifestation, this is classified as the Wind or wandering blockage syndrome, the Cold or pain blockage syndrome, and the Dampness or adherent blockage syndrome. Additionally, if there is a constitutional Excess of Yang and Vital Energy, or hyperactivity of Yang due to Deficiency of Yin, the Wind, Cold and Dampness may transform into Heat and lead to Heat blockage syndrome.

Diagnosis & Treatment

1. Wandering arthralgia

Signs & Symptoms: Wandering pain in limbs and joints, difficulty in flexion and extension, may be accompanied by External Syndrome such as fever or aversion to Wind. *Tongue:* white, thin fur. *Pulse:* superficial.

Therapeutic Principle: Expel Wind, dredge Collaterals.

A. Arms

Principal Measure: Roll arms with pushing and grasping, pinch arms with nipping and kneading, arrange the shoulders.

Subordinate Measure: Knead Jianyu (LI 15), Tianzong (SI 11), Quchi (LI 11) and Shousanli (LI 10); grasp Jianjing (GB 21), Jianliao (TW 14) and Binao (LI 14); nip Neiguan (Per 6), Waiguan (TW 5) and Shaohai (H 3).

B. Legs

Principal Measure: Push Six Meridians of the Foot, grasp and revolve the patella, revolve the buttocks, knead the popliteal fossa, roll the legs.

Subordinate Measure: Press Jimai (Liv 12), Jimen (Sp 11) and Futu (St 32); knead both Xiyan (Ex-LE 2); nip Zusanli (St 36), Jiexi (St 41) and Xuanzhong (GB 39).

C. Head and torso

Principal Measure: Stroke and caress the head, nip Zanzhu (UB 2), lift and grasp Fengchi (GB 20), push the back with pinching and grasping, deep-press the spine with kneading and revolving, pluck the tendons of the spine, rub the back and waist.

Subordinate Measure: Nip Touwei (St 8), Baihui (GV 20) and Fengfu (GV 16); knead Dazhui (GV 14) and Lingtai (GV 10).

2. Pain arthralgia

Signs & Symptoms: A more serious pain in a fixed spot but without any sensation of heat, difficult flexion and extension, symptoms are aggravated when body is cooled, alleviated when warmed. *Tongue:* white fur. *Pulse:* stringy, tense.

Therapeutic Principle: Disperse Cold, relieve pain.

A. Arms

Principal Measure: Pinch the arms with nipping and kneading, pull the arm with rotating and rectifying, twist the arm with rocking and jerking.

Subordinate Measure: Press Jianyu (LI 15), Yunmen (Lu 2), Zhongfu (Lu 1), Bingfeng (SI 12), Jianwaishu (SI 14) and Binao (LI 14); knead Quchi (LI 11), Chize (Lu 5), Yangxi (LI 5), Laogong (Per 8) and Outer Laogong.

B. Legs

Principal Measure: Push the Six Meridians of the Foot, drag the legs with plucking and grasping, roll the legs with revolving and pinching, rub Yongquan (K 1), knead the popliteal fossa, roll the legs.

Subordinate Measure: Knead Biguan (St 31), Xuehai (Sp 10), Huantiao (GB 30), Chengfu (UB 36) and Weizhong (UB 40); nip Yinlingquan (Sp 9), Sanyinjiao (Sp 6), Zhaohai (K 6) and Kunlun (UB 60); rub Yongquan (K 1).

C. Head and torso

Principal Measure: Stroke and caress the head, grasp Jianjing (GB 21), deep-press the spine with kneading and revolving, push the back with pinching and grasping, pluck Collaterals with knocking and scratching, revolve Shenshu (UB 23) and Zhishi (UB 52) with your forearm.

Subordinate Measure: Knead Dazhui (GV 14), Shendao (GV 11), Lingtai (GV 10), Jizhong (GV 6), Mingmen (GV 4), Yaoyangguan (GV 3) and Shenshu (UB 23); rub Eight Liao (UB 31-34, both sides).

3. Adherent arthralgia

Signs & Symptoms: Fixed pain with sensation of weight, numbness or swelling; weakness and flaccidity of limbs, difficulty in movement. *Tongue:* white, greasy fur. *Pulse:* soft, floating, moderate.

Therapeutic Principle: Eliminate Dampness, dredge Collaterals.

A. Arms

Principal Measure: Pinch the arms with nipping and kneading, roll the arm with pushing and grasping, twist the arm with rocking and jerking, arrange the shoulder, rectify the fingers.

Subordinate Measure: Knead Yunmen (Lu 2), Jianyu (LI 15) and Binao (LI 14); press Quepen (St 12), Shaohai (H 3), Shousanli (LI 10), Neiguan (Per 6), Waiguan (TW 5), Laogong (Per 8) and Outer Laogong.

B. Legs

Principal Measure: Push the Six Meridians of the Foot, drag the leg with plucking and grasping, roll the leg with revolving and pinching, pull the leg with knocking and vibrating, knead the leg with rotating and round-rubbing, pinch the calf, roll the legs.

Subordinate Measure: Knead Biguan (St 31), Jimen (Sp 11), Yinbao (Liv 9), Xuehai (Sp 10) and Liangqiu (St 34); grasp Dubi (St 35) and both Xiyan (Ex-LE 2); nip Zusanli (St 36), Yanglingquan (GB 34), Yinlingquan (Sp 9) and Sanyinjiao (Sp 6); grasp Kunlun (UB 60).

C. Head and torso

Principal Measure: Stroke and caress the head, grasp Jianjing (GB 21), pluck Collaterals with knocking and scratching, push the back with pinching and grasping, knock the back and waist, strengthen the waist by rolling and rubbing, relieve the chest by dotting and vibrating, relax the chest by pressing and kneading, push and wipe to divide the ribs, push the abdomen with round-rubbing and revolving, grasp the abdomen with lifting and jerking.

Subordinate Measure: Knead Dazhui (GV 14), Taodao (GV 13), Feishu (UB 13), Xinshu (UB 15), Ganshu (UB 18), Pishu (UB 20), Dachangshu (UB 25) and Shenshu (UB 23); rub Eight Liao (UB 31-34, both sides).

4. Heat arthralgia

Signs & Symptoms: Redness, swelling, tenderness and wandering joint pain; symptoms are alleviated when cooled; inability to move, possible local subcutaneous accumulation and stasis of hemorrhage; fever, thirst, perspiration, aversion to Wind, short-temper, feeling of weight, nausea. *Tongue:* dry yellow fur. *Pulse:* slippery, rapid.

Therapeutic Principle: Clear Heat, dredge Collaterals, expel Wind, dry Dampness.

Principal Measure: Stroke and caress the head, pluck, vibrate and knock the back; nip Zanzhu (UB 2), lift and grasp Fengchi (GB 20), relieve the chest by dotting and vibrating, push and wipe to divide the ribs, grasp the abdomen with lifting and jerking, roll the abdomen with knocking and vibrating, Taiji round-rub the abdomen, pluck Collaterals with knocking and scratching, push the back with pinching and grasping. Additionally, select routine techniques to massage the diseased joints.

Subordinate Measure: Knead Fengchi (GB 20), Fengfu (GV 16), Taiyang (Ex-HN 4), Tiantu (CV 22), Dazhui (GV 14), Taodao (GV 13), Lingtai (GV 10), Shenzhu (GV 12), Xinshu (UB 15), Feishu (UB 13), Ganshu (UB 18), Geshu (UB 17), Dachangshu (UB 25) and Weizhong (UB 40).

Facial paralysis

This is often encountered in young people and those in the prime of life, usually at the end of autumn and the beginning of winter.

Etiology: Facial Collaterals of Yangming Meridian are attacked by exogenous Wind, or attacked by endogenous Wind due to violent rage; stagnation of Vital Energy due to emotional depression; starvation of facial muscles due to Deficiency of Vital Energy and Blood; obstruction of Collaterals due to accumulation of Phlegm.

Diagnosis & Treatment

1. Attack of exogenous Wind

Signs & Symptoms: Sudden onset of deviation of the eye and mouth, facial paresthesia, headache, stuffy nose, stiff neck and nape, occasional twitching of facial muscles, the eye on the affected side cannot be closed, facial lines become shallow or flat. *Tongue:* white thin fur. *Pulse:* superficial.

Therapeutic Principle: Expel Wind, disperse Cold.

Principal Measure: Open Passes and dredge Apertures; stroke and caress the head; pull, push and knead the neck; pluck, vibrate and knock the neck, pluck Collaterals with knocking and scratching.

Subordinate Measure: Nip and knead Fengfu (GV 16), rub Fengchi (GB 20) with joined hands, knead and press Quepen (St 12); nip Neiguan (Per 6), Waiguan (TW 5), Quchi (LI 11) and Hegu (LI 4).

2. Deficiency of Vital Energy and Blood

Signs & Symptoms: Deviation of the eye and mouth, forehead lines become shallow or flat, the eye on the affected side cannot be closed, lacrimation, drooling, leakage of food from the mouth while chewing, shortness of breath, withdrawal. *Tongue:* pale and tender with thin white fur. *Pulse:* thready, feeble.

Therapeutic Principle: Nourish Blood, expel Wind.

Principal Measure: Open Passes and dredge Apertures; stroke and caress the head; pull, push and knead the neck; pluck, vibrate and knock the neck; pinch and lift both ears; lift, drag and rock both ears (Beat Heaven's Drum); Taiji round-rub the abdomen, rectify the limbs and fingers.

Subordinate Measure: Knead Neiguan (Per 6), Waiguan (TW 5), Quchi (LI 11), Hegu (LI 4), Zusanli (St 36), Sanyinjiao (Sp 6) and Tiaokou (St 38).

3. Depression and stagnation of Liver Energy

Signs & Symptoms: Sudden onset of the paralysis, facial lines become flat, the eye on the affected side cannot be closed, photophobia, lacrimation, swelling and pain at the base of the ear, sighing, feeling of fullness and distress in the chest and rib cage, loss of appetite, occasional grief and crying. *Tongue:* white thin fur. *Pulse:* stringy.

Therapeutic Principle: Relieve depression, activate Collaterals.

Principal Measure: Stroke and caress the head, open Passes and dredge Apertures, press and push the supraclavicular fossa, relax the chest by pressing and kneading, push the abdomen with round-rubbing and revolving, press the abdomen with deep-pressing and kneading, grasp the abdomen with lifting and jerking, revolve Huantiao (GB 30) with your elbow.

Subordinate Measure: Knead Wangu (GB 12), Fengchi (GB 20), Tianyou (TW 16) and Waiguan (TW 5); nip Yaoyangguan (GV 3), Yangjiao (GB 35) and Qiuxu (GB 40).

Hypertension

In Traditional Chinese Medicine, hypertension corresponds to headache, dizziness and hyperactivity of Liver Yang.

Etiology: The hyperactivity of Liver Yang is often due to mental strain, overeating rich foods, or excessive drinking of alcohol. It may be accompanied by endogenous Wind or Phlegm. In its early stage, there is a Deficiency of Kidney; later, there will be a Deficiency of Liver Yin and Excess of Liver Yang. As time goes on, there will ultimately be a Deficiency of both Yin and Yang. We may regard Kidney as the root of hypertension and Liver as its branch, since Kidney and Liver influence each other.

Diagnosis & Treatment

1. Flaming up of Liver Fire

Signs & Symptoms: Vertigo, dizziness, headache, stiff neck, reddened complexion, conjunctival congestion, bitter taste in the mouth, general anxiety, constipation, deep-colored urine. *Tongue:* red with yellow fur. *Pulse:* stringy.

Therapeutic Principle: Quell Liver, reduce Fire.

Principal Measure: Pinch and grasp the Three Yin Meridians of the Hand (both sides), nip Three Yang Meridians of the Hand (both sides), pluck

Collaterals with knocking and scratching, revolve Huantiao (GB 30) with your elbow (all reducing).

Subordinate Measure: Knead Yongquan (K 1); nip Quchi (LI 11), Zusanli (St 36) and Sanyinjiao (Sp 6) (all both sides).

2. Hyperactivity of Yang due to Deficiency of Yin

Signs & Symptoms: Headache, vertigo, dizziness, tinnitus, memory loss, short-temper, heat at palms and soles of feet, palpitation, insomnia, soreness and weakness of the waist and knees. *Tongue:* red with thin fur. *Pulse:* stringy, thready, rapid.

Therapeutic Principle: Foster Yin, retrieve Yang.

Principal Measure: Stroke and caress the head, lift and grasp Fengchi (GB 20), grasp Jianjing (GB 21), round-rub rib cage, Taiji round-rub the abdomen, revolve lower abdomen with your forearm, revolve both Huantiao (GB 30) with your elbow.

Subordinate Measure: Grasp Weizhong (UB 40) and Chengshan (UB 57), nip Taichong (Liv 3), push Yongquan (K 1) (both sides).

3. Deficiency of both Yin and Yang

Signs & Symptoms: Vertigo, dizziness, headache, tinnitus, palpitation, feebleness, shortness of breath, labored breathing during physical activity, soreness and weakness of the waist and knees, insomnia, dreaminess, twitching muscles and tendons. *Tongue:* pale or red with white fur. *Pulse:* stringy, thready.

Therapeutic Principle: Foster Yin, support Yang.

Principal Measure: Pluck, vibrate and knock the neck; lift and grasp Fengchi (GB 20); grasp Jianjing (GB 21) with pinching and grasping; push and wipe to divide the ribs, Taiji round-rub the abdomen, revolve the lower abdomen with your forearm, revolve both Huantiao (GB 30) with your elbow.

Subordinate Measure: Revolve Mingmen (GV 4) with your forearm, nip Weizhong (UB 40) and Sanyinjiao (Sp 6), push Yongquan (K 1) (both sides).

4. Accumulation of Phlegm-Dampness

Signs & Symptoms: Vertigo, dizziness, headache, feeling of weight in the head, heaviness in the chest, palpitation, labored breathing, wheezing from retention of Phlegm, poor appetite, nausea, vomiting sputum and saliva. *Tongue:* white greasy fur. *Pulse:* slippery.

Therapeutic Principle: Eliminate Phlegm, resolve Dampness.

Principal Measure: Stroke and caress the head, push the back with pinching and grasping, relieve the chest by dotting and vibrating, relax the chest by pressing and kneading, rectify the fingers, push the abdomen with round-rubbing and revolving, revolve both Huantiao (GB 30) with your elbow.

Subordinate Measure: Nip Fenglong (St 40) and Sanyinjiao (Sp 6), knead Yongquan (K 1).

Epilepsy

This describes convulsive attacks usually accompanied by loss of awareness.

Etiology: This is primarily caused by the covering up of Clear Apertures by Phlegm-Turbidity and the turmoil of endogenous Wind. Congenital predisposition, emotional depression, strain and overeating are involved in its pathogenesis.

Diagnosis & Treatment

1. During onset

Signs & Symptoms: Vertigo, dizziness, headache, syncope, pale complexion, lockjaw, frothing saliva, rolling up of the eyes to show the whites, twitching limbs, shrill cries, incontinence. After this period, the patient falls into a lethargic sleep. Aside from persistence of the headache, the symptoms disappear after the episode. The patient is exhausted. *Tongue:* white greasy fur. *Pulse:* stringy, slippery.

Therapeutic Principle: Suppress convulsions, eliminate Phlegm.

Principal Measure: First Aid — open Passes and dredge Apertures. After resuscitation — stroke and caress the head, relieve the chest by dotting and vibrating, scratch the back, revolve Huantiao (GB 30) with your elbow.

Subordinate Measure: Nip Shanglian (LI 9), Lower Lianquan (CV 23), the Twelve Jing Points, and Hegu (LI 4); rub Yongquan (K 1).

2. Prevention of epileptic seizure

Signs & Symptoms: Before the seizure, there is usually an aura lasting from several seconds to several hours. The aura may occur intermittently or regularly. Dizziness, short-temper, feeling of heaviness in the chest, labored breathing, weariness, feebleness. *Pulse:* deep, stringy.

Therapeutic Principle: Preventive therapy should be done to clear the Heart, eliminate Phlegm.

Principal Measure: Open Passes and dredge Apertures, relieve the chest by dotting and vibrating, relax the chest by pressing and kneading, push and wipe to divide the ribs, scratch the back, revolve both Huantiao (GB 30) with your elbow, pinch the spine, grasp the tendons of the back.

Subordinate Measure: Nip Neiting (St 44), Fenglong (St 40), Hegu (LI 4) and Neiguan (Per 6); nip Shixuan (Ex UE 9) or Bafeng (Ex LE-3) heavily.

Surgery

Thromboangiitis obliterans (Buerger's disease)

Thromboangiitis obliterans is a chronic, progressive, recurring vascular disease of the extremities. In Traditional Chinese Medicine, it is called gangrene of the finger or toe. In the early stage, there is coldness, loss of arterial pulse and excruciating pain. Later, there may be necrosis and loss of the diseased part. In the early and intermediate stages of this disease, massage may be moderately effective.

Etiology: Depressed evil Fire exhausts Yang and cannot be controlled due to Yin Deficiency; exogenous Dampness-Heat obstructs Meridians and Collaterals resulting in Vital Energy stagnation and Blood stasis.

Diagnosis & Treatment

1. Insufficient Yang leads to accumulation of Cold

Signs & Symptoms: Pale, cold limbs; numbness, pain, aversion to cold; longing for warmth — pain intensifies when exposed to cold. The anterior tibial pulse is thready or cannot be felt. Symptoms progress to burning pain, local skin color changes from dim purple to black, and ultimately, tendons and bones putrefy. *Tongue:* pale red with thin white fur. *Pulse:* deep, thready.

Therapeutic Principle: Warm Meridians, dredge Collaterals, regulate and harmonize Nutrient and Blood Systems.

Principal Measure: Push the back with pinching and grasping, deep-press the spine with kneading and revolving, scratch the back along Governor Vessel and Urinary Bladder Meridians, revolve the back with your forearm, pinch the spine, roll the back, revolve Shenshu (UB 23) and Zhishi (UB 52), grasp Kunlun (UB 62).

Subordinate Measure: Knead Yinlian (Liv 11), Futu (St 32), Zusanli (St 36), Ligou (Liv 5), Shanglian (LI 9), Xialian (LI 8), Juegu (GB 39), Fengfu (GV 16), Dazhui (GV 14), Chengfu (UB 36), Yinmen (UB 37), Weizhong (UB 40), Heyang (UB 55), Chengshan (UB 57), Fuyang (UB 59) and Shenmai (UB 62)

2. Accumulation of Dampness-Heat

Signs & Symptoms: Distending pain, resistance to pressure; heaviness, feebleness, redness; swelling, pain and heat at locale; erythema; intermittently appearing nodular or elongated lumps; anterior tibial pulse is thready. *Tongue:* red with slippery and greasy fur. *Pulse:* rapid.

Therapeutic Principle: Clear Heat, eliminate Dampness, activate Blood, resolve stasis.

Principal Measure: Revolve Huantiao (GB 30) with your elbow, pinch and grasp Six Meridians of the Foot, knead the legs with rotating and round-rubbing, roll the legs with revolving and pinching, nip and grasp Kunlun (UB 60) and Taixi (K 3), nip and knead Zusanli (St 36), revolve the popliteal fossa with your forearm, push Yongquan (K 1).

Subordinate Measure: Knead Yanglingquan (GB 34), Juegu (GB 39) and Sanyinjiao (Sp 6).

3. Accumulation of evil Heat

Signs & Symptoms: Excruciating and burning pain, localized redness and swelling, symptoms intensified at night, aversion to heat, desire for coolness, anterior tibial pulse is indistinct, localized ulceration or gangrene with discharge of pus and foul odor, possible fever and chills. *Tongue:* red or crimson with yellow greasy fur. *Pulse:* slippery, rapid, energetic.

Therapeutic Principle: Nourish Yin, depress Fire, activate Blood, detoxify evils.

Principal Measure: Deep-press the spine with kneading and revolving, push the back with pinching and grasping, pluck Collaterals with knocking and scratching on the back, nip and grasp Weizhong (UB 40), revolve Huantiao (GB 30), nip and grasp the Six Meridians of the Foot, grasp Chengshan (UB 57), roll the legs with your hands, push Yongquan (K 1) (all reducing).

Subordinate Measure: Nip Zusanli (St 36), Kunlun (UB 60) and Taixi (K 3).

4. Deficiency of Vital Energy and Blood

Signs & Symptoms: Weak constitution, localized dry and peeling skin, anterior tibial pulse is thready and weak, nails are thick and loose, protruding scabbing on wound surface, small amount of discharge of watery pus. *Tongue:* pale and tender with thin yellow fur. *Pulse:* thready, weak.

Therapeutic Principle: Strengthen the immune system, eliminate pathogenic factors, invigorate Vital Energy, benefit Blood.

Principal Measure: Stroke and caress the head; pluck, vibrate and knock the neck; push the abdomen with round-rubbing and revolving; roll the abdomen with knocking and vibrating; roll the arms with pushing and grasping; push the back with pinching and grasping; deep-press the spine with kneading and revolving; strengthen the waist by rolling and rubbing; pluck Collaterals with knocking and scratching on the back. Be careful to perform these techniques more gently than usual.

Subordinate Measure: Nip Zusanli (St 36), Fuyang (UB 59), Juegu (GB 39), Kunlun (UB 60), Taixi (K 3), Yongquan (K 1) (all invigorating).

Intestinal obstruction from ascarides

Etiology: This is a mechanical obstruction caused by an entangled mass of ascarides, usually seen in children under the age of 6. In TCM, it is categorized with abdominal pain from parasitic infestation, and may be accompanied by vomiting.

Diagnosis & Treatment

Signs & Symptoms: Random occasions of abdominal colic; fullness and distension of the abdomen; elongated lump may be seen or felt, sometimes changing shape; nausea, vomiting which may include ascarides, constipation, pityriasis alba on face, blue-grey spots on conjunctivae, protruding spots on inner lower lip, red papillary spots on the tip and sides of the tongue.

Therapeutic Principle: Relieve constipation, loosen bowels, promote the flow of Vital Energy, dissipate stagnation.

Principal Measure: Relax the chest by pressing and kneading, push and wipe to divide the ribs, push the abdomen with round-rubbing and revolving, press the abdomen with deep-pressing and knocking, grasp the abdomen with lifting and jerking, roll the abdomen with kneading and vibrating, roll the legs with revolving and pinching, knead the legs with twisting and round-rubbing, pinch and grasp Chengshan (UB 57).

Subordinate Measure: Nip Quchi (LI 11), Hegu (LI 4), Zusanli (St 36), Yanglingquan (GB 34), Neiting (St 44), Dadun (Liv 1) and Xingjian (Liv 2) (all both sides).

N.B. Therapeutic effect is improved when a laxative is administered with the massage.

Intestinal adhesion

This is usually a complication after surgery or sequela to peritonitis. In TCM, it is in the category of abdominal pain from Cold stagnation or Blood stasis.

Etiology: Pus-producing infection, traumatic or surgical injury to organs in the abdomen; Deficiency of Spleen Yang brings accumulation of endogenous Cold; adhesion of intestines due to Vital Energy stagnation and Blood stasis.

Diagnosis & Treatment

1. Deficiency of Vital Energy and Blood

Signs & Symptoms: Varying pain in abdomen, desire to be pressed, borborygmus, abdominal distension, coldness in abdomen, poor appetite, weariness, afternoon fever, loose stools. *Tongue:* red with white fur. *Pulse:* deep, uneven.

Therapeutic Principle: Regulate Vital Energy, consolidate Origin, dissipate stasis, disperse Cold.

Principal Measure: Push the abdomen with round-rubbing and revolving, grasp the abdomen with lifting and jerking, roll the abdomen with knocking and vibrating, push and wipe to divide the ribs, revolve middle and lower abdomen with your forearm, push the back with pinching and grasping, pinch the spine, pluck Collaterals with knocking and scratching, revolve Huantiao (GB 30) with the elbow, grasp the popliteal fossae.

Subordinate Measure: Knead Zusanli (St 36) and Sanyangjiao (opposite Sanyinjiao), nip Ququan (Liv 8) and Xingjian (Liv 2).

2. Vital Energy stagnation and Blood stasis

Signs & Symptoms: Fullness and heaviness in the abdomen, agglomeration in the intestine, fixed pain and tenderness in the abdomen, poor appetite, hiccups, intermittent fever, short-temper, thirst without desire for drink; during defecation, first stool is dry, thereafter, loose; pain in abdomen eased after defecation.

Therapeutic Principle: Regulate Vital Energy, activate Blood, dissipate stasis, loosen agglomeration.

Principal Measure: Relieve the chest by dotting and vibrating, push and wipe to divide the ribs, push the abdomen with round-rubbing and revolving, press the abdomen with deep-pressing and kneading, grasp the abdomen with lifting and jerking, roll the abdomen with knocking and vibrating, revolve Huantiao (GB 30) with your elbow, pinch the spine, pluck Collaterals with knocking and scratching on the back and waist, deep-press the spine with kneading and revolving, push the back with pinching and grasping.

Subordinate Measure: Dot Weizhong (UB 40) and Chengshan (UB 57); nip Zusanli (St 36), Neiting (St 44), Dadun (Liv 1) and Xingjian (Liv 2) (all on both sides).

Volvolus

This refers to the twisting of the stomach along its major axis, resulting in epigastric pain, fullness, distension and vomiting. It is often seen in the newborn and the elderly. Definite diagnosis is established by X- ray. In TCM, it corresponds to Deficiency of Stomach Yin or disharmony of Stomach Energy.

Etiology: Relaxation of stomach ligaments from Deficiency of Spleen and Stomach, brought on by incessant vomiting or sudden change of body posture.

Diagnosis & Treatment

Signs & Symptoms: Serious epigastric pain and spasms with feeling of distension and fullness, nausea, vomiting, difficulty in eating, vague pains in back and rib cage, constipation, emaciation, listlessness, withered and sallow complexion, dry mouth. *Tongue:* red with thin white fur. *Pulse:* deep, thready, weak.

Therapeutic Principle: Harmonize Stomach, depress the adverse uprising, nourish Yin, foster Stomach.

Principal Measure: Relieve the chest by dotting and vibrating, relax the chest with pressing and kneading, push and wipe to divide the ribs, push the abdomen with round-rubbing and revolving, grasp the abdomen with lifting and jerking, roll the abdomen with knocking and vibrating, revolve upper and middle abdomen with your forearm, roll the legs with revolving and pinching, pinch the spine, strengthen the waist by rolling and rubbing.

Subordinate Measure: Grasp Tianshu (St 25); knead Daheng (Sp 15), Pishu (UB 20), Weishu (UB 21) and Shenshu (UB 23); nip and knead Zusanli (St 36).

Hypertrophic spondylitis

This is also called proliferating spondylitis or retrograde degenerative spondylitis, and is common, to one degree or another, in people over the age of 50. The principal physiological changes include retrograde degeneration of vertebral articular cartilage, ossification at points of ligament attachment, and the formation of osteophytes. Clinical manifestations include protracted lumbago, stiffness of the waist involving the sacral area and sometimes the legs, causing neuralgia of the hip. In TCM, its is categorized with Wind-Dampness lumbago and Kidney Deficiency lumbago.

Etiology: Kidney resides in the waist. After middle age, Kidney Energy and Kidney Yang weaken and decline. Generally, hypertrophic spondylitis is the result of prolonged strain on the spine, attack on Governor Vessel Meridian and Urinary Bladder Meridian at the waist by Wind-Cold-Dampness; adhesion of lumbar tendons and vertebrae due to Vital Energy stagnation and Blood stasis.

Diagnosis & Treatment

1. Lumbago due to Wind-Cold-Dampness

Signs & Symptoms: Continuous dull pain in the waist, often accompanied by pain at the buttocks, the sacrum, and side of the thigh. Symptoms are worst on awaking, alleviated after physical activity or warming. Symptoms are aggravated in cold, wet weather, in autumn and winter. *Tongue:* white, thin fur. *Pulse:* deep, stringy or tense.

Therapeutic Principle: Warm Meridians, disperse Cold, relax Tendons, rectify joints.

Principal Measure: Push the back with pinching and grasping, deep-press the spine with kneading and revolving, pluck Collaterals with knocking and scratching, pull the waist with jerking and dragging, revolve the back along Urinary Bladder Meridian with your forearm, drag the leg with plucking and grasping, jerk and drag to relax the waist, bend and deep-press to tug the waist, rock the knee to twist the hip, strengthen the waist by rolling and rubbing.

Subordinate Measure: Knead Feishu (UB 13), Ganshu (UB 18), Shenshu (UB 23) and Dachangshu (UB 25); deep-press Huantiao (GB 30) and Chengfu (UB 36) with the elbow; knead Fengshi (GB 31), Futu (St 32) and Weizhong (UB 40) with the fingers; nip and knead Jiexi (St 41).

2. Lumbago from adhesion of Dampness

Signs & Symptoms: Heaviness and weighty aching of the waist, difficulty in movement, weariness, feebleness, inability to walk or sit for extended periods, aversion to cold and dampness with aggravated symptoms on wet days. *Tongue:* white, thick or greasy fur. *Pulse:* deep, moderate.

Therapeutic Principle: Warm Meridians, disperse Cold, regulate Middle Warmer, dry Dampness.

Principal Measure: Push the back with pinching and grasping, pinch the spine, revolve the waist and the back with your forearm; knock, clap and pound the back; twist circularly to restore the waist, jerk and drag to relax the waist; roll the leg with revolving and pinching; drag the leg with plucking and grasping; push the abdomen with round-rubbing and revolving; roll the abdomen with knocking and vibrating; knock Shenque (CV 8).

Subordinate Measure: Knead Feishu (UB 13), Ganshu (UB 18), Pishu (UB 20), Weishu (UB 21), Shenshu (UB 23) and Dachangshu (UB 25); revolve Eight Liao (UB 31-34, both sides) with the forearm; deep-press and knead Huantiao (GB 30) and Chengfu (UB 36) with your elbow; nip and knead Zusanli (St 36).

3. Lumbago due to Deficiency of Kidney

Signs & Symptoms: Continuous vague pain alleviated by bed rest, aggravated by work; heaviness in the body; cold limbs, hunched back; longing for warmth/aversion to cold; shortness of breath; clear and long-passing urine; constipation or loose stools; dreaminess, seminal emission in males — irregular menstruation in females. *Tongue:* pale or tender with little fur. *Pulse:* deep, thready.

Therapeutic Principle: Dredge Meridians, activate Collaterals, warm Kidney, invigorate Yang.

Principal Measure: Strengthen the waist by rolling and rubbing, push the back with pinching and grasping, pluck Collaterals with knocking and scratching, push the back pausing intermittently, pinch the spine, jerk and drag to relax the waist, bend and deep-press the leg to tug the waist, revolve Shenshu (UB 23) and Zhishi (UB 52) with your forearm, rub the waist, push the abdomen with round-rubbing and revolving, roll the abdomen with knocking and vibrating, roll the leg with revolving and pinching.

Subordinate Measure: Knead Feishu (UB 13), Ganshu (UB 18), Pishu (UB 20) and Dachangshu (UB 25); revolve Eight Liao (UB 31-34, both sides) with the forearm; revolve Huantiao (GB 30) with your elbow; nip and knead Weizhong (UB 40), Zusanli (St 36) and Sanyinjiao (Sp 6).

Rheumatoid arthritis

Rheumatoid arthritis is a chronic, progressive, systemic disease characterized by damage of joint structures. In the early stages, there is wandering pain and symmetrical swelling of joints; in the advanced stages, there will be atrophy of muscles, rigidity or deformity of the joints, and even disability. Generally, the onset is either peripheral — in the small joints of the extremities, spreading inward to the larger joints; or central — in the lumbosacral joints, spreading to include the entire spine and sometimes also the jaw. Onset may vary, but is most common in middle age. In TCM, it belongs to Bone blockage syndrome.

Etiology: There is no consensus about the cause of this disease. Constitutional weakness, weariness, malnutrition, Deficiency of Vital Energy and Blood, and attack of Wind-Cold-Dampness may be involved. Exogenous evils take advantage of the Deficiency situation, invade the fasciae, periostea and Meridians, and block the flow of Vital Energy and Blood. Heat is produced when Healthy Energy struggles against evils, resulting in fever, swelling and pain in joints and fascial spaces. Ultimately, there will be hypertrophy and deformity.

Diagnosis & Treatment

1. Central

Signs & Symptoms: Pain, stiffness and numbness of the lumbosacral area; weighty pain and difficulty in movement on awakening. Symptoms are aggravated after work or in wet weather. Progressive stiffness of the back leading to advanced stages where there will be rigidity, deformity of the spine and possibly scoliosis.

Therapeutic Principle: Dredge Meridians, activate Collaterals, soften Tendons, ease joints, strengthen Kidney, invigorate Spleen.

Principal Measure: Push the back with pinching and grasping; pluck Collaterals with knocking and scratching; deep-press the spine with kneading and revolving; revolve Eight Liao (UB 31-34, both sides) with the forearm; rock the knee to twist the hip; jerk and drag to relax the waist; revolve the back along Governor Vessel Meridian and Urinary Bladder Meridian with the forearm; pluck, vibrate and knock the neck; lift and grasp Fengshi (GB 20), shoulder, and neck; rub the back and the waist; scratch the back and the waist.

Subordinate Measure: Nip and knead Fengfu (GV 16) and Dazhui (GV 14); nip and grasp Quchi (LI 11) and Neiguan (Per 6); knead Hegu (LI 4); revolve Huantiao (GB 30) and Chengfu (UB 36) with the elbow; grasp Weizhong (UB 40), Chengjin (UB 56) and Kunlun (UB 60); nip and grasp Zusanli (St 36); pinch and grasp Sanyinjiao (Sp 6); nip Yongquan (K 1).

2. Peripheral

Signs & Symptoms: Symmetrical redness, swelling, heat and pain in the small joints of the extremities. Ultimately, the wrist, elbow, ankle or knee joints become involved with hypertrophy and stiffness of joints with muscular atrophy.

Therapeutic Principle: Dredge Meridians, activate Collaterals, dissipate stasis, lubricate and ease joints.

Principal Measure: Pull, push and knead the neck; push the back with pinching and grasping, pinch the shoulder with nipping and kneading, support the elbow to twist the shoulder, twist and rock the elbow, rectify the wrist, roll the arm with pinching and grasping, pull the arm with twisting and rectifying, strengthen the waist by rolling and rubbing, revolve Eight Liao (UB 31-34, both sides) with the forearm, revolve Huantiao (GB 30) with the elbow, roll the leg with revolving and pinching, rock the knee to twist the hip, push and knead the knee joint, drag and rock the ankle, pinch and grasp the ankle and Achilles tendon, knead the leg with rotating and round-rubbing.

Begin these techniques gently, gradually increasing force, but never to the point of harshness or violence.

Acute mastitis

Stomach Meridian is in charge of the breast, and Liver Meridian is in charge of the nipple.

Etiology: Emotional depression leads to stagnation of Liver Energy, impeding lactation; accumulated Stomach Heat concentrates milk, which further obstructs lactation; trauma or crushing injury.

Diagnosis & Treatment

1. Stagnation of Vital Energy

Signs & Symptoms: Persistent diffuse swelling and distension with pain in the breast; poor and impeded lactation; feeling of heaviness in the chest; feeling of fullness, pain and distension in rib cage; anxiety. *Tongue:* pale with white or yellowish fur. *Pulse:* stringy.

Therapeutic Principle: Disperse and rectify Liver Energy, eliminate stasis, resolve swelling.

Principal Measure: Push and wipe to divide the ribs, push the abdomen with round-rubbing and revolving, relieve the chest by dotting and vibrating, pinch and grasp Three Yin Meridians of the Hand, relax the chest by pressing and kneading, round-rub and knead the peri-mammary area with your fingers, comb the breast. (Stretch out all five fingers and press the pads firmly to the breast. Draw your fingers together from the perimeter of the breast to the nipple. Continue this technique repeatedly, gradually increasing the strength applied, but avoid painful squeezing. If milk drains off freely, the swelling mass will disappear.)

Subordinate Measure: If there is fever and headache, also stroke and caress the head, grasp and knead both Fengchi (GB 20), revolve Huantiao

(GB 30) with the elbow, nip Waiqiu (GB 36), Diwuhui (GB 42) and Xiaxi (GB 43).

2. Retention of milk

Signs & Symptoms: Hardened lump with feeling of distension in the breast, viscous milk, difficult lactation, thirst, anxiety, loss of appetite. Later, burning heat, swelling and pain in the breast, aversion to cold, decrease in urination, deep colored urine. *Tongue:* red with greasy yellow fur. *Pulse:* stringy, rapid.

Therapeutic Principle: Disperse Liver Energy, clear Stomach Heat, resolve retention, dredge Collaterals.

Principal Measure: Push and wipe to divide the ribs, comb the breast, roll the Three Yin Meridians of the Hand with your hands, relax the chest by pressing and kneading, roll the abdomen with knocking and vibrating, relieve the chest by dotting and vibrating, stroke and caress the head, knead and grasp both Fengchi (GB 20), nip and knead Diwuhui (GB 42) and Xiaxi (GB 43).

Subordinate Measure: Nip Neiguan (Per 6), Laogong (Per 8), Yanglingquan (GB 34), Yangjiao (GB 35), Sanyinjiao (Sp 6), and Xingjian (Liv 2) (all on both sides).

3. Blood stasis

Signs & Symptoms: Hardened tissue in the breast with fixed stabbing pain, impaired lactation. Later stage includes reddening and swelling, fever, aversion to cold. *Tongue:* dim and pale with thin white fur. *Pulse:* stringy, uneven.

Therapeutic Principle: Activate Blood, resolve stasis, dredge lactation, dissipate stagnation.

Principal Measure: Push and wipe to divide the ribs, round-rub and knead the periphery of the hardened area with your fingers, relax the chest by pressing and kneading, comb the breast, stroke and caress the head, grasp and knead both Fengchi (GB 20), nip and knead Waiqiu (GB 36), Diwuhui (GB 42) and Xiaxi (GB 43); relieve the chest by dotting and vibrating.

Subordinate Measure: Nip both Neiguan (Per 6) and both Laogong (Per 8).

These techniques should begin gently and slowly, gradually increasing force. If the fever flares up, the pain becomes serious, the hardening expands or there is suppuration, massage is contraindicated.

Osteochondritis of the sternum

This occurs at the juncture of the manubrium and the sternal body. In TCM, it is in the category of blockage syndrome from Cold.

Etiology: Injury due to constant overwork; attack of Wind-Cold; clogging of stagnated Vital Energy and Blood.

Diagnosis & Treatment

Signs & Symptoms: Sudden onset of localized swelling and distending pain, feeling of heaviness in the chest, pain restricts respiratory motion, labored breathing, cough, anxiety. *Tongue:* thin white fur. *Pulse:* superficial, tense.

Therapeutic Principle: Warm Meridians, dredge Collaterals, activate Blood, resolve stasis.

Principal Measure: Relax the chest by pressing and kneading, push and wipe to divide the ribs, lift and grasp Fengchi (GB 20), relieve the chest by dotting and vibrating, knead Shencang (K 25) and Lingxu (K 24) with your palms.

Subordinate Measure: Knead Tiantu (CV 22), Yunmen (Lu 2), Zhongfu (Lu 1) and Zhangmen (Liv 13).

Sternocostal chondritis

Usually occurs at the juncture of the sternum and the second rib — an aching bulge protrudes. Often seen in women.

Etiology: Injury due to constant overwork; attack on Lung Meridian by Wind-Heat; clogging of Vital Energy, Blood and exogenous evils.

Diagnosis & Treatment

Signs & Symptoms: (generally on the left side) Onset of serious pain followed by localized redness and swelling, resistance to pressing. The pain may radiate to the back and restrict respiratory movement and movement of the shoulder. Ultimately, the protrusion will harden. *Tongue:* white thin fur or greasy yellow fur. *Pulse:* stringy, rapid.

Therapeutic Principle: Clear Heat, expel Wind, resolve stasis, dredge Collaterals.

Principal Measure: Relieve the chest by dotting and vibrating, push and wipe to divide the ribs, knead the local area with fingers or palms, relax the chest by pressing and kneading, knead and pinch the arm along Three Yin Meridians of the Hand, push the back with pinching and grasping.

Subordinate Measure: Knead Xuanji (CV 21), Huagai (CV 20), Qishe (St 11), Qihu (St 13), Yunmen (Lu 2), Ganshu (UB 18), Danshu (UB 19). If patient has fever, add Open Passes and Dredge Apertures and revolve Huantiao (GB 30) with the elbow (all on both sides).

Gynecology

Irregular menstruation

Irregular menstruation refers to abnormal or pathological changes in frequency, quantity, quality, and color. Changes of frequency may be classified as premature, delayed and irregular. Changes of quantity may be classified as excessive or lacking, the former often associated with premature menstruation, the latter with delayed. Changes in quality and color of menstrual blood must also be taken into account in clinical practice.

Etiology: Deficiency of Vital Energy and Blood; Vital Energy stagnation and Blood stasis; retention and obstruction of Dampness-Phlegm; bleeding due to Blood-Heat; insufficiency of Liver and Kidney; emotional depression.

Diagnosis & Treatment

1. Premature menstruation

This refers to menstruation more than 7 days prior to the due date or even 2 menses in 1 month. There are 2 types.

A. Deficiency of Vital Energy

Constitutional weakness, malnutrition, Spleen impaired by mental or physical overwork, debility of Vital (Chong) Meridian. (The Vital Meridian is not included in the brief discussion of 14 Meridian Paths in the beginning of this book.)

Signs & Symptoms: Excessive flow is watery with pale color, palpitations, shortness of breath, listlessness, weariness, empty and sinking feeling in lower abdomen, insensitivity to taste. *Tongue:* pale with thin white fur. *Pulse:* thready, weak.

Therapeutic Principle: Invigorate Vital Energy, conserve Blood.

Principal Measure: Knead Feishu (UB 13), Jueyinshu (UB 14) and Xinshu (UB 15) with fingers (all both sides); strengthen the waist by rolling and rubbing; stroke and caress the head; push and wipe to divide the ribs; push the abdomen with round-rubbing and revolving; Taiji round-rub the abdomen; roll the abdomen with knocking and vibrating.

Subordinate Measure: Grasp both Jianjing (GB 21).

Herbal Preparation: Cinnamon Twig (Gui Zhi) decoction.

B. Blood-Heat

This may be classified as Deficient Heat, Excess Heat, and Heat produced by Liver depression. Clinically, Deficient Heat due to Liver Depression is most frequently encountered.

Signs & Symptoms: Abundant loss of sticky, purple blood mixed with clots; irritability, short temper, bitter taste in mouth, dry stools. *Tongue:* red with thin yellow fur. *Pulse:* stringy, rapid.

Therapeutic Principle: Clear Heat, cool Blood. Massage should be done after menstruation is completed.

Principal Measure: Press and push the supraclavicular fossa; nip and knead Laogong (Per 8); push and rub Yongquan (K 1); knead both Jueyinshu (UB 14), Xinshu (UB 15), Ganshu (UB 18) and Danshu (UB 19) with your fingers (all both sides); strengthen the waist by rolling and rubbing; push the back with pinching and grasping; roll the abdomen with knocking and vibrating; relax the chest by pressing and kneading; push and wipe to divide the ribs; stroke and caress the head; revolve Dantian with your forearm.

Subordinate Measure: Grasp Neiguan (Per 6), Quchi (LI 11) and Sanyinjiao (Sp 6) (both sides).

Herbal Preparation: Radix Scutellariae (Huang Qin) decoction.

2. Delayed menstruation

The menses is delayed by more than 7 days. This falls into 3 categories: Blood Cold, Vital Energy depression, and Phlegm clogging.

A. Blood Cold

This is caused by constitutional deficiency of Yang and/or invasion of Cold evil during menstruation.

Signs & Symptoms: Scanty menses with pale color, coldness and pain in lower abdomen, desire to be warmed and pressed, pale complexion. *Tongue:* pale with thin white fur. *Pulse:* deep, slow or tense.

Therapeutic Principle: Warm Meridians, disperse Cold. Massage should be done prior to menstruation.

Principal Measure: Knead Baihui (GV 20) with your fingers; pinch and grasp Fengchi (GB 20); revolve Shenshu (UB 23); Zhishi (UB 52) and the Upper, Second, Middle Liao (UB 31-33, both sides) with the forearm; strengthen the waist by rolling and rubbing; pluck Collaterals with knocking and scratching; press the abdomen with deep-pressing and kneading;

push the abdomen with round-rubbing and revolving, Taiji round-rub the abdomen.

Subordinate Measure: Knead and grasp Sanyinjiao (Sp 6) and Xuehai (Sp 10), rub both Yongquan (K 1).

Herbal Preparation: Decoction of Fructus Evodiae (Wu Zhu Yu) and Cinnamon Twig (Gui Zhi).

B. Vital Energy Depression

Emotional depression impairs Liver and impedes the Energy flow in Vital and Conception Vessel Meridians.

Signs & Symptoms: Scanty menses with dim color, distension and pain in the lower abdomen, fullness and heaviness in chest and rib cage. *Tongue:* dim. *Pulse:* stringy, uneven.

Therapeutic Principle: Relieve depression, promote the flow of Vital Energy, activate Blood, regulate menstruation.

Principal Measure: Revolve Huantiao (GB 30) with the elbow, knead and grasp Weizhong (UB 40), both on both sides; relax the chest by dotting and vibrating, grasp the abdomen with lifting and jerking, roll the abdomen with knocking and vibrating, rub the spine, open Passes and dredge Apertures.

Subordinate Measure: Nip and knead Yanglingquan (GB 34), grasp and knead Sanyinjiao (Sp 6) and Xuehai (SP 10).

C. Phlegm Clogging

Constitutional obesity or overeating of rich foods resulting in accumulation and retention of Phlegm.

Signs & Symptoms: Dizziness, heaviness in chest and epigastrium, morbid leukorrhea, mass in abdomen, scanty menses with sticky discharge. *Tongue:* white, greasy fur. *Pulse:* stringy, slippery.

Therapeutic Principle: Resolve Phlegm, rectify Vital Energy, activate Blood, regulate menstruation.

Principal Measure: Pinch and grasp Three Yin Meridians of the Hand (both sides), deep-press the spine with kneading and revolving, pluck Collaterals with knocking and scratching, relax the chest by pressing and kneading, relieve the chest by dotting and vibrating, push and wipe to divide the ribs, press the abdomen with deep-pressing and kneading, roll the abdomen with knocking and vibrating.

Subordinate Measure: Grasp Weizhong (UB 40), Chengshan (UB 57), Fenglong (St 40) (all both sides).

Herbal Preparation: Ginger Juice (Sheng Jiang).

3. Irregular menstruation

This is usually classified as Spleen Deficiency, Liver depression and Kidney Deficiency.

A. Spleen Deficiency

Signs & Symptoms: Listlessness, lassitude, pale complexion, palpitations, shortness of breath, cold limbs, edema, somnolence, desire to stay in bed, abdominal distension, desire to be pressed, loose stools, leukorrhea. *Tongue:* pale with white or greasy fur. *Pulse:* moderate, weak.

Therapeutic Principle: Invigorate Spleen, benefit Vital Energy.

Principal Measure: Revolve Pishu (UB 20), Weishu (UB 21), Shenshu (UB 23) and the Upper, Second, Middle Liao (UB 31-33) with the forearm, all both sides; rub the back and waist, push the abdomen with round-rubbing and revolving, Taiji round-rub the abdomen.

Subordinate Measure: Press and knead Zusanli (St 36) and Sanyinjiao (Sp 6), both on both sides.

Herbal Preparation Decoction of ginger (Sheng Jiang) and cinnamon twig (Gui Zhi).

B. Liver depression

Signs & Symptoms: Heaviness and distension in the chest and rib cage, distended pain in the lower abdomen, belching, poor appetite. *Tongue:* red fringe with thin or slightly yellow fur. *Pulse:* stringy.

Therapeutic Principle: Rectify Vital Energy, relieve depression, nourish Blood, regulate menstruation.

Principal Measure: Revolve Ganshu (UB 18), Danshu (UB 19), Hunmen (UB 47) and Yanggang (UB 48) with the forearm, all both sides; relieve the chest by pressing and kneading; push and wipe to divide the ribs; roll the abdomen with knocking and vibrating; press the abdomen with deep-pressing and kneading, pluck Collaterals with kneading and scratching.

Subordinate Measure: Revolve Huantiao (GB 30) with the elbow; nip and knead Yanglingquan (GB 34), Yangjiao (GB 35), Xuehai (Sp 10) and Neiguan (Per 6).

C. Kidney Deficiency

Constitutional Kidney Deficiency, sexual overindulgence, repeated pregnancies or childbirth.

Signs & Symptoms: Scanty menses with pale watery bleeding; dim complexion; vertigo, dizziness, tinnitus; soreness and weakness of the waist and legs; empty, sinking feeling in the lower abdomen; loose stools, frequent urination at night, night sweats, dreaminess. *Tongue:* pale with thin fur. *Pulse:* deep, weak.

Therapeutic Principle: Strengthen the waist, invigorate Kidney, nourish Blood, regulate menstruation.

Principal Measure: Revolve Sanjiaoshu (UB 22), Shenshu (UB 23), Huangmen (UB 51) and Zhishi (UB 30) (invigorating, all on both sides); Baihuanshu (UB 30), Eight Liao (UB 31- 34, both sides) with the forearm; strengthen the waist by rolling and rubbing, pluck Collaterals with kneading and scratching; roll the abdomen with knocking and vibrating; push the abdomen with round-rubbing and revolving.

Subordinate Measure: Nip and knead Zusanli (St 36), push and rub Yongquan (K 1), knead Xuehai (Sp 10).

Herbal Preparation: Decoction of Ginger (Sheng Jiang) and Cinnamon Twig (Gui Zhi).

Dysmenorrhea

Dysmenorrhea refers to pain in the lower abdomen and the waist around or during menstruation. It may be accompanied by systemic symptoms such as vomiting, diarrhea, lower back pain, distended and painful breasts. Primary dysmenorrhea is usually seen in sexually inactive women, secondary dysmenorrhea in sexually active women.

Etiology: Dysmenorrhea is principally due to the impeded flow of Vital Energy and Blood, and may be divided into four types: Deficiency of Vital Energy and Blood; Vital Energy stagnation and Blood stasis; accumulation and retention of Cold-Dampness; depletion and impairment of Liver-Kidney.

Diagnosis & Treatment

1. Deficiency of Vital Energy and Blood

Signs & Symptoms: Continuous pain in lower abdomen during or after menstruation, pale and watery menses, pale complexion, listlessness, tiredness. *Tongue:* pale with thin fur. *Pulse:* deficient, thready.

Therapeutic Principle: Invigorate Vital Energy, nourish Blood.

Principal Measure: Pinch and grasp Jianjing (GB 21); revolve Feishu (UB 13), Jueyinshu (UB 14), Xinshu (UB 15), Shenshu (UB 23) and Zhishi (UB 52) with the forearm, all both sides, all invigorating; knead Guanyuan (CV 4) and both Dahe (K 12) with the palms (invigorating); strengthen the waist by rolling and rubbing; push the abdomen with round-rubbing and revolving.

Subordinate Measure: Nip and knead Zusanli (St 36) (invigorating).

Herbal Preparation: Ginger Juice (Sheng Jiang).

2. *Vital Energy stagnation and Blood stasis*

Signs & Symptoms: Distension and pain in lower abdomen before or during menstruation with notable tenderness, reduced flow, the menses is purple and mixed with clots, pain is relieved by discharge of clots. These symptoms may be accompanied by headache, distending pain in the breasts, chest and rib cage. *Tongue:* purple with or without petechiae at the fringe. *Pulse:* deep, stringy.

Therapeutic Principle: Promote the flow of Vital Energy, activate Blood, eliminate stasis, relieve pain.

Principal Measure: Knead Zhongji (CV 3), Guanyuan (CV 4), Second Liao (UB 32), Diji (Sp 8), both sides, and Xuehai (Sp 10) with the fingers; relieve the chest by dotting and vibrating; roll the abdomen with knocking and vibrating; press the abdomen with deep-pressing and kneading.

Subordinate Measure: Revolve Huantiao (GB 30) with the elbow, pull and grasp Weizhong (UB 40), both on both sides, both reducing.

Herbal Preparation: Decoction of Radix Angelicae Sinensis (Dang Gui) and Rhizoma Ligustici Wallichii (Chuan Xiong).

3. *Accumulation and retention of Cold-Dampness*

Signs & Symptoms: Cold pain in lower abdomen before or during menstruation involving the back and waist; pain may be alleviated by warmth; impeded menses is scanty, dim red and mixed with clots; aversion to cold, loose stools. *Tongue:* pale with white or greasy fur. *Pulse:* deep, tense.

Therapeutic Principle: Disperse Cold, eliminate Dampness, resolve retention, relieve pain.

Principal Measure: Knead Qihai (CV 6) with the fingers, revolve Tianshu (St 25) and Weidao (GB 28) with the forearm, both sides; nip and knead both Juliao (GB 29); deep-press the spine with kneading and revolving; revolve Eight Liao (UB 31-34, both sides); pluck Collaterals with kneading and scratching; push the abdomen with round-rubbing and revolving; roll the abdomen with kneading and vibrating.

Subordinate Measure: Dot Sanyinjiao (Sp 6), grasp Weizhong (UB 40).

Herbal Preparation: Decoction of Cinnamon Bark (Rou Gui) and Ginger (Sheng Jiang).

4. Depletion and impairment of Liver-Kidney

Signs & Symptoms: Pale, scanty menses; vague pain in lower abdomen after menstruation; dizziness, tinnitus; soreness of back and waist; tiredness and weakness of legs and knees. *Tongue:* pale red with thin fur. *Pulse:* deep, thready.

Therapeutic Principle: Nourish and rectify Liver-Kidney.

Principal Measure: Knead Ligou (Liv 5), Shuiquan (K 5), Zhaohai (K 6), Taixi (K 3), Zhongdu (Liv 6), Ququan (Liv 8), Siman (K 14) and Zhongzhu (K 15) with the fingers, all both sides; knead Mingmen (GV 4) with the palms; deep-press the spine with kneading and revolving; strengthen the waist by rolling and rubbing; roll the abdomen with knocking and vibrating; push the abdomen with round-rubbing and revolving.

Subordinate Measure: Revolve Shenshu (UB 23) and Zhishi (UB 52) with the forearm, on both sides; knead and nip Baihui (GV 20).

Amenorrhea

Primary amenorrhea refers to failure of appearance of menarche by age 18. Secondary amenorrhea indicates cessation of menstruation for more than three months for reasons other than pregnancy. Primary amenorrhea is beyond the scope of massage therapy.

Etiology: There are various causes, but generally, they belong to either Deficiency or Excess. Most Deficiency amenorrhea is caused by insufficient Liver-Kidney or Deficiency of Vital Energy and Blood. Most of Excess amenorrhea is caused by Vital Energy stagnation and Blood stasis or the retention and obstruction of Phlegm-Dampness.

Diagnosis & Treatment

1. Deficient Liver-Kidney

Signs & Symptoms: Amenorrhea, or the onset of menarche occurs considerably later than normal with scanty pinkish menses, gradually decreasing to actual amenorrhea. Dim complexion, vertigo, dizziness, tinnitus, soreness and weakness of the waist and knees, irritability, heat at palms and soles of feet, agitated fever, perspiration. *Tongue:* red or pale with minimal fur. *Pulse:* thready, stringy/thready, uneven.

Principal Measure: Knead Pishu (UB 20)) with your fingers; revolve Shenshu (UB 23) and Zhishi (UB 52) with the forearm, both on both sides; knead Qihai (CV 6) with the fingers; nip and knead Zusanli (St 36), invigorating on both sides; knead Mingmen (GV 4) with your palms; strengthen the waist by rolling and rubbing; deep-press the spine with kneading and revolving; push and wipe to divide the ribs; roll the abdomen with knocking and vibrating; push the abdomen with round-rubbing and revolving.

Subordinate Measure: Dot both Sanyinjiao (Sp 6), revolve Eight Liao (UB 31-34, both sides) with the forearm.

2. Deficiency of Vital Energy and Blood

Signs & Symptoms: Delayed menstruation with minimal menses gradually becoming amenorrhea. Pale, withered or sallow complexion; dizziness, palpitations, shortness of breath, listlessness; weak limbs, poor appetite, loose stools. *Tongue:* pale with pale lips. *Pulse:* thready, weak; or thready, moderate, feeble.

Therapeutic Principle: Benefit Vital Energy, nourish Blood, regulate menstruation.

Principal Measure: Pinch and grasp Jianjing (GB 21); revolve Feishu (UB 13), Jueyinshu (UB 14), Xinshu (UB 15), Shenshu (UB 23), Zhishi (UB 52), all invigorating, all both sides; Eight Liao (UB 31-34, both sides) and Mingmen (GV 4) with the forearm; strengthen the waist by rolling and scratching; push and wipe to divide the ribs; push the abdomen with round-rubbing and revolving.

Subordinate Measure: Nip and knead Zusanli (St 36), dot Taixi (K 3), knead Xuehai (Sp 10).

3. Vital Energy stagnation and Blood stasis

Signs & Symptoms: Amenorrhea for several months, emotional depression, listlessness, anxiety, irritability, distension and fullness in the chest and rib cage, distension and pain in the lower abdomen, resistance to pressing. *Tongue:* dim purple possibly with petechiae. *Pulse:* deep, stringy; or deep, uneven.

Therapeutic Principle: Promote the flow of Vital Energy, activate Blood, eliminate stagnancy, resolve stasis.

Principal Measure: Knead Zhongji (CV 3) and Shimen (CV 5) with the fingers; nip and knead Hegu (LI 4), reducing, both sides; dot Xuehai (Sp 10); pull and grasp Weizhong (UB 40), both sides, reducing; push the back with pinching and grasping; pluck Collaterals with kneading and scratching; relax the chest by pressing and kneading; roll the abdomen with knocking and vibrating.

Subordinate Measure: Dot Sanyinjiao (Sp 6) and Xingjian (Liv 2).

4. Retention and obstruction of Phlegm-Dampness

Signs & Symptoms: Obesity, fullness and heaviness in the chest and rib cage, nausea, vomiting, excessive sputum, weariness, feebleness, abundant leukorrhea. *Tongue:* pale with greasy white fur. *Pulse:* stringy, slippery.

Therapeutic Principle: Eliminate Phlegm, dry Dampness, promote the flow of Vital Energy, induce menstruation.

Principal Measure: Revolve Yuzhong (K 26), Shencang (K 25), Lingxu (K 24), Kufang (St 14), Wuyi (St 15), Yingchuang (St 16) and Neiguan (Per 6) with your forearm, all both sides, all reducing; knead Tiantu (CV 22), push and wipe to divide the ribs, grasp the abdomen with lifting and jerking; relieve the chest by dotting and vibrating; roll the abdomen with knocking and vibrating.

Subordinate Measure: Dot Qihai (CV 6) and Xuehai (Sp 10), both sides, and Sanyinjiao (Sp 6), both sides, purging.

Leukorrhea

A small discharge of mucus from the vagina, increasing around menstruation or the beginning of pregnancy is normal. Leukorrhea refers to a continuous or profuse discharge of white mucus, like nasal discharge. When there is blood mixed with it, it is referred to as leukorrhea with red discharge.

Etiology: Deficiency of Spleen results in accumulation of Dampness; downward flow of Dampness-Heat; Deficiency of Kidney from sexual overindulgence or multiple abortions; attack on uterine Collaterals from noxious Dampness.

Diagnosis & Treatment

1. Deficiency of Spleen

Signs & Symptoms: Continuous white, sticky discharge without fetid odor; glossy white or withered sallow complexion, cold limbs; weariness, feebleness, possibly obesity, edema at face and extremities; poor appetite; loose stools. *Tongue:* pale and enlarged with white or greasy fur. *Pulse:* moderate, weak.

Therapeutic Principle: Strengthen Spleen, eliminate Dampness, stop discharge.

Principal Measure: Revolve the middle abdomen around Zhongwan (CV 12) with your forearm; knead Qihai (CV 6) and Guanyuan (CV 4) with the fingers; revolve both Daimai (GB 26) with the forearm; knead both Baihuanshu (UB 30) with the fingers; roll the abdomen with knocking and vibrating; push and wipe to divide the ribs; push the abdomen with round-rubbing and revolving.

Subordinate Measure: Press both Yinlingquan (Sp 9) with the fingers, invigorating.

2. Deficiency of Kidney

Signs & Symptoms: Cold, clear, abundant discharge like egg white, dripping every day; dim complexion, listlessness, serious lower back pain, feeling of coldness in lower abdomen; frequent urination. *Tongue:* pale with white fur. *Pulse:* deep, thready.

Therapeutic Principle: Benefit Kidney, foster Primordium, consolidate and constrict uterine Collaterals, stop discharge.

Principal Measure: Revolve Shenshu (UB 23), Zhishi (UB 52), both sides, invigorating, and Mingmen (GV 4) with the forearm; push and wipe to divide the ribs; roll the abdomen with knocking and vibrating; deep-press the spine with kneading and revolving; strengthen the waist by rolling and rubbing.

Subordinate Measure: Revolve the middle abdomen around Zhongwan (CV 12) with the forearm.

3. Noxious Dampness

Signs & Symptoms: Abundant sticky discharge with fishy and fetid odor, or mixed with blood, or cloudy, like rice-water; itching of the pudenda; dizziness, heaviness in the head, thirst without desire to drink; pain in lower abdomen; difficult urination, deep colored urine; bitter taste in the mouth, dry throat. *Tongue:* red with yellow fur. *Pulse:* soft, floating and rapid or slippery.

Therapeutic Principle: Clear Heat, detoxify noxious evil, eliminate Dampness.

Principal Measure: Knead Baihuanshu (UB 30), both sides, and Qihai (CV 6) with the fingers; dot both Sanyinjiao (Sp 6); push and wipe to divide the ribs; push the abdomen with round-rubbing and revolving; grasp the abdomen with lifting and jerking; roll the abdomen with knocking and vibrating; relieve the chest by dotting and vibrating.

Subordinate Measure: Nip and knead Xingjian (Liv 2), Yanglingquan (GB 34) and Zusanli (St 36); knead Pishu (UB 20), Weishu (UB 21) and Danshu (UB 19).

Leukorrhagia (Spontaneous emission)

This occurs in women who dream about sexual activity at night, discharging white or yellow mucus from the vagina, like nocturnal emission in men.

Etiology: Constitutional weakness, mental overexertion, emotional depression, hyperactivity of Ministerial Fire, Deficiency of Liver-Kidney Yin.

Diagnosis & Treatment

1. Hyperactivity of Heart-Kidney Fire

Signs & Symptoms: Pale yellow and sticky vaginal discharge after dreaming of sex; dizziness, fever, anxiety, thirst, dry throat; aching in the waist, feebleness; decreased amount of urine, deep-colored urine, hot sensation in urethra during urination, dry stools. *Tongue:* red with yellow, thin or greasy fur. *Pulse:* thready, rapid.

Therapeutic Principle: Nourish Yin, clear Fire, consolidate and constrict uterine Collaterals, stop vaginal discharge.

Principal Measure: Knead Guanyuan (CV 4), Dahe (K 12), Xinshu (UB 15), Shenmen (H 7) and Neiguan (Per 6) with the fingers; revolve Shenshu (UB 23) and Zhishi (UB 52), both on both sides, and Mingmen (GV 4) and Eight Liao (UB 31-34, both sides) with the forearm; stroke and caress the head; push the abdomen with round-rubbing and revolving; push and wipe to divide the ribs; roll the abdomen with knocking and vibrating.

Subordinate Measure: Nip Zusanli (St 36) and Taixi (K 3), both on both sides.

2. Deficiency of Liver-Kidney Yin

Signs & Symptoms: Watery discharge, dizziness, tinnitus, flushing of the cheeks, irritability, hotness at palms and soles of feet, agitated fever, night sweats, thirst without desire for drink, soreness and weakness of the waist and knees, distending pain in lower abdomen, frequent urination. *Tongue:* red with little fur. *Pulse:* thready, rapid or stringy.

Therapeutic Principle: Nourish Liver, invigorate Kidney, consolidate and constrict uterine Collaterals, stop vaginal discharge.

Principal Measure: Dot Xingjian (Liv 2), Taichong (Liv 3), Zhongfeng (Liv 4), Rangu (K 2), Zhaohai (K 6) and Taixi (K 3), all both sides, all reducing; revolve Shenshu (UB 23) Mingmen (GV 4) and Eight Liao (UB 31-34, both sides) with the forearm; roll the abdomen with knocking and vibrating; push and wipe to divide the ribs; strengthen the waist by rolling and rubbing.

Subordinate Measure: Push Yongquan (K 1), knead Ququan (Liv 8) with the fingers.

Abdominal mass (Zhen and Jia)

Zhen and Jia indicate abdominal masses in TCM. Zhen refers to a palpable, distending, immovable mass with fixed pain in the abdomen, and belongs to Blood syndrome. Jia refers to an indefinite, movable mass which appears intermittently with wandering pain, and belongs to Vital Energy syndrome. These must be diagnosed unequivocally with current gynecological techniques. Massage can be effective in treatment of functional, benign masses, but is contraindicated with organic, malignant ones.

Etiology: Depression and stagnation of Energy Mechanism from emotional disturbance; attack on uterine Collaterals during postpartum or menstruation by Wind-Cold; stasis and obstruction of semen and blood from sexual overindulgence; accumulation and retention of Phlegm and fluids.

Diagnosis & Treatment

1. Vital Energy stagnation (Jia)

Signs & Symptoms: Intermittently present soft mass, emotional depression, feeling of fullness in rib cage, belching, dim cyanotic complexion. *Tongue:* red margin or petechiae with thin fur. *Pulse:* deep, stringy.

Therapeutic Principle: Promote the flow of Vital Energy, eliminate stagnation.

Principal Measure: Nip Neiguan (Per 6); knead Chengman (St 20) and Shangqu (K 17); dot Weicang (UB 50) and Huangmen (UB 51), both on both sides, purging; relieve the chest by dotting and vibrating; press the abdomen with round-rubbing and revolving; push and wipe to divide the ribs; grasp the abdomen with lifting and jerking; press the abdomen with deep-pressing and kneading; relax the chest by pressing and kneading.

Subordinate Measure: Nip and knead Xingjian (Liv 2) and Neiting (St 44), both on both sides, both reducing.

2. Blood stasis (Zhen)

Signs & Symptoms: Mass in lower abdomen with fixed pain, resistance to pressing, dark complexion, dry skin, irregular menstruation and menstrual blood loss, menses unwholesome color. *Tongue:* dim purple or petechiae. *Pulse:* deep, uneven.

Therapeutic Principle: Corrupt Blood stasis, eliminate mass in abdomen.

Principal Measure: Press and knead Xiawan (CV 10), Qihai (CV 6), Guanyuan (CV 4), Siman (K 14) and Qixue (K 13), all both sides and reducing; push and wipe to divide the ribs; grasp the abdomen with lifting and jerking; roll the abdomen with knocking and vibrating; push the abdomen with round-rubbing and revolving.

Subordinate Measure: Knead and grasp Sanyinjiao (Sp 6), nip and knead Xingjian (Liv 2), both on both sides, reducing.

3. Retention of Phlegm

Signs & Symptoms: Obesity with immovable hardened mass in the abdomen, pale complexion, heaviness in the chest, nausea, vomiting, delayed menstruation or amenorrhea, profuse leukorrhea. *Tongue:* pale with white greasy fur. *Pulse:* slippery.

Therapeutic Principle: Eliminate and dissipate Phlegm retention.

Principal Measure: Dot Yuzhong (K 26), Lingxu (K 24), Bulang (K 22), Huagai (CV 20), Zigong (CV 19) and Yutang (CV 18) and nip Neiguan (Per 6) — all both sides, all purging; relieve the chest by dotting and vibrating; nip and knead Tiantu (CV 22); relax the chest by pressing and kneading; revolve the abdomen with the forearm; grasp the abdomen with lifting and jerking; push the abdomen with round-rubbing and revolving.

Morning sickness (Hyperemesis gravidarum)

In the second and third month of pregnancy, about half of women suffer a period of dizziness, nausea and vomiting, known as Morning Sickness. These symptoms usually disappear by themselves after 1-3 weeks. If they persist for a much longer time and the woman cannot take food, there will be depletion of Vital Energy and Blood, damaging the health of the woman and impairing the development of the fetus.

Etiology: Uterine Collaterals connect with the opening of the Stomach. Common causes are Deficiency of Spleen and Stomach leading to harassment of the harmonizing and descending mechanism; Liver attacks Stomach from emotional depression, resulting in adverse uprising of Vital Energy.

1. Deficiency of Spleen and Stomach

Signs & Symptoms: Constitutional weakness, nausea, vomiting, no appetite, listlessness, weariness. *Tongue:* pale with white fur. *Pulse:* moderate, slippery.

Therapeutic Principle: Strengthen Spleen, harmonize Stomach, depress the adverse uprising, stop vomiting.

Principal Measure: Knead the middle and upper abdomen with the palms; roll the Three Yin Meridians of the Hand with the hands, both sides; push and wipe to divide the ribs.

Subordinate Measure: Knead Neiguan (Per 6) (both sides), Tiantu (CV 22), Zusanli (St 36) (both sides).

2. Disharmony between Liver and Stomach

Signs & Symptoms: Sour or bitter watery vomitus, belching, heaving sighs, irritability, full sensation in the head, feeling of fullness and heaviness in the chest and rib cage. *Tongue:* red with slightly yellow fur. *Pulse:* stringy, slippery.

Therapeutic Principle: Disperse Liver Energy, harmonize Stomach, depress the adverse uprising, stop vomiting.

Principal Measure: Knead the middle and upper abdomen, Qimen (Liv 14), Riyue (GB 24) and Zhangmen (Liv 13) with the palms; push and wipe to divide the ribs; knead Tiantu (CV 22).

Subordinate Measure: Nip and knead Zusanli (St 36).

N.B. These techniques should be done very gently.

Adverse uprising of Fetal Energy (Fetal dysphoria)

This is most often encountered in the middle or later stages of pregnancy. In serious cases, there may be labored breathing, pain and restlessness.

Etiology: Constitutional weakness of Spleen and Stomach; depressed Liver attacks Spleen; the growing fetus impedes normal functions of the woman's internal organs.

Diagnosis & Treatment

Signs & Symptoms: Feeling of heaviness and distension in the chest and abdomen with aggravation of symptoms after eating; anxiety, insomnia, potential miscarriage. *Tongue:* thin yellow fur. *Pulse:* stringy, slippery.

Therapeutic Principle: Disperse Liver Energy, strengthen Spleen, rectify Vital Energy, remove stasis.

Principal Measure: Knead Qimen (Liv 14), Riyue (GB 24) and Zhangmen (Liv 13) with the thenar mound, all on both sides; roll Three Yin and Yang Meridians of the Hand with your hands; roll Stomach and Liver Meridians of the Foot with the hands.

Subordinate Measure: Round-rub and revolve the abdomen around Zhongwan (CV 12) with the hands.

N.B. These techniques should be done very gently.

Persistent cough during pregnancy

This refers to an intractable cough, irritability, hotness at palms and soles of feet, and possible miscarriage. If the cough persists for an extended time and is accompanied by agitated fever, night sweats, blood-tinged sputum, lassitude and severe weight loss, it is called tubercular cough.

Etiology: Flaming uprising of Deficient Fire due to Deficiency of Lung-Kidney Yin is the usual cause, although attack of exogenous Wind-Cold may be a factor.

Diagnosis & Treatment

Signs & Symptoms: Intractable cough without sputum or with blood-tinged sputum, dizziness, dry throat, flushed cheeks, hotness at palms and soles of feet, intermittent low fever. *Tongue:* red with minimal fur or yellow and dry with thin fur. *Pulse:* thready, rapid, slippery.

Therapeutic Principle: Nourish Yin, moisten Lung, stop cough, calm fetus.

Principal Measure: Knead Tanzhong (CV 17) and Feishu (UB 13) with your fingers, nip Lieque (Lu 7), nip and knead Taiyuan (Lu 9), knead Zhangmen (Liv 13) with the fingers, nip and knead Chize (Lu 5), revolve Shenshu (UB 23) and Zhishi (UB 52) with the forearm, nip Fenglong (St 40) and Yanglingquan (GB 34) on both sides, relax the chest by pressing and kneading, relieve the chest by dotting and vibrating.

Subordinate Measure: Nip and knead Zusanli (St 36), Taibai (Sp 3) and Taixi (K 3), all on both sides.

Involuntary spasms of the legs and foot during pregnancy

Spasms, twitching and cramping of the lower leg and the foot are often encountered in the later stages of pregnancy.

Etiology: Malnutrition of Tendons and Vessels of the mother because Essence and Blood are being absorbed by the fetus.

Diagnosis & Treatment

Signs & Symptoms: Those mentioned above are more frequent and more serious at night; difficulty in walking.

Therapeutic Principle: Nourish Liver, soften Tendons.

Principal Measure: Pinch and grasp Chengshan (UB 57) and Chengjin (UB 56), knead the legs with rotating and round-rubbing, or pinch the calf.

Subordinate Measure: Revolve both Weizhong (UB 40) with the forearm.

N.B. These techniques should be done gently.

Pantalgia or arthralgia after childbirth

Etiology: Depletion of Vital Energy and Blood after delivery; attack on Meridians by Wind-Cold-Dampness from inattention to health.

Diagnosis & Treatment

1. Deficiency of Blood

Signs & Symptoms: Glossy pale or sallow, withered complexion; listlessness, weariness, dizziness, palpitations; joint pain, numbness in the limbs, difficult flexion and extension; symptoms may be alleviated by pressing and kneading. Tongue: pale red with little fur. Pulse: thready, stringy.

Therapeutic Principle: Benefit Vital Energy, nourish Blood, relax Tendons, dredge Collaterals.

Principal Measure: Stroke and caress the head, grasp Jianjing (GB 21) on both sides; nip and knead Shousanli (LI 10) and Waiguan (TW 5), both invigorating, both sides; roll arms with pushing and grasping; pluck Collaterals with knocking and scratching; push the back with pinching and grasping; roll the legs with revolving and pinching.

Subordinate Measure: knead and grasp Zusanli (St 36) and Zhaohai (K 6), both invigorating, both sides.

2. Exogenous attack

Signs & Symptoms: Pantalgia, especially noticeable at the joints of four limbs; difficult flexion and extension; pain wanders and varies in intensity; possible swelling and numbness; aversion to Wind and Cold, desire to be warmed. Tongue: pale with thin white fur. Pulse: thready and moderate or stringy and swift.

Therapeutic Principle: Nourish Blood, expel Wind, disperse Cold, dry Dampness.

Principal Measure: Rub Fengchi (GB 20); nip and knead Chize (Lu 5), Quchi (LI 11), Hegu (LI 4) and Yin Pool (opposite of Yangchi) with the forearm, all on both sides; nip Renzhong (GV 26); revolve Guanyuan (CV 4) and Fengshi (GB 31) with the forearm on both sides; nip and knead Dubi (St 35) on both sides; knead Shenzhu (GV 12) and Shenshu (UB 23) on both sides; roll the arms with pushing and grasping; pull the arms with rolling and rectifying; push the back with pinching and grasping; pluck Collaterals with knocking and scratching; roll the legs with revolving and pinching; knead the legs with rotating and round-rubbing.

Subordinate Measure: Nip and knead Yanglingquan (GB 34) and Kunlun (UB 60) on both sides.

Postpartum lumbago

Postpartum lumbago is often accompanied by pain in the heel. Before delivery, lumbago is caused by conception. After delivery, it may be resolved with careful nursing, and massage therapy is unnecessary. If the lumbago persists after lochia has stopped, this is an indication for massage.

Etiology: Three Yin Meridians of the Foot pass by the heel, and Kidney resides in the lumbar region. After delivery, there is depletion of Vital Energy and Blood and Deficiency of Kidney Energy. Lumbago may also be caused by an attack of Wind-Cold.

Diagnosis & Treatment

1. Deficiency of Kidney

Signs & Symptoms: Lumbago; definite tenderness on both sides of lumbar vertebrae, but without muscle rigidity; the lumbago involves the lower abdomen; feeling of heaviness, soreness and weakness at the waist and legs; dizziness, weariness, pale complexion, frequent urination. *Tongue:* pale red with thin white fur. *Pulse:* deep, thready.

Therapeutic Principle: Benefit Kidney, strengthen the waist.

Principal Measure: Revolve Shenshu (UB 23) and Zhishi (UB 52) with the forearm on both sides, knead Mingmen (GV 4) with the fingers, relax the chest by pressing and kneading, push the back with pushing and grasping, pluck Collaterals with knocking and scratching, strengthen the waist by rolling and rubbing, Taiji round-rub the abdomen, roll the abdomen with knocking and vibrating.

Subordinate Measure: Knead both Taixi (K 3).

2. Exogenous attack

Signs & Symptoms: Lumbago with feeling of soreness, heaviness and weakness; difficulty in turning left or right; inability to sit or stand for extended time; symptoms respond to warmth, are aggravated by cold and damp weather; rigidity of lumbar muscles; slow reflexes. *Tongue:* pale with thin white fur. *Pulse:* deep, thready, stringy.

Therapeutic Principle: Strengthen the waist, invigorate Kidney, activate Collaterals, relieve pain.

Principal Measure: Revolve Yaoyangguan (GV 3), Shenshu (UB 23) and Zhishi (UB 52) with the forearm, all on both sides; push the back with pinching and grasping; pluck Collaterals with knocking and scratching; deep-press the spine with kneading and revolving.

Subordinate Measure: Pull and grasp Weizhong (UB 40), pinch Kunlun (UB 60), all on both sides.

Postpartum abdominal pain

This generally occurs at the epigastrium or the lower abdomen in multiple births.

Etiology: Deficiency and depletion of Vital Energy and Conception Vessel Meridians due to loss of blood during delivery; Blood stasis due to attack of exogenous Cold; stagnation of Vital Energy from emotional depression; retention of lochia.

Diagnosis & Treatment

1. Deficiency of Blood

Signs & Symptoms: Continuous pain in lower abdomen, alleviated when pressed; scanty lochia with pale color; dizziness, tinnitus, dry stool. *Tongue:* pale red with thin fur. *Pulse:* deficient, thready.

Therapeutic Principle: Nourish Blood, benefit Vital Energy, relieve pain.

Principal Measure: Knead both Jueyinshu (UB 14) and Xinshu (UB 15) with the fingers; revolve Guanyuan (CV 4), Shimen (CV 5) and Yinjiao (CV 7) with the forearm, all invigorating; round-rub rib cage; roll the abdomen with knocking and vibrating; push the abdomen with round-rubbing and revolving; Taiji round-rub the abdomen.

Subordinate Measure: Nip both Zusanli (St 36), knead both Zhongdu (Liv 6) and Baihui (GV 20), invigorating.

2. Blood stasis

Signs & Symptoms: A resistant mass may be felt in the lower abdomen, abdominal pain with a cold sensation which alleviates with warmth; pale and cyanotic complexion, cold limbs. The abdominal pain may be complicated by distending pain in the chest and rib cage, scant lochia or lochia with dull-colored clots. *Tongue:* slightly purple with slippery white fur. *Pulse:* deep and tense, or stringy and uneven.

Therapeutic Principle: Activate Blood, disperse Cold, relieve pain.

Principal Measure: Revolve Guanyuan (CV 4), Shimen (CV 5), Yinjiao (CV 7), Dahe (K 12), Qixue (K 13) and Siman (K 14) with the forearm (manipulate these points gently on the same side[s] as the pain); push and wipe to divide the ribs; round-rub rib cage; roll the abdomen with knocking and vibrating; grasp the abdomen with lifting and jerking; Taiji round-rub the abdomen.

Subordinate Measure: Knead both Zhongdu (Liv 6) and Neiting (St 44).

Prolapse of the uterus (Hysteroptosia)

This indicates the protrusion of the uterus at the opening of the vagina, usually after childbirth. In mild or moderate cases (the uterus not fully protruded), massage therapy may be effective. In serious cases, massage is less successful.

Etiology: Deficiency of Vital Energy, Deficiency of Kidney.

1. Deficiency of Vital Energy

Signs & Symptoms: Weighty sensation in the lower abdomen, palpitations, shortness of breath, listlessness, weariness, pale complexion, frequent urination, clear urine, watery leukorrhagia, symptoms aggravated by physical labor. *Tongue:* pale with thin fur. *Pulse:* superficial, deficient.

Therapeutic Principle: Strengthen Middle Warmer, benefit and lift Vital Energy.

Principal Measure: Knead Baihui (GV 20), grasp both Jianjing (GB 21), knead Qihai (CV 6), revolve Dahe (K 12) and Weidao (GB 28) with the forearm, all on both sides; round-rub rib cage; Taiji round-rub the abdomen; roll the abdomen with knocking and vibrating; revolve Zhongji (CV 3), Guanyuan (CV 4) and Yinjiao (CV 7) with the forearm.

Subordinate Measure: Knead Taichong (Liv 3) and Zhaohai (K 6), both invigorating, both sides.

2. Deficiency of Kidney

Signs & Symptoms: Soreness and weakness of the waist and knees, weighty sensation in the lower abdomen, frequent urination, dizziness, tinnitus. *Tongue:* pale red with thin white fur. *Pulse:* deep, thready.

Therapeutic Principle: Invigorate Kidney, benefit and lift Vital Energy.

Principal Measure: Knead Baihui (GV 20) and Qihai (CV 6); revolve Dahe (K 12), Weidao (GB 28), Shenshu (UB 23) and Zhishi (UB 52) with the forearm, all invigorating, all both sides; strengthen the waist by rolling and rubbing; push and wipe to divide the ribs; revolve the middle and lower abdomen with the forearm; push the abdomen with round-rubbing and revolving.

Subordinate Measure: Knead Taixi (K 3), Taichong (Liv 3) and Zhaohai (K 6), all invigorating, all on both sides.

Postpartum convulsions

This indicates twitching of limbs, stiffness of the nape and back, even lockjaw and opisthotonos.

Etiology: Failure of nourishing and moistening of Tendons and Vessels due to loss of blood and body fluids after childbirth; attack of exogenous Wind evil.

Diagnosis & Treatment

1. Deficiency of Blood

Signs & Symptoms: Excessive loss of blood during delivery, sudden onset of convulsions, stiffness of neck and nape, lockjaw, twitching limbs, pale or sallow withered complexion. *Tongue:* pale red with no fur. *Pulse:* thready, stringy.

Therapeutic Principle: Nourish Blood, foster Yin, soften Liver, cease Wind.

Principal Measure: Nip Renzhong (GV 26) and Xiaguan (St 7); knead Jiache (St 6) with the fingers; nip Quchi (LI 11) and Hegu (LI 4); knead Xinshu (UB 15), Ganshu (UB 18) and Danshu (UB 19) with the fingers; dot Xingjian (Liv 2), all on both sides. Rectify limbs, lift and grasp Fengchi (GB 20), stroke and caress the head.

Subordinate Measure: Revolve Huantiao (GB 30) with the elbow, rub Yongquan (K 1).

2. Attack of exogenous Wind

Signs & Symptoms: Stiffness and pain of the neck and head, fever, aversion to Wind and Cold, aching trunk and waist, lockjaw, possible rigidity of the nape and back, opisthotonos. *Tongue:* white thin fur. *Pulse:* superficial, stringy.

Therapeutic Principle: Expel Wind, calm convulsions, nourish Blood, moisten Tendons.

Principal Measure: Pinch Duiduan (GV 27); rub Fengchi (GB 20) with joined hands; knead Jiache (St 6), Shousanli (LI 10) and Waiguan (TW 5); nip and knead Quze (Per 3) and Hegu (LI 4), all on both sides; open Passes and dredge Apertures; pinch and grasp the neck and nape; pull, push and knead the neck; push and wipe to divide the ribs; pluck Collaterals with knocking and scratching; chop the legs with joined hands.

Subordinate Measure: Revolve Huantiao (GB 30) with the elbow, grasp Weizhong (UB 40) and Kunlun (UB 60) on both sides.

Postpartum constipation

This indicates constipation after childbirth despite the mother eating and drinking normally. In serious cases, there may be deep anxiety and depression, fever, possibly delirium.

Etiology: Depletion of Blood and body fluids during childbirth; dryness of intestinal tract from flaming uprising of Deficient Fire; Excess Fire from exogenous evils.

Diagnosis & Treatment

1. Deficiency of Blood

Signs & Symptoms: Constipation, difficult bowel movements without pain or distension, withered and sallow complexion, dry skin, normal appetite. When Deficiency of Blood is accompanied with Heat, there is also dizziness, palpitations and dry mouth. *Tongue:* pale red with minimal fur. *Pulse:* thready, uneven.

Therapeutic Principle: Nourish Blood, moisten intestinal dryness, relax bowels.

Principal Measure: Revolve Feishu (UB 13), Jueyinshu (UB 14), Xinshu (UB 15), Pishu (UB 20) and Weishu (UB 21) with the forearm, all invigorating, both sides; knead Dachangshu (UB 25) and Tianshu (St 25) with the fingers, both sides; nip and knead Zhigou (TW 6), grasp the abdomen with lifting and jerking; push the abdomen with round-rubbing and revolving; push Eight Liao (UB 31-34, both sides) downward.

Subordinate Measure: Knead Shangjuxu (St 37) and Dadun (Liv 1) on both sides.

2. Excess with dry stool

Difficult and painful bowel movement, fever, anxiety, hardness and pain in the epigastrium and lower abdomen, fever increases toward evening, halitosis, desire for cold food. *Tongue:* red with dry yellow fur. *Pulse:* deep, replete, energetic.

Therapeutic Principle: Clear Heat, nourish Blood, relax bowels.

Principal Measure: Revolve Shiguan (K 18), Shangqu (K 17), Huangshu (K 16), Zhongzhu (K 15) and Tianshu (St 25) with the forearm; nip and knead Quchi (LI 11), Zhigou (TW 6) and Hegu (LI 4) (all reducing, both sides), grasp the abdomen with lifting and jerking; roll the abdomen with knocking and vibrating.

Subordinate Measure: Pinch the spine, nip and knead Shangjuxu (St 37), both sides, reducing.

Postpartum anuria

This refers to a desire to urinate after childbirth but without production, resulting in retention of urine and distension of the lower abdomen.

Etiology: Excessive depletion of Vital Energy during delivery leads to Deficiency of Lung and Spleen; Deficiency of Kidney Yang and diminished function of Urinary Bladder; obstruction of urinary pathway from Liver depression.

Diagnosis & Treatment

1. Depletion of Vital Energy

Signs & Symptoms: Postpartum anuria, desire to urinate, distension of lower abdomen, anxiety, shortness of breath, remoteness, pale complexion, feebleness. Tongue: pale with minimal fur. Pulse: moderate, weak.

Therapeutic Principle: Invigorate Vital Energy, promote urination.

Principal Measure: Grasp both Jianjing (GB 21); knead Shimen (CV 5), Qihai (CV 6) and Guanyuan (CV 4); knead and nip Shuiquan (K 5); push Yongquan (K 1), all on both sides. Push the abdomen with round-rubbing and revolving.

Subordinate Measure: Scratch the Shu-points on the back.

2. Deficiency of Kidney

Signs & Symptoms: Anuria; feeling of distension, fullness and pain in lower abdomen; soreness and weakness of the waist and knees; restlessness; dark complexion; possibly loose stools or diarrhea. Tongue: pale red with white fur. Pulse: deep, slow.

Therapeutic Principle: Invigorate Kidney Yang.

Principal Measure: Revolve Sanjiaoshu (UB 22), Shenshu (UB 23), and Eight Liao (UB 31-34, both sides) with the forearm; knead Qixue (K 13), Daju (St 27) and Shuidao (St 28, all on both sides; knead Mingmen (GV 4) and Shimen (CV 5) with the fingers; strengthen the waist by rolling and rubbing.

Subordinate Measure: Nip and knead Weiyang (UB 39) and Yingu (K 10), push Yongquan (K 1).

3. Vital Energy stagnation from emotional depression

Signs & Symptoms: Anuria, distension of the lower abdomen, difficult/painful bowel movements, possible loss of consciousness. *Tongue:* red with minimal or white fur. *Pulse:* stringy, tense.

Therapeutic Principle: Rectify Vital Energy, eliminate distension, disperse stagnation, promote urination.

Principal Measure: Knead Dashu (UB 11), Feishu (UB 13) and Sanjiaoshu (UB 22), all on both sides, also Shuifen (CV 9) and Qihai (CV 6); knead Guanyuan (CV 4) and Shimen (CV 5) with the fingers; relax the chest by pressing and kneading; press the abdomen with deep-pressing and kneading.

Subordinate Measure: Pinch and grasp Yanglingquan (GB 34) and Sanyinjiao (Sp 6).

Postpartum pollakiuria and urinary incontinence

The symptoms of pollakiuria and urinary incontinence are different, but their causes are identical, so similar therapeutic techniques are used. Since there is no pain during urination, they should be distinguished from infectious diseases of the urinary system.

Etiology: Deficiency of Vital Energy and Blood due to exhaustive fatigue in childbirth from constitutional weakness; Deficiency of Lung and Kidney causing deterioration of Urinary Bladder function; injury to the pudenda during childbirth.

Diagnosis & Treatment

1. Deficiency of Vital Energy

Signs & Symptoms: Pollakiuria or incontinence after delivery, urine is watery and clear, shortness of breath, listlessness, feeling of weight and distension in the lower abdomen. *Tongue:* pale with thin fur. *Pulse:* deficient, moderate.

Therapeutic Principle: Invigorate Vital Energy, consolidate and conserve the urethral sphincter.

Principal Measure: Stroke and caress the head; revolve Shenshu (UB 23), Zhishi (UB 52), Guanyuanshu (UB 26), Xiaochangshu (UB 27) and Pangguangshu (UB 28) with the forearm, all on both sides; knead Guanyuan (CV 4) and Zhongji (CV 3); roll the abdomen with knocking and vibrating; push the abdomen with round-rubbing and revolving.

Subordinate Measure: Grasp both Jianjing (GB 21), push and wipe to divide the ribs, nip Yangjiao (GB 35).

2. Deficiency of Kidney

Signs & Symptoms: Pollakiuria or incontinence, dark complexion, cold limbs, soreness and weakness of the waist and knees. *Tongue:* pale red with thin damp fur. *Pulse:* deep, slow.

Therapeutic Principle: Invigorate Kidney, consolidate and conserve the urethral sphincter.

Principal Measure: Knead Shenshu (UB 23), Pangguangshu (UB 28) and Sanjiaoshu (UB 22), all on both sides, also Mingmen (GV 4); revolve Guanyuan (CV 4) and Shimen (CV 5); round-rub rib cage; strengthen the waist by rolling and rubbing.

Subordinate Measure: Nip and knead Taixi (K 3), Zhaohai (K 6) and Sanyinjiao (Sp 6), all on both sides.

N.B. Injury to the pudenda should be treated surgically.

Galactostasis

This refers to any interference with the secretion of milk including diminished secretion, complete absence, or impeded secretion.

Etiology: Constitutional weakness, loss of Vital Energy and Blood during delivery, frequent pregnancies; stagnation of Vital Energy from emotional depression or anger.

Diagnosis & Treatment

1. Deficiency of Vital Energy and Blood

Signs & Symptoms: Little or no secretion; no distension or pain in the breast; dim, sallow or pale complexion; listlessness, lassitude, dry skin; dizziness, palpitations, poor appetite. *Tongue:* pale with thin fur. *Pulse:* deficient, weak.

Therapeutic Principle: Invigorate Vital Energy, benefit Blood, dredge Meridians, promote lactation.

Principal Measure: Knead Rugen (St 18) on both sides, and Tanzhong (CV 17), Tianxi (Sp 18); nip Shaoze (SI 1) and Pishu (UB 20), both invigorating, both sides; relax the chest by pressing and kneading; round-rub rib cage; push the abdomen with round-rubbing and revolving; Taiji round-rub the abdomen; strengthen the waist by rolling and rubbing.

Subordinate Measure: Knead and nip both Zusanli (St 36), invigorating; knead both Sanyinjiao (Sp 6) with your fingers, invigorating.

2. Stagnation of Liver Energy

Signs & Symptoms: Failure of breast feeding, distension and fullness in the chest and rib cage, distending pain in breast, possible fever. *Tongue:* red with white or yellow fur. *Pulse:* stringy.

Therapeutic Principle: Disperse Liver Energy, eliminate stagnation, dredge Meridians, promote lactation.

Principal Measure: Knead Tanzhong (CV 17), Rugen (St 18) and Tianxi (Sp 18); nip Shaoze (SI 1); knead Qimen (Liv 14); dot Ganshu (UB 18). (Do all on both sides.) Round-rub rib cage, roll the abdomen with knocking and vibrating, push and wipe to divide the ribs.

Subordinate Measure: Revolve Huantiao (GB 30) with the elbow, dot Xingjian (Liv 2).

Postpartum insomnia

Etiology: Depletion of Vital Energy and Blood resulting in malnutrition of Heart; over-fatigue or fright after delivery; mental stress.

Diagnosis & Treatment

1. Deficiency of Blood

Signs & Symptoms: Pale complexion, dizziness, palpitations, insomnia, dreaminess, easily awakened, weariness, desire to lie in bed, poor appetite. *Tongue:* pale with thin fur. *Pulse:* thready, weak.

Therapeutic Principle: Invigorate Vital Energy, nourish Blood, tranquilize the mind.

Principal Measure: Stroke and caress the head; knead Xinshu (UB 15), Pishu (UB 20), Shenshu (UB 23), and Shenmen (H 7)with the fingers, all invigorating, all on both sides; round-rub rib cage; Taiji round-rub the abdomen; strengthen the waist by rolling and rubbing.

Subordinate Measure: Knead and grasp Zusanli (St 36), Sanyinjiao (Sp 6) and Taixi (K 3), all invigorating, both sides.

2. Stagnation of Vital Energy

Signs & Symptoms: Insomnia, easily awakened, absent-mindedness, melancholy, heavy sighs, fullness and heaviness in the chest and rib cage, anxiety. *Tongue:* pale red with thin fur. *Pulse:* stringy.

Therapeutic Principle: Disperse and rectify Liver Energy, nourish Heart, tranquilize the mind.

Principal Measure: Knead Shenting (GV 24) with the fingers; revolve the middle abdomen with the forearm; nip Lingdao (H 4), Shenmen (H 7) and

Neiguan (Per 6), all on both sides; relieve the chest by dotting and vibrating; push and wipe to divide the ribs; relax the chest by pressing and kneading; roll the abdomen with knocking and vibrating; push the abdomen with round-rubbing and revolving.

Subordinate Measure: Revolve Huantiao (GB 30) with the elbow; dot Taixi (K 3) and Xingjian (Liv 2), all on both sides.

Hysteria

Signs and symptoms of hysteria are absent-mindedness, extreme depression and anxiety or sadness, mercurial temper and frequent yawning. This is common after delivery.

Etiology: Constitutional weakness, depletion of Heart Yin from extended worry, depression of Liver Energy, damage of Spleen from overexertion, upward harassment of Fire transformed from Five Emotions.

Diagnosis & Treatment

Signs & Symptoms: Absent-mindedness, crying without cause, continuous yawning, anxiety, suspiciousness, jumpiness, irregular sleeping, lethargy or insomnia, dry mouth, nausea, constipation. *Tongue:* red or tender and red with minimal fur. *Pulse:* weak or stringy and thready.

Therapeutic Principle: Soften Liver, strengthen Spleen, calm Heart, tranquilize the mind.

Principal Measure: Nip Renzhong (GV 26); dot Ganshu (UB 18), Jianshi (Per 5), Daling (Per 7) and Hegu (LI 4); nip Shaochong (H 9), all purging, both sides. Open Passes and dredge Apertures, push and wipe to divide the ribs, Taiji round-rub the abdomen.

Subordinate Measure: Nip Xingjian (Liv 2), rub Yongquan (K 1), knead Neiguan (Per 6) and Waiguan (TW 5).

Alternate Prescription

Principal Measure: Pinch Duiduan (GV 27); knead and nip Neiguan (Per 6), Shenmen (H 4) and Laogong (Per 8), all on both sides; stroke and caress the head.

Subordinate Measure: Knead and grasp Sanyinjiao (Sp 6) and Taichong (Liv 3), all on both sides.

In serious cases, use both prescriptions together as one.

Trauma

Injury to upper limbs

Dislocation of the long head of the Biceps brachii muscle tendon

This is frequently encountered in shoulder trauma. It is characterized by the tearing away of this tendon and its shifting slip to the inside of the tuberculum minus humeri. Signs and symptoms are swelling and pain at the front of the shoulder and restricted motor function of the shoulder joint. In TCM, it belongs to the category of tendon trauma.

Etiology: Sudden sprain and bruising while the forearm is in a position of abduction-supination; the forearm is dragged revolvingly backward with violent force causing dislocation of the Hand Taiyin Tendon at the front tip of the shoulder, becoming trapped in the fissure of the bones; flaccidity and weakness of tendons due to Deficiency of Vital Energy and Blood, old age, or childhood.

Diagnosis & Treatment

Signs & Symptoms: The arm hangs down and cannot be raised or turned outward; swelling, spasm and pain at the front of the shoulder, Jianyu (LI 15), Yunmen (Lu 2) and Zhongfu (Lu 1); the protruding part is resistant to pressing.

Therapeutic Principle: Rectify and reposition the tendon, relax Tendinomuscular Meridians, dredge and promote the flow of Vital Energy and Blood, nourish and consolidate Tendons and muscles.

Principal Measure: Pinch the arm with nipping and kneading, roll the arm with pushing and grasping, pull the arm and abduct the shoulder while kneading with the fingers, twist the arm with rocking and jerking, pluck and pinch to shift and reposition the tendon.

Subordinate Measure: Pinch and grasp Fengchi (GB 20), Yunmen (Lu 2), Tianliao (TW 15), Zhongfu (Lu 1), Jianyu (LI 15), Jiquan (H 1), Binao (LI 14), Qingling (H 2) and Tianfu (Lu 3); knead Bingfeng (SI 12), Tianzong (SI 11), Jianzhen (SI 9), Quchi (LI 11) and Hegu (LI 4) with the fingers.

Tendosynovitis of the long head of the biceps brachii muscle

Principal signs and symptoms are swelling and pain of the front of the shoulder and restricted abduction of the arm. In TCM, it is also called stickiness or lengthening of Tendon Collaterals.

Etiology: Direct impact or bruising of the front of the shoulder joint; tugging or wrenching of Tendon Collaterals around the shoulder joint; stagnation of Vital Energy and Blood, body fluid stasis from persistent overwork or repeated trauma; attack of Wind-Cold-Dampness.

Diagnosis & Treatment

1. Stagnation of Vital Energy and stickiness of Tendon Collaterals

Signs & Symptoms: Protruding and stringy tightening of Tendon Collaterals at the front tip of the shoulder, tenderness, pain, spasm, weighted sensation, feebleness. The tendon is hard, thick and ridged. When raised, the arm drops weakly. Pain is alleviated when the arm is raised and supported. There is tenderness at Yunmen (Lu 2) and Zhongfu (Lu 1).

Therapeutic Principle: Dredge Meridians, activate Collaterals, relax spasm, relieve pain.

Principal Measure: Pinch the arm with nipping and kneading; knead and grasp Three Yin Meridians of the Hand, twist the arm with rocking and jerking, pull the arm to abduct the shoulder, pull the arm with rotating and rectifying.

Subordinate Measure: Pinch and grasp Fengchi (GB 20) 20; knead Dazhui (GV 14), Jianjing (GB 21), Bingfeng (SI 12), Jianzhen (SI 9), Yunmen (Lu 2) and Zhongfu (Lu 1) with the fingers; nip and grasp Quze (Per 3), Quchi (LI 11) and Hegu (LI 4).

2. Blood stasis and lengthening of Tendon Collaterals

Signs & Symptoms: Swelling, weighted pain and tenderness at the front of the shoulder, requiring support and immobilization; alleviation in the day and aggravation at night — the pain is not relieved by rest or lying in bed; feebleness, restricted physical activity, the tendon is lengthened, sometimes with lumps or nodes.

Therapeutic Principle: Activate Blood, resolve stasis, soften and toughen Tendon Collaterals.

Principal Measure: Pinch the arm with nipping and kneading, roll the arm with pushing and grasping, knead the shoulder with both hands, round-rub the periphery of the shoulder with your hand, pinch and grasp the Three Yang Meridians of the Hand, pull the arm with rotating and rectifying.

Subordinate Measure: Pinch and grasp Fengchi (GB 20), Yunmen (Lu 2), Bingfeng (SI 12), Jiquan (H 1) and Binao (LI 14); knead Jianjing (GB 21), Jugu (LI 16), Jianyu (LI 15), Jianzhongshu (SI 15), Jianwaishu (SI 14) and Tianzong (SI 11) with the fingers.

Traumatic syndrome of the supraspinatus muscle

Among the muscles around the shoulder joint, the supraspinatus is the most susceptible to injury from an outside force or to suffer degenerative changes. The traumatic syndrome includes traumatic tendinitis, localized pain below the acromion from partial laceration or calcification, intense/crushing pain when the arm is abducted near or past horizontal, restricted range of movement. In TCM, it is called tendon spasm or tendon nodulation.

Etiology: Injury or laceration of tendons from exertion resulting in Vital Energy stagnation and Blood stasis. Protracted stagnation leads to rigidity of tendons and muscles, even tendon nodulation.

Diagnosis & Treatment

1. Tendon spasm from stagnation of Vital Energy

Signs & Symptoms: Weighty pain in the shoulder, especially at Jianyu (LI 15); cramping along Yangming Tendinomuscular Meridian of the Hand from the neck, shoulder and lateral upper arm to Zhouliao (LI 12); when palpated, the tendon is stringy and tight; tenderness at Bingfeng (SI 12) and Fufen (UB 41); restricted abduction of arm because of pain.

Therapeutic Principle: Relax Tendon, rectify Vital Energy, eliminate spasm, relieve pain.

Principal Measure: Pinch the arm with nipping and kneading; roll the arm with pushing and grasping; twist the shoulder joint by supporting the elbow; pluck and grasp Three Yang Meridians of the Hand; drag, tug and stretch the elbow; rotate the arm and rectify the fingers; rub the periphery of the shoulder with joined hands.

Subordinate Measure: Pinch and grasp Fengchi (GB 20), Jiquan (H 1), Binao (LI 14), Qingling (H 2), Shouwuli (LI 13), Shaohai (H 3) and Quchi (LI 11); knead and vibrate Jianwaishu (SI 14), Quyuan (SI 13), Bingfeng (SI 12) and Tianzong (SI 11); nip and knead Yangxi (LI 5) and Hegu (LI 4).

2. Tendon nodulation from Blood stasis

Signs & Symptoms: Aching with feeling of weight at Jianyu (LI 15), lateral upper arm, the neck, the shoulder, and the back of the shoulder where the tendon protrudes. Restricted ability to raise the arm, with stabbing or crushing pain at Jianyu (LI 15) when the arm is abducted. Pain increases as the arm is raised higher. If the arm has been abducted above the horizontal, or if it is helped and lifted, the pain may disappear or diminish, but as soon as help is withdrawn, the arm drops and the pain returns. When palpated, the tendon is ridged, thick, rigid and stringy. There is tenderness at Bingfeng (SI 12) and Fufen (UB 41).

Therapeutic Principle: Dredge Meridians, activate Collaterals, promote Blood flow, resolve stasis, soften Tendons, dissipate nodules, ease joints and apertures.

Principal Measure: Pinch the arm with nipping and kneading, twist the arm with rocking and jerking, pluck points around the shoulder with the fingers, pluck and grasp Three Yang Meridians of the Hand, pull the arm with rotating and rectifying, round-rub the local area with the hands.

Subordinate Measure: Nip and grasp Fengchi (GB 20); knead Fengfu (GV 16), Dazhui (GV 14), Fengmen (UB 12), Bingfeng (SI 12), Jianliao (TW 14) and Jianzhen (SI 9) with the fingers; nip and knead Quchi (LI 11) and Hegu (LI 4).

Subacromial bursitis

This inflammation is usually the result of trauma. Swelling and pain restrict the rotating and abduction of the arm.

Etiology: Yangming and Taiyin Tendinomuscular Meridians connect with Shaoyang Tendinomuscular Meridian and pass by Jianyu (LI 15); various Tendon Collaterals are attached to the shoulder joint, which is one of the Eight Void Apertures. The normally smooth and free movement is due to the moistening and lubricating action of the synovial fluid and the abundant supply of Vital Energy and Blood. When stagnation of Vital Energy and stasis of Blood persist, adhesion and rigidity of tendons and muscles follow, resulting in restricted movement.

Diagnosis & Treatment

Signs & Symptoms: When palpated, the swollen deltoid muscle is round and plump as if pumped with air; occasional pressure-resistant stringy tightness and protrusion of the tendon at the front of the upper arm, under the shoulder tip. Abduction, adduction and rotating of the arm are restricted.

Therapeutic Principle: Resolve Tendons, rectify joints, activate Blood, remove stasis, relax spasm, relieve pain.

Principal Measure: Pinch the arm with nipping and kneading, knead the arm with pushing and grasping, hold the arm to drag the shoulder joint, pull the arm to abduct the shoulder joint, twist the arm with rocking and jerking, knead and pinch Six Meridians of the Hand.

Subordinate Measure: Pinch and grasp Fengchi (GB 20), Yunmen (Lu 2), Tianliao (TW 15), Zhongfu (Lu 1), Jianjing (GB 21), Qingling (H 2) and Binao (LI 14); knead Jugu (LI 16), Jianyu (LI 15), Bingfeng (SI 12), Tianzong (SI 11), Naoshu (SI 10) and Jianzhen (SI 9) with the fingers.

Traumatic omoarthritis

This is a very commonly encountered disorder. Injury to the soft tissue around the shoulder joint, its capsule, or the synovial membrane from outside force brings an inflammatory reaction and a series of signs and symptoms.

Etiology: Impact, spraining or violent tugging of the shoulder results in stagnation and stasis of Vital Energy, Blood and fluids in a localized area. Without proper treatment, injured tissues may stick together and become hardened and rigid.

Diagnosis & Treatment

Signs & Symptoms: Intense pain at the shoulder joint with fear of moving it; the arm droops beside the body and needs help and support; swelling is most prominent at the front edge of the armpit; fullness in the supraclavicular fossa or Quepen (St 12) and Tianchi (Per 1); cramping and stringy tightness of tendons and muscles around the shoulder tip, which are resistant to pressing.

Therapeutic Principle: Relax spasm, relieve pain, dredge Meridians, activate Collaterals, resolve Tendons, rectify joints, promote Blood flow, remove stasis.

Early Stage

Principal Measure: Pinch the arm with nipping and kneading; knead the arm with pushing and grasping; hold the arm to drag the shoulder joint and pluck Collaterals; pluck, vibrate, and knock the neck; push the back with pinching and grasping; knead and round-rub points around the shoulder; twist the arm with rocking and jerking; twist and rectify the Six Meridians of the Hand.

Subordinate Measure: Pinch and grasp Fengchi (GB 20), Yunmen (Lu 2), Tianliao (TW 15), Zhongfu (Lu 1), Jianjing (GB 21), Qingling (H 2), Binao (LI 14), Jianzhen (SI 9) and Jianyu (LI 15); pluck Naoshu (SI 10) and Bingfeng (SI 12) with the fingers; vibrate Jianzhongshu (SI 15), Jianwaishu (SI 14), Tianzong (SI 11) and Fufen (UB 41) with the palms.

Intermediate Stage

Principal Measure: Knead the arm with pushing and grasping; knead, rub and round-rub the shoulder; pinch, grasp and knead the neck; push, rub and press the back; revolve Shenshu (UB 23) and Mingmen (GV 4) with the forearm; pull the arm with rotating and rectifying; twist the arm with rocking and jerking.

Subordinate Measure: Knead and pinch Fengchi (GB 20), Quepen (St 12) and Jianjing (GB 21), Zhongfu (L 1) and Jugu (LI 16), Tianzong (SI 11) and Jianliao (TW 14), Jianzhen (SI 9) and Jianyu (LI 15); grasp Quchi (LI 11) and Xiaohai (SI 8); dot Zusanli (St 36), Waiguan (TW 5) and Hegu (LI 4).

For treatment in the Advanced Stage, refer below to Shoulder joint adhesion.

Shoulder joint adhesion

Adhesion of the shoulder joint is often encountered in people of middle age and older. It is characterized by difficulty in raising the arm, possible rigidity of the shoulder, and chronic pain around the periphery. In addition to disorders of the joint itself, it is caused by injuries to peripheral tissues or by other factors, such as Cold, overexertion, or prolonged immobility. By the time a patient realizes there is impairment to the shoulder joint, it is often too late to learn the exact time or cause of the onset.

Etiology: Tendons connect with joints, and joints belong to bones. Kidney is in charge of bones, but its function declines in middle age. After that time, Kidney may not produce sufficient essence to nourish bones, joints and Tendons, and also nourish Liver. In this situation, trauma, persistent overwork, or attack of exogenous evils may lead to adhesion of the shoulder joint.

Diagnosis & Treatment

1. Rigidity of the joint from Blood stasis

Signs & Symptoms: Weighty aching and swelling of the shoulder, spasm in related tendons and muscles; reluctance to move, the joint is sticky and no longer smooth, gradual decrease in range of motion of the arm; pain is alleviated only by letting the arm hang and is more intense at night. Inability to lie on the diseased side or sleep well. Tenderness at Yunmen (L 2), Jianjing (GB 21), Quyuan (SI 13), Tianzong (SI 11), Jianyu (LI 15) and Naoshu (SI 10). Attempts to move the arm passively in a wider-than-usual range moves the shoulder but not the arm, and aggravates pain.

Therapeutic Principle: Relax Tendons and muscles, activate Blood, eliminate stasis, slacken the joint, dredge adhesion.

Principal Measure: Pinch the arm with nipping and kneading, knead the arm with holding and grasping, pull the arm and knead points around the shoulder with your fingers, rotate and rectify the Six Meridians of the Hand, twist the arm with rocking and jerking, revolve the back and the waist with the forearm, scratch the back.

Subordinate Measure: Pluck Fengfu (GV 16), Yunmen (Lu 2), Jianyu (LI 15), Jianliao (TW 14), Jianzhen (SI 9) and Naoshu (SI 10) with the fingers; pinch and grasp Fengchi (GB 20), Qingling (H 2), Binao (LI 14), Jiquan (H 1), Tianfu (Lu 3), Quchi (LI 11), Shaohai (H 3), Neiguan (Per 6), Waiguan (TW 5), Hegu (LI 4) and Houxi SI 3).

2. Adhesion of the joint from stagnation of Vital Energy

Signs & Symptoms: Localized pain in the shoulder, stringy spasm of related tendons and muscles; restricted movement but with definite range of motion remaining; migratory mild pain; minimal pain when patient carries something with the arm down; discomfort in sleep only when local area is pressed; desire to move slowly; passive movement of the arm may temporarily increase range of comfortable motion.

Therapeutic Principle: Slacken the joint, dredge the stagnated Vital Energy.

Principal Measure: Pinch the arm with nipping and kneading, pull the arm with rotating and rectifying, knead the shoulder with both hands, twist the arm with rocking and jerking, pull the arm to abduct the shoulder joint, support the elbow to twist the shoulder joint, hold the arm to drag the shoulder joint, roll the arm with pushing and grasping.

Subordinate Measure: Knead and pinch Fengchi (GB 20), Yunmen (Lu 2), Tianliao (TW 15), Zhongfu (Lu 1), Jianyu (LI 15) and Jianzhen (SI 9); nip and knead Jiquan (H 1), Qingling (H 2), Zhouliao (LI 12), Quchi (LI 11) and Hegu (LI 4).

3. Adhesion of the joint from exogenous attack

Signs & Symptoms: Weighty pain in the shoulder, desire for warmth, aversion to cold; pain is progressively aggravated on wet days; symptoms increase at night; atrophy of muscles and stiffness of connective tissue at localized area; spasm, joint rigidity and restricted range of motion; chilly sensation inside joint; insomnia from intense pain.

Therapeutic Principle: Warm Meridians, dredge Collaterals, expel Wind and Cold, relieve spasm and pain, slacken the shoulder joint.

Principal Measure: Pinch the arm with nipping and kneading, grab and grasp the joint, pluck and grasp the Six Meridians of the Hand, roll the arm with pushing and grasping, hold the arm to drag the joint, support the elbow to twist the shoulder, pull the arm to abduct the shoulder, twist the arm with rocking and jerking, pull the arm with rotating and rectifying, scratch the back.

Subordinate Measure: Pinch and grasp Fengchi (GB 20), Yunmen (Lu 2), Jianjing (GB 21), Zhongfu (Lu 1), Bingfeng (SI 12), Jiquan (H 1), Binao (LI 14), Qingling (H 2) and Tianfu (Lu 3); knead Jianzhongshu (SI 15), Jianwaishu (SI 14), Quyuan (SI 13), Tianzong (SI 11), Naoshu (SI 10), Quchi (LI 11) and Hegu (LI 4) with your fingers.

In slackening the adhesion of a shoulder joint, the force applied should be proportionate to the condition, the patient's constitutional state and ability to endure the manipulations. Before proceeding, explain the techniques to be used and aggravation of pain which will occur. After the techniques are completed, instruct the patient in subsequent exercise of the joint — raising the hand to reach a high object 2-3 times daily is useful to relieve pain and improve the range of motion.

Traumatic brachial plexus neuritis

This is usually caused by tugging of the shoulder and neck, or injury to the minor articulations of the cervical vertebrae. The injury involves or directly damages the brachial plexus, resulting in intense radiating pain at the neck, shoulder and arm, or partial paralysis. In TCM, it is called the Quepen (St 12) Syndrome.

Etiology: Quepen is a converging point of Tendons and Meridians, and an Aperture with abundant Vital Energy and Blood. If the neck is twisted or bent abruptly, or the shoulder and neck are sprained by impact, or the arm is hyper-extended, there will be Vital Energy stagnation and Blood stasis at Quepen.

Diagnosis & Treatment

1. Injury to Tendinomuscular Meridians

Signs & Symptoms: Weighty distress of the shoulder and neck with spasms of sharp, intolerable pain radiating along the neck, shoulder and arm; swelling and fullness at Quepen, the subclavicular fossa and the front edge of the armpit which are resistant to pressing. Generally, the head inclines toward the afflicted side. If the neck and shoulder are disturbed suddenly or there is uncoordinated respiratory motion, there is very severe pain, which leads to disorder of Heart Energy, anxiety, restlessness, shortness of breath, palpitations and spontaneous perspiration.

Therapeutic Principle: Relax Tendons and muscles, relieve spasms and pain, resolve stasis, dredge to reduce stagnation.

Principal Measure: Knead and pinch Fengchi (GB 20); pull, push and knead the neck; pluck, vibrate, and knock the neck; pinch the arm with nipping and kneading; knead the arm with pushing and grasping; press and push the clavicular fossae; pull the arm with rotating and rectifying; push and rub the back and waist.

Subordinate Measure: Knead Fengfu (GV 16), Yamen (GV 15), Dazhui (GV 14), Fengmen (UB 12), Bingfeng (SI 12), Jianjing (GB 21), Jianyu (LI 15), Jianzhen (SI 9), Zhongfu (Lu 1), Yunmen (Lu 2) and Qihu (St 13) with the fingers; grasp Jiquan (H 1), Qingling (H 2), Shaohai (H 3), Quchi (St 13) and Hegu (LI 4).

2. Injury to Meridians and Collaterals

Signs & Symptoms: Vague, weighty pain and aching, or no pain in the affected part; the arm hangs loosely by the side; widened articular cavity of the shoulder; atrophy and flaccidity of related tendons and muscles; feebleness of the arm; numbness or tingling at the fingertips; the neck is stiff and held erect. Distress and numbness are aggravated if the neck is rotated or bent to either side.

Principal Measure: Pull, push and knead the neck; pluck, vibrate, and knock the neck; knead the arm with pushing and grasping; twist the arm with rocking and jerking; push and press the clavicular fossae; revolve the back and waist with the forearm; rectify the fingers; pinch and grasp the Six Meridians of the Hand.

Subordinate Measure: Knead Fengchi (GB 20), Fengfu (GV 16), Yamen (GV 15), Dazhui (GV 14), Fengmen (UB 12), Tianliao (TW 15), Jianjing (GB 21), Zhongfu (Lu 1), Yunmen (Lu 2) and Bingfeng (SI 12) with the fingers; pinch and grasp Jianyu (LI 15) and Jianzhen (SI 9), Qingling (H 2) and Shouwuli (LI 13), Quchi (LI 11) and Shaohai (H 3).

N.B. Prior to treatment, clavicular fracture and numbness due to other causes should be ruled out carefully through clinical examination.

Dislocation of the shoulder

When the shoulder is dislocated, the caput humeri is displaced either into the armpit, under the front of the shoulder tip, or under the clavicle.

Dislocation of the shoulder is often accompanied by laceration or fracture of the bone. These should be identified carefully in clinical practice. Posterior and superior dislocation of the caput humeri are beyond the scope of manual repositioning and should be treated orthopedically.

Etiology: The shoulder joint is enclosed, tough and rich in Vital Energy and Blood, with a wide range of motion. It is solidified by excessive Yang, but is Deficient in compactness of Yin, since the armpit beneath it is empty. Falling, sudden strain or tugging may damage the solidity of the Yang. In those who are old and weak, in whom Yang solidity is impaired, abduction or stretching the arm may cause dislocation of the shoulder.

Diagnosis & Treatment

1. Complete dislocation

Signs & Symptoms: Depression at Jianyu (LI 15), protrusion of the acromion, spasm and pain in the tendons and muscles around the shoulder, reluctance to move; the caput humeri may be felt in the armpit, or in the subclavicular fossa, or under the front of the shoulder tip. In serious cases, there may be numbness of the fingers. The arm hangs or is held slightly out, requiring support and immobilization.

Therapeutic Principle: Reposition the joint, relieve pain.

Prescription: There are three approaches to use, the choice depending on the extent of injury and the patient's constitution.

A. Face the patient who is sitting in a stable posture.

Press one arm into the armpit of the affected shoulder and hold and lift the joint with your elbow. Pinch and grasp the dislocated part and reposition the caput humeri while abducting the upper arm.

B. With the patient sitting, stand on the side of the affected shoulder.

Raise one knee to prop the caput humeri up, tug the arm with one hand, pinch and grasp the dislocated part with the other to reposition by lifting while abducting.

C. Sit beside the patient who is supine.

Press up into the armpit with your heel and tug the arm with both hands. If the dislocation is downward, tug the arm outward. If it is a forward dislocation, tug the arm downward and reposition the caput humeri while stretching and rotating the arm in or out, whichever is the appropriate direction.

N.B. The caput humeri can only be properly repositioned by first pulling the joint apart.

2. Partial dislocation

Signs & Symptoms:: The arm is usually held out from the body and needs support from the other hand. Pain is usually localized at the front of Jianyu (LI 15) and beneath the armpit. There is reluctance to move and no obvious deformation of the shoulder.

Therapeutic Principle: Slacken the joint, relax Tendons, relieve spasm.

Prescription: Essentially the same as above, but the technique of supporting the elbow to rotate the arm should be done with less force. Techniques such as "Hold the arm to stretch the shoulder," and "Pull the arm to relax the shoulder" may also be used. After repositioning, round-rub the periphery of the joint to relieve pain.

Injury to the acromioclavicular joint

This is often seen in young and middle-aged people, and involves some tearing of the joint capsule and soft-tissue damage. There is swelling and pain above the acromion and restricted motion of the shoulder.

Etiology: The acromioclavicular joint is connected to Collaterals of Yangming and Taiyin Tendinomuscular Meridians of the Hand. It is made of cartilage and is rich in fluids and Deficient in Blood. When it is injured by an outside force, there is spasm, swelling and localized pain, and fluid retention within the joint. Without proper treatment, a firm repositioning is difficult. After healing, a local protuberance persists.

Diagnosis & Treatment

1. Joint adhesion

Signs & Symptoms: Localized hardened swelling at Jugu (LI 16); pain increases when joint is moved. Abduction of the arm brings crushing or sharp pain.

Therapeutic Principle: Divide Tendons, rectify the joint, activate Blood, resolve stasis, relieve spasm and pain.

Principal Measure: Pluck, vibrate, and knock the neck; roll the arm with pushing and grasping; twist the arm and pluck the periphery of the shoulder with the fingers; knead the shoulder with both hands; pull the arm with rotating and rectifying; hold the arm to stretch the shoulder.

Subordinate Measure: Pinch and grasp Fengchi (GB 20), Yunmen (Lu 2) and Jianjing (GB 21), Zhongfu (Lu 1) and Jugu (LI 16), Jianyu (LI 15) and Jianzhen (SI 9); knead and vibrate Dazhui (GV 14), Bingfeng (SI 12), Naoshu (SI 10) and Jianliao (TW 14); pluck and grasp Six Meridians of the Hand.

2. Joint malposition

Signs & Symptoms: Swelling at Jianyu (LI 15) and the shoulder periphery. The shoulder protrudes forward from the prominent lateral condyle of the clavicle. The arm is feeble and hangs by the side, requiring support from the other hand; reluctance to move; marked localized tenderness; palpation presents a floating sensation. The pain may radiate along the shoulder and side of the neck. Range of motion is restricted.

Therapeutic Principle: Divide Tendons, rectify and reposition the joint, activate Blood, resolve stasis, relieve spasm and pain.

Principal Measure: Pluck, vibrate, and knock the neck; knead the shoulder with both hands; press and push the clavicular fossa; pull the arm to abduct the shoulder. After these techniques are done, rectify the shoulder and reposition the joint: stretch and lift the arm slightly out from the body; deep-press the end of the clavicle with the thumb of one hand while continuing to stretch the arm and raise it to the horizontal. After this, gradually let it return to hang down freely while pressing it in to reposition the clavicle.

Subordinate Measure: After repositioning, gently pinch and knead Zhongfu (Lu 1), Yunmen (Lu 2), Jianjing (GB 21), Jugu (LI 16), Qingling (H 2), Binao (LI 14), Quze (Per 3) and Quchi (LI 11) .

After reduction: Movement such as raising the arm should be strictly avoided to prevent recurrence. After a complete dislocation, immobilize the arm at a horizontally-abducted angle. Pad a soft pillow under the armpit and wind a cloth 6 cm wide around the shoulder, including the pillow. The joint should be immobile for 1-2 weeks. Examine it every 5 days. (In some cases, the joint dislocates again and cannot be completely restored.) Massage after 2 weeks (see Joint adhesion). Even though some deformity remains, this does not necessarily affect the function of the joint, and does not require repeating a major repositioning effort.

Arthritis of the acromioclavicular joint

This is characterized by swelling, pain and heat at the joint, followed by local hyperplasia and protrusion. At times, the pain will inhibit respiration, coughing and movement of the arm. This condition is often seen in young or middle-aged women. Except in cases of obvious trauma, it is often associated with strain or rheumatism.

Etiology: The acromioclavicular joint is rich in fluids and Deficient in Blood; it is closely connected and relatively immobile. Contusion or strain can damage the joint, resulting in spasm of tendons and muscles, and accumulation of Vital Energy and fluids. Also, attack of Wind-Cold-Dampness may lead to localized heat, swelling and pain.

Diagnosis & Treatment

1. Joint stickiness from Vital Energy stagnation and Blood stasis

Signs & Symptoms: In addition to those mentioned above, there is a sharp pain at the joint which may be alleviated by pressing.

Therapeutic Principle: Divide Tendons, rectify the joint, dredge and promote the flow of Vital Energy and Blood, resolve stasis, relieve pain.

Principal Measure: Pull, push and knead the neck; hold the arm to stretch the shoulder; pinch the arm with nipping and kneading; pull the arm and pluck the periphery of the shoulder with the fingers; grab and grasp the shoulder joint; twist the arm with rocking and jerking; relieve the chest by dotting and vibrating.

Subordinate Measure: Knead Qishe (SI 11), Qihu (St 13), Yunmen (Lu 2) and Zhongfu (Lu 1) with the fingers; press and push Quepen (St 12); pinch and grasp Jianjing (GB 21) and Tianliao (TW 5), Jugu (LI 16) and Bingfeng (SI 12), Fengchi (GB 20) (both sides), Fengfu (GV 16) and Tianyou (TW 16).

2. Joint adhesion from attack of Cold-Dampness.

Signs & Symptoms: In addition to those above, the area is resistant to pressing, the pain radiates along the Shaoyang Tendinomuscular Meridian of the Foot to the pectoral, or along Taiyin Tendinomuscular Meridian of the Hand to Quepen (St 12) and the front edge of the armpit. Usually accompanied by fever and aversion to cold.

Therapeutic Principle: Expel Cold, eliminate Dampness, dredge Meridians, activate Collaterals, divide Tendons, rectify joints, relieve spasm and pain.

Principal Measure: Pluck, vibrate, and knock the neck; lift and grasp the two major tendons of the shoulder; press and push the clavicular fossa, pull the arm to abduct the shoulder joint; round-rub the periphery of the shoulder with the hands; scratch the back; relax the chest by pressing and kneading.

Subordinate Measure: Knead Tianyou (TW 16), Tianchuang (SI 16), Tianding (LI 17), Qishe (St 11), Qihu (St 13), Yunmen (Lu 2), Zhongfu (Lu 1), Fengfu (GV 16), Dazhui (GV 14) and Fengmen (UB 12) with the fingers; pinch and grasp Fengchi (GB 20), Jianjing (GB 21) and Quyuan (SI 13), Jugu (LI 16) and Bingfeng (SI 12).

Traumatic arthritis of the elbow

The elbow is composed of three small joints — the humeroulnar, the humeroradial, and the radioulnar. Serious swelling or hematoma may occur from trauma because its blood supply is abundant. Injury to one joint may give rise to inflammatory changes of the others, complicating the original problem. The principal manifestations of traumatic arthritis of the elbow are swelling, hematoma, pain, spasm, and restricted range of motion.

Etiology: The elbow joint is one of the Eight Voids of the body and is rich in Vital Energy and Blood. It also connects with the Three Yin and Three Yang Tendinomuscular Meridians of the hand.

Diagnosis & Treatment

Signs & Symptoms: Swelling and pain of the joint, especially at the cubital fossa (connecting with the Jueyin Tendinomuscular Meridian of the Hand), at the medial epicondyle of the humerus (connecting with the Shaoyin Tendinomuscular Meridian of the Hand), and at the olecranon fossa (connecting with the Taiyang Tendinomuscular Meridian of the Hand); fullness or bulging of these normally concave regions; resistance to pressing; stringy spasm of related tendons and muscles; rigid flexion of the elbow; reluctance to move; aggravation of pain when the tendons are stretched.

Therapeutic Principle: In the stage of Vital Energy stagnation and Blood stasis, divide Tendons, rectify joints, relieve spasm and pain. In the stage of tissue generation and stasis elimination, dredge Meridians, activate Collaterals, promote the flow of Blood, resolve stasis, relieve pain and spasm.

A. Stage of Vital Energy stagnation and Blood stasis (Prescription 1)

Principal Measure: Pinch and grasp Six Meridians of the Hand, knead and pinch the elbow joint.

Subordinate Measure: Nip and grasp Jiquan (H 1) and Binao (LI 14), Qingling (H 2) and Shouwuli (LI 13), Shaohai (H 3) and Quchi (LI 11), Quze (Per 3) and Zhouliao (LI 12), Chize (Lu 5) and Tianjing (TW 10), Neiguan (Per 6) and Waiguan (TW 5).

B. Stage of tissue generation and stasis elimination (Prescription 2)

Principal Measure: Knead and pinch the elbow joint; pull the elbow with pinching and grasping; hold and rotate the arm; twist and rock the elbow; hold, grasp and bend the elbow; stretch, drag and tug the elbow; rectify the fingers.

Subordinate Measure: Pinch and knead Jiquan (H 1), Tianquan (Per 2) and Binao (LI 14), Qingling (H 2) and Shouwuli (LI 13), Xiaohai (SI 8) and Chize (Lu 5), Shaohai (H 3) and Quchi (LI 11), Tianjing (TW 10) and Quze (Per 3), Neiguan (Per 6) and Waiguan (TW 5); nip Hegu (LI 4) and Yangchi (TW 4).

Adhesion of the elbow after trauma

Improper or neglected treatment after injury to the elbow can result in fibrous adhesion through return of inflammation. The joint remains rigid, and range of motion is restricted or absent.

Etiology: Extended immobilization or suspension of the injured elbow leads to stickiness of blood and fluids within the joint.

Diagnosis & Treatment

1. Injury to the elbow and Blood stasis

Signs & Symptoms: Prolonged, persistent and diffused swelling of the joint; fullness, distension and hardness at the cubital fossa; localized dampness and heat; aversion to cold, desire for warmth. Pain subsides by day and increases at night.

Therapeutic Principle: Divide Tendons, rectify the joint, dredge and promote the flow of Vital Energy, activate Blood, resolve stasis.

Principal Measure: Pull the elbow with pushing and grasping; stretch, drag and tug the elbow; round-rub the elbow with the hands; knead the arm along the Three Yin Meridians of the Hand with your fingers, from Tianfu (Lu 3) to Kongzui (Lu 6), from Qingling (H 2) to Shenmen (H 7), and from Tianquan (Per 2) to Neiguan (Per 6) respectively, until the tendons are flexible and the pain is relieved.

Subordinate Measure: Pinch and grasp Quze (Per 3) and Zhouliao (LI 12), Shaohai (H 3) and Quchi (LI 11), Chize (Lu 5) and Tianjing (TW 10), Hegu (LI 4) and Houxi (SI 3).

2. Spasm of Tendons and rigidity of elbow

Signs & Symptoms: No evident swelling of the joint except localized tumescence at the cubital fossa; stringy spasm of tendons and muscles with distinct space between bones; rigidity and thickening likely at the spot where Jueyin or Taiyin Tendinomuscular Meridians connect; pain and tenderness; resistance to pressing; restricted range of motion.

Therapeutic Principle: Relax Tendons and muscles, activate Blood, resolve stasis, slacken the joint, relieve spasm, benefit the elbow.

Principal Measure: Knead and pinch the elbow joint; hold and rotate the arm; stretch, drag and tug the elbow; round-rub the elbow with your hands; lay stress on the cubital fossa where Jueyin, Taiyin and Shaoyin Tendinomuscular Meridians connect.

Subordinate Measure: Nip and grasp Jiquan (H 1) and Binao (LI 14), Tianfu (Lu 3) and Xiaoluo (TW 12), Qingling (H 2) and Shouwuli (LI 13),

Shaohai (H 3) and Quchi (LI 11), Xiaohai (SI 8) and Chize (Lu 5), Neiguan (Per 6) and Waiguan (TW 5), Hegu (LI 4) and Houxi (SI 3).

Traumatic fascitis of the elbow

This is characterized by swelling and spasm of the fascia at the cubital fossa, and restricted range of motion due to pain.

Etiology: Fascial injury or strain from tugging, overexertion or continual flexion. Most injuries occur at Taiyang and Jueyin Tendinomuscular Meridians of the Hand at the cubital fossa, and pain is localized there.

Diagnosis & Treatment

Signs & Symptoms: The elbow joint is usually stretched or slightly flexed; mild swelling; stringy spasm and aching of cubital tendons and muscles; small, broken tubers or nodules may be felt on the surface of the tendons. There is intense cutting pain when the patient attempts to move the joint, which subsides after bending and stretching. After this, the pain gradually increases and range of movement is restricted. When the elbow is moved passively, there is no feeling of stiffness, and repeated passive flexion and extension causes a decreasing amount of pain.

Therapeutic Principle: Relax Tendons and muscles, dredge and promote the flow of Vital Energy and Blood, relieve spasm and pain.

Principal Measure: Nip and knead the elbow joint, pinch and grasp the Three Yin and Three Yang Meridians of the Hand, rectify the arm, restore the elbow, rectify the fingers.

Subordinate Measure: Knead Jianjing (GB 21), Jianyu (LI 15), Quchi (LI 11), Shaohai (H 3), Zhouliao (LI 13), Chize (Lu 5), Quze (Per 3), Xiaohai (SI 8) and Neiguan (Per 6).

Tennis elbow

Injury of the radial elbow joint is named for its occurrence in tennis players, but is common with people who use their elbows in their work. It brings local swelling and pain and restricted motion and ability to lift objects. It may be classified as lateral humeral epicondylitis, inflammation or strain of the extensor carpi radialis muscle, or radiohumeral arthritis.

Etiology: Yangming Tendinomuscular Meridian connects and joins the elbow on the lateral side. When this tendon is injured by impact, tugging, wrenching or strain, or attacked by Wind-Cold-Dampness, tennis elbow occurs.

Diagnosis & Treatment

1. Blood stasis and tendon adhesion

Signs & Symptoms: Swelling and protrusion at Quchi (LI 11) or the lateral end of the transverse crease of the elbow; intermittent dull pain or weighty aching; aversion to cold, desire for warmth; stringy spasm of tendons and muscles; bending the elbow causes pain; clenching the fists and rotating the forearm causes cutting pain. Ultimately, tendon adhesion develops into a hardened protrusion, and is extremely painful when pressed.

Therapeutic Principle: Dredge Meridians, activate Collaterals, relieve spasm and pain, promote the flow of Blood, eliminate stasis, soften Tendons, dissipate adhesion.

Principal Measure: Pinch and grasp points on the Three Yin and Three Yang Meridians of the Hand; nip and grasp the elbow joint; restore the elbow; rectify the arm; rotate the elbow with the hands; stretch, drag and tug the elbow joint.

Subordinate Measure: Knead and pinch Zhouliao (LI 12), Shouwuli (LI 13), Quze (Per 3), Shaohai (H 3), Tianying (Ashi point), Quchi (LI 11), Shousanli (LI 10), Shanglian (LI 9), and Xialian (LI 8) sequentially; lay stress on Quchi (LI 11), and repeat manipulations until tendon adhesion softens and pain has been relieved.

2. Vital Energy stagnation and tendon stickiness

Signs & Symptoms: Weighty aching on the outside of the forearm or along the pathway of the Yangming Tendinomuscular Meridian; feebleness in flexion of the joint; clenching the fist, flexing the wrist or rotating the forearm causes intense pain; boat-shaped hardened tumescence of tendons and muscles, and sometimes nodules or tubercles, may be felt by palpation; desire for being pressed. Ultimately, the tendons and muscles rise, become thick and rigid.

Therapeutic Principle: Soften Tendons, ease joint, dredge Meridians, activate Collaterals, relieve spasm and pain.

Principal Measure: Nip and grasp the elbow joint; rectify the arm; restore the elbow; rectify fingers; stretch, drag and tug the elbow; twist and rock the elbow; hold the hand to bend the elbow.

Subordinate Measure: Knead Jianyu (LI 15), Zhouliao (LI 12), Shousanli (LI 10), Shaohai (H 3), Quchi (LI 11), Quze (Per 3) and Waiguan (TW 5).

3. Blood stasis and joint stickiness

Signs & Symptoms: Elbow is slightly flexed, and extension is restricted by pain; passive stretching causes crushing pain, especially intense when the forearm is forcibly rotated; palpation reveals indistinct joint interspace; thickness and roughness of fascia; tenderness along the lateral side of the elbow, particularly at Quchi (LI 11), Zhouliao (LI 12) and Xiaohai (SI 8).

Therapeutic Principle: Slacken the joint, dredge and promote the flow of Vital Energy and Blood, divide Tendons, rectify joint, relieve spasm and pain.

Principal Measure: Restore the elbow; pinch and grasp the Three Yin and Three Yang Meridians of the Hand; rectify the arm; rectify the fingers; nip and grasp the elbow joint; rotate the elbow with the hands; roll the elbow with the hand and revolve with the forearm; stretch, drag and tug the elbow joint.

Subordinate Measure: Nip and grasp Tianyang (Ashi point), Shouwuli (LI 13), Shaohai (H 3), Zhouliao (LI 12), Jianyu (LI 15) and Jianjing (GB 21).

Dislocation of the elbow joint

This is often seen clinically, is caused by outside force, and is characterized by swelling, joint pain and loss of range of motion.

Etiology: Responding to outside force, the lower end of the humerus shifts forward while the upper end of the radius and ulna shift back, resulting in dislocation. If Tendon or Meridian Collaterals are stretched or obstructed, there is numbness of the hand and forearm.

Diagnosis & Treatment

Signs & Symptoms: The elbow is in a forced, slightly flexed position; there is swelling in the anterior cubital region where palpation reveals stringy spasm of tendons and protruding bones; the posterior of the elbow is depressed and the olecranon is pushed backwards; passive movement of the joint shows abnormal motion and impeded sensation.

Therapeutic Principle: Soften Tendons, ease joint, reposition.

Principal Measure: To relieve spasm before repositioning, pinch the arm with nipping and kneading. Hold, grasp and bend the elbow to reposition it. After this, soften the tendons and ease the joint by pulling the arm with rotating and rectifying. Instruct the patient in gentle, slow flexion-extension exercise to prevent adhesion and rigidity.

Subordinate Measure: Knead Quchi (LI 11), Chize (Lu 5), Xiaohai (SI 8), Shaohai (H 3), Shousanli (LI 10) and Hegu (LI 4) with the fingers.

Traumatic fibromyositis of the forearm flexor

This is characterized by swelling and spasm of the medial forearm with restriction of motion.

Etiology: The Three Yin Meridians of the Hand are rich in Vital Energy and Blood, and pass along the medial forearm. They are tough, thick and flexible. After injury, swelling and pain result from Vital Energy stagnation and Blood stasis. Ultimately, this results in stickiness, adhesion and rigidity of tendons and muscles.

Diagnosis & Treatment

Signs & Symptoms: Aching tendons and muscles on the medial forearm, with numbness, distension and disability; diminished ability to hold objects; exertion aggravates pain; symptoms may be relieved by flexing fingers. Later, stringy spasm and rigidity of tendons and muscles, sometimes with roughness, thickness, hardness and even tubercles discernible through palpation. Pain intensifies when affected locale is touched or pressed; fingers usually slightly bent, with flexion restricted.

Therapeutic Principle: Soften Tendons, dissipate adhesion, dredge and promote the flow of Vital Energy and Blood.

Principal Measure: Pinch and grasp the Three Yin Meridians of the Hand; restore the elbow, rectify the fingers, rectify the arm.

Subordinate Measure: Nip and knead Quze (Per 3), Shaohai (H 3), Kongzui (Lu 6) and Neiguan (Per 6).

Traumatic tendinitis of extensor carpi radialis

This is also called peripheral inflammation of the extensor carpi radialis muscle. Its principal manifestation is pain during flexion of the wrist, with restricted range of motion.

Etiology: Yangming Tendinomuscular Meridian of the Hand passes obliquely up along the forearm from Yinxi (opposite of Yangxi) and connects with Quchi (LI 11). Strain from repeated turning of the wrist, or injury from an outside force may cause Vital Energy stagnation and Blood stasis. Ultimately, there will be stickiness of tendons and muscles.

Diagnosis & Treatment

Signs & Symptoms: Swelling and pain of the tendon along the radial forearm from Pianli (LI 6) to Wenliu (LI 17); resistance to pressing; reluctance to flex the wrist; roughness, thickness and protrusion of the tendon may be felt by palpation, and crepitation may be heard.

Therapeutic Principle: Relax Tendons and muscles, activate Blood, resolve stasis, relieve spasm and pain.

Principal Measure: Rectify the wrist; pinch the arm with nipping and kneading; roll, push and grasp the arm; pull the arm with rotating and rectifying; rectify fingers; twist the arm with rocking and jerking.

Subordinate Measure: Nip and knead Jianyu (LI 15), Shouwuli (LI 13), Binao (LI 14), Quchi (LI 11), Shousanli (LI 10) and Hegu (LI 4).

Injury to the distal radioulnar articulation

This is also called injury to the ligament of the triquetral bone. It is characterized by the inability to pronate the hand or bend the wrist because of resultant pain.

Etiology: The radioulnar joint of the wrist connects and joins with the Taiyang Tendinomuscular Meridian of the Hand at Yanggu (SI 5), the Shaoyang Tendinomuscular Meridian of the Hand at Yangchi (TW 4), and the Shaoyin Tendinomuscular Meridian of the Hand at Yinxi (H 6). This joint may be injured by over-rotating the wrist while holding an object in the hand or breaking a fall by extending the hand, resulting in dislocation, Vital Energy stagnation and Blood stasis.

Diagnosis & Treatment

Signs & Symptoms: Pain at the ulnar joint with sense of weight and disability; diminished ability to hold objects; dorsiflexion and pronation intensify the pain; palpation demonstrates a floating or rocking motion of the joint. When Shenmen (H 7) is pressed, pain radiates up the ulnar side of the forearm along the Shaoyin Tendinomuscular Meridian of the Hand.

Therapeutic Principle: Divide and relax Tendons, rectify and strengthen joint, activate Blood, resolve stasis, relieve spasm and pain.

Principal Measure: Rectify the wrist, rectify the arm, rectify fingers, pull the arm with rotating and rectifying, twist the arm with rocking and jerking.

Subordinate Measure: Nip Shenmen (H 7), Tongli (H 5), Yinxi (H 6) and Shaohai (H 3).

After the manipulations described above, full recovery will be helped by wrapping the wrist to hold the caput ulnae firmly in towards the palm of the hand. Use a band of cloth 4.5 cm wide or a handkerchief.

Traumatic arthritis of the wrist

Etiology: The wrist is rich in Vital Energy, Deficient in Blood. It is the starting point of the Three Yin and Three Yang Tendinomuscular Meridians of the Hand. Signs and symptoms of traumatic arthritis vary.

Diagnosis & Treatment

1. Tendon injury

This is usually due to tugging or wrenching the wrist.

Signs & Symptoms: Swelling and pain at Yangchi (TW 4), Wangu (SI 4) and Yangxi (LI 5) where they join with the Three Yang Tendinomuscular Meridians; or at Daling (Per 7), Shenmen (H 7) and Taiyuan (Lu 9) where they join the Three Yin Tendinomuscular Meridians. These points are resistant to pressing. The hand has little strength for holding, and restricted range of motion.

Therapeutic Principle: Relax Tendons and muscles, dredge and promote the flow of Vital Energy and Blood, relieve spasm and pain.

Principal Measure: Rectify the wrist, rotate the hand, rectify the fingers, rectify the arm, twist the arm with rocking and jerking.

Subordinate Measure: Nip and knead Yangxi (LI 5), Neiguan (Per 6), Tongli (H 5), Quze (Per 3), Xiaohai (SI 8) and Qingling (H 2).

2. Joint injury

This is usually due to direct bruising.

Signs & Symptoms: Noticeable swelling and intense pain on the back of the hand, accompanied by tendon spasm involving the forearm; movement of fingers brings acute pain; restricted range of motion; protuberance of bone on the back of the wrist from dislocation; the affected area is resistant to pressing.

Therapeutic Principle: Divide Tendons, rectify joint, relax Tendons and muscles, resolve stasis, relieve pain.

Principal Measure: First, knead points connected to Tendinomuscular Meridians around the wrist to relax spasm; drag and stretch the fingers with one hand and press, grasp, deep-press and extend the injured joint with the other to assist and accomplish the repositioning. After that, rotate the hand and rectify fingers. Caution the patient to avoid holding or carrying anything of weight.

Subordinate Measure: Nip and knead Quchi (LI 11) and Chize (Lu 5); pluck Shaohai (H 3) with the fingers; knead Yangxi (LI 5), Lieque (Lu 7), Neiguan (Per 6) and Hegu (LI 4) with the fingers.

3. Joint stickiness

This is usually the result of strain.

Signs & Symptoms: Mild swelling and aching of the wrist, feebleness, restricted range of motion.

Therapeutic Principle: Slacken the joint, dredge and promote the flow of Vital Energy and Blood.

Principal Measure: Rectify the wrist, knead points around the wrist where the Six Tendinomuscular Meridians of the Hand connect with the fingers, twist the arm with rocking and jerking, pinch the arm with nipping and kneading, pull the arm with rotating and rectifying, rectify the fingers.

Subordinate Measure: Nip and grasp Jianliao (TW 14), Jianzhen (SI 9), Binao (LI 14), Shousanli (LI 10) and Hegu (LI 4).

Constrictive tenosynovitis at the styloid process of the radius.

This is a constriction of tendon sheaths of the abductor pollicis longus and extensor pollicis brevis muscles due to fibrosis from injury, resulting in restricted range of motion of the wrist and thumb.

Etiology: The Yangming Tendinomuscular Meridian of the Hand joins the styloid process of the radius. Injury from tugging or strain of the thumb can result in tenosynovitis. Ultimately, there will be constriction of the tendon sheaths.

Diagnosis & Treatment

1. Tendon stickiness

Signs & Symptoms: Swelling and pain at the back of Yuji (Lu 10) or at the styloid process of the radius; pain increases when the thumb is extended or flexed; range of motion is restricted; fullness at Yangxi (LI 5) which resists pressing; the pain may radiate up or down along the Yangming Tendinomuscular Meridian of the Hand to Xialian (LI 8), Shousanli (LI 10), Kongzui (Lu 6) and Yuji (Lu 10).

Therapeutic Principle: Relax Tendons and muscles, dredge and promote the flow of Vital Energy and Blood.

Principal Measure: Pinch and grasp the Three Yin Meridians of the Hand; pinch and grasp the Three Yang Meridians of the Hand; rectify the arms; hold the hand to stretch the wrist, bending it to the ulnar side; knead Yangxi (LI 5) with the fingers; roll the arm with pushing and grasping; twist the arm with rocking and jerking; pinch the arm with nipping and kneading.

Subordinate Measure: Pinch and grasp Tianfu (Lu 3) and Xiabai (Lu 4); nip Chize (Lu 5), Taiyuan (Lu 9), Quchi (LI 11) and Binao (LI 14).

2. Tendon adhesion

Signs & Symptoms: Swelling at the back of Yuji (Lu 10); the thumb cannot be bent or abducted; thickening of tendons and muscles may be felt by palpation; there may be an immovable, hardened protuberance on the bone at Yangxi (LI 5); intense pain and tenderness.

Therapeutic Principle: Soften Tendons, dissipate adhesion, resolve stasis, relieve pain.

Principal Measure: Pinch the arm with nipping and kneading, hold the thumb to stretch and tug it, knead Yangxi (LI 5) and the hardened protuberance with your fingers, pull the arm with rotating and rectifying, roll the arm with pushing and grasping, rectify the arm, rotate the hand, rectify the fingers.

Subordinate Measure: Pinch and grasp Tianfu (Lu 3), Xiabai (Lu 4), Chize (Lu 5), Kongzui (Lu 6), Yuji (Lu 10), Jianyu (LI 15), Shousanli (LI 10) and Hegu (LI 4).

Injury to metacarpophalangeal joints

In this disorder, injury to the thumb is the most commonly seen.

Etiology: Laceration of tendons or malposition of joints is generally caused by bruising, tugging or wrenching.

Diagnosis & Treatment

1. Injury to tendons and joints

Signs & Symptoms: Localized swelling and pain, spasm of Tendon Collaterals, localized tenderness; finger movement is restricted; stretching a finger intensifies pain.

Therapeutic Principle: Divide Tendons, rectify joints, dissipate stasis, relieve pain.

Principal Measure: Pinch the arm with nipping and kneading, pull the arm with rotating and rectifying, rectify digits. Manipulation should be done slowly and gently.

Subordinate Measure: Nip and knead Xiabai (Li 4), Binao (LI 14), Quchi (LI 11), Chize (Lu 5), Shousanli (LI 10) and Neiguan (Per 6).

2. Malposition or dislocation of finger joints

Signs & Symptoms: Deformed, shortened, swollen finger with intense pain, inability to bend or stretch.

Therapeutic Principle: Reposition, dissipate stasis, relieve pain.

Prescription: Knead and rectify the finger to relieve spasm, then rectify and stretch it with one hand, pinch and grasp the dislocated joint to reposition it. The force used should be appropriate, in order to prevent further injury through over-stretching. After repositioning, caution the patient to avoid contact with cold water, and to resist rocking, kneading or pinching the affected area.

Constrictive tenosynovitis of flexor digitorum

This refers to the sliding shift of a tendon with a snapping sound when the finger is moved, accompanied by a sliding shift of a nodule on the tendon at the palmar side of the metacarpophalangeal joint. It is also called snapping or cracking or trigger finger.

Etiology: Frequently seen in middle-aged women, especially those who work with their hands. Strained or injured tendons stick together, and gradually tendon sheaths constrict and nodules appear. This is most often seen at the thumb, the middle finger and the ring finger.

Diagnosis & Treatment

1. Early stage

Signs & Symptoms: Movement of the finger is difficult on arising, with distension and stabbing pain at the affected joint; after appropriate exercise, symptoms may ease. As the condition progresses, however, there is progressive impediment to flexion and extension, accompanied by a snapping sound and pain, and exercise has no therapeutic effect. A nodule on the palmar side of the joint which slides up or down along with the stretching or bending of the digit may be felt by palpation. A trigger or squeezing sensation may be felt.

Therapeutic Principle: Dredge and promote the flow of Vital Energy and Blood, soften Tendons, ease joints.

Principal Measure: Rectify fingers, rotate the hand, rectify the arm with nipping and kneading, roll the arm with pushing and grasping, rectify the arm.

Subordinate Measure: Nip and knead Yuji (LI 10), Hegu (LI 4), Taiyuan (Lu 9), Quchi (LI 11), Chize (Lu 5), Jianyu (LI 15) and Tianfu (Lu 3).

2. Intermediate stage

Signs & Symptoms: Passive pulling becomes necessary to start the stretching/bending of the finger, and this is accompanied by a snapping sound and pain. Symptoms are especially pronounced on waking. A bean-shaped, hardened nodule protrudes where the tendons stick together. It resists pressing and moves along with flexion and extension.

Therapeutic Principle: Dredge and promote the flow of Vital Energy and Blood, relax Tendons, soften the nodule.

Principal Measure: Pinch and grasp the Three Yin Meridians of the Hand, nip and grasp the Three Yang Meridians of the Hand, rectify the arm, pull the finger and knead the local area, roll the arm with pushing and grasping, rectify the fingers, rotate the hand.

Subordinate Measure: Nip and knead Yangxi (LI 5), Jingqu (Lu 8), Shousanli (LI 10), Xiabai (Lu 4), Binao (LI 14) and Jianyu (LI 15).

3. Late Stage

Signs & Symptoms: Spasm and rigidity of tendons force the finger into a permanently crooked posture. Stretching or bending can only be accomplished by strenuous pulling. There is a hardened nodule at the metacarpophalangeal joint with prominent local swelling and resistance to pressing.

Therapeutic Principle: Dredge and promote the flow of Vital Energy and Blood, divide Tendons, rectify joints, dissipate stasis, relieve pain.

Principal Measure: Rock fingers, rectify fingers, rotate the hand, rectify the arm, pinch and grasp the Three Yin Meridians of the Hand, nip and grasp the Three Yang Meridians of the Hand, pinch the arm with nipping and kneading, roll the arm with pushing and grasping, pull the arm with rotating and rectifying, twist the arm with rocking and jerking.

Subordinate Measure: Nip and knead Yuji (LI 10), Taiyuan (Lu 9), Hegu (LI 4), Shousanli (LI 10), Kongzui (Lu 6), Chize (Lu 5), Zhouliao (LI 12), Shouwuli (LI 13), Xiabai (Lu4) and Tianfu (Lu 3).

Injury to the neck and nape

Careless bending, turning, stretching or bruising to the neck may injure related tendons and muscles, or even joint Apertures, resulting in pain, wryneck, restricted motion, etc.

Sprained neck muscles

Etiology: Tendons and muscles of the neck may be injured by stretching, wrenching, sprain, bruising, prolonged bending of the neck or hyperextension of the arm and shoulder.

Diagnosis & Treatment

It is important to distinguish between the signs and symptoms caused by disorders of Vital Energy and Blood and those from injury to various Tendinomuscular Meridians.

A. Tendon injury and Vital Energy stagnation

Signs & Symptoms: Spasm and acute pain of tendons and muscles of the neck, wryneck which cannot be turned.

Therapeutic Principle: Relieve spasm and pain, soften Tendons, rectify Vital Energy.

B. Tendon injury and Blood stasis

Signs & Symptoms: Spasm and swelling of tendons and muscles of the nape and back, the neck cannot be turned.

Therapeutic Principle: Relax Tendons and muscles, activate Blood, resolve stasis, relieve spasm and pain.

1. Injury to the neck branch of Foot Taiyang Tendinomuscular Meridian

Signs & Symptoms: The neck is turned, bending slightly upwards and inclined to the injured side; spasm and pain or weighty sensation of tendons and muscles extends along the major tendon on the affected side of the nape. Swallowing may also be restricted.

Principal Measure: Pinch and grasp the neck (principally the Taiyang Tendinomuscular Meridian of the Foot), pull the neck, press and push the clavicular fossae; pull, push and knead the neck; pluck, vibrate and knock the neck; push and knead the shoulder and the back and Lingtai (GV 10).

Subordinate Measure: Grasp Weizhong (UB 40), Heyang (UB 55), Chengjin (UB 56), Chengshan (UB 57) and Kunlun (UB 60), all on both sides.

2. Injury to the neck branch of the Foot Shaoyang Tendinomuscular Meridian

Signs & Symptoms: The neck turns slightly and bends toward the affected side; spasm and pain of tendons and muscles extends on a line along the major tendon below the mastoid to the interior of the chest.

Principal Measure: Pull the neck; twist the neck; pull, push and knead the neck (primarily Shaoyang Tendinomuscular Meridian of the Foot); pluck, vibrate and knock the neck; revolve Huantiao (GB 30) with the elbow; press and push the clavicular fossae.

Subordinate Measure: Nip and grasp Fengchi (GB 20), Fengshi (GB 31), Xiyangguan (GB 33), Yanglingquan (GB 34), Waiqiu (GB 36), Xuanzhong (GB 39) and Qiuxu (GB 40), all on both sides.

3. Injury to the neck branch of Foot Yangming Tendinomuscular Meridian

Signs & Symptoms: The neck bends down and turns obliquely toward the affected side; spasm and pain of tendons and muscles extend along the front side of the neck and pass through Quepen (St 12) into the chest; respiratory movement is inhibited because of pain within the chest.

Principal Measure: Pull up the neck; twist the neck; press and push the clavicular fossae; arrange the shoulder; pull, push and knead the neck (primarily the Yangming Tendinomuscular Meridian of the Foot); push and knead Lingtai (GV 10) and Yingchuang (St 16).

4. Injury to the neck branch of Foot Shaoyin Tendinomuscular Meridian

Signs & Symptoms: The head is bent slightly backward and inclines toward the affected side; spasm and weighty pain of tendons and muscles extending along the major tendon of the nape to the shoulder and the back, and involving the interior of the spine; movement of the arms and shoulders is restricted.

Principal Measure: Pinch and grasp the cervical vertebrae; knead and grasp the side of the neck, (primarily Shaoyin Tendinomuscular Meridian of the Foot); twist the neck; pull up the neck; arrange the shoulder; push and knead Lingtai (GV 10).

Subordinate Measure: Knead Yuzhong (K 26), Lingxu (K 24) and Bulang (K 22); grasp Yingu (K 10), Zhubin (K 9), Fuliu (K 7) and Taixi (K 3), all on both sides.

5. Injury to the neck branch of Hand Taiyang Tendinomuscular Meridian

Signs & Symptoms: The neck bends backward and inclines toward the affected side; spasm and weighty pain of tendons and muscles extending along the back side of the neck to the back side of the arm; movement is restricted.

Principal Measure: Pull the neck; twist the neck; press and push the clavicular fossae; arrange the shoulder; restore the elbow; push and knead Lingtai (GV 10).

Subordinate Measure: Nip Houxi (SI 3), Yanglao (SI 6), Xiaohai (SI 8), Tianzong (SI 11), Jianzhen (SI 9), Shaoze (SI 1), Quyuan (SI 13) and Jianwai-shu (SI 14), all on both sides.

6. Injury to the neck branch of Hand Shaoyang Tendinomuscular Meridian

Signs & Symptoms: The neck is bent toward the injured side; spasm and pain of tendons and muscles characterized by a weighty sensation extends along the side of the neck to the shoulder and the side of the arm; fullness, distension, pain and spasm at Quepen (St 12); sore throat, restricted movement.

Principal Measure: Nip and grasp the cervical vertebrae; pinch and grasp the side of the neck; grasp both shoulders; arrange the shoulder; pull up the neck; pluck Collaterals with knocking and scratching; press and push the clavicular fossae.

Subordinate Measure: Nip Yemen (TW 2), Yangchi (TW 4), Sanyangluo (TW 8), Tianjing (TW 10), Xiaoluo (TW 12), Jianliao (TW 14) and Tianliao (TW 15), all on both sides.

7. Injury to the neck branch of Hand Yangming Tendinomuscular Meridian

Signs & Symptoms: The neck bends forward and turns toward the injured side; weighty spasm and pain of tendons and muscles extends along the major tendon on the front side of the neck to the shoulder at its connecting spot, continuing along the back, the spine and the side of the upper arm.

Principal Measure: Pull the neck; twist the neck; pull up the neck; pull, push and knead the neck; pluck, vibrate and knock the neck; push the back with pinching and grasping (principally Yangming Tendinomuscular Meridian of the Hand).

Subordinate Measure: Push and grasp Futu (LI 18), Tianding (LI 17), Jianyu (LI 15), Shouwuli (LI 13), Shousanli (LI 10), Wenliu (LI 7) and Hegu (LI 4), all on both sides.

Malposition of the minor articulations of the cervical vertebrae

This is frequently encountered in clinical practice.

Etiology: The spine is developed from the Governor Vessel Meridian, making it rich in Vital Energy and flexible. When tendons and muscles become slack and joint Apertures become loose in old age, and/or when one suffers an injury to the neck from stretching, wrenching, dodging or bumping, there will be some malposition of the minor articulations of the cervical vertebrae. Signs and symptoms are swelling, spasm, localized pain and restricted motion.

Diagnosis & Treatment

1. Malposition of articulations

Signs & Symptoms: Most malposition occurs at the 2d - 3rd or 5th - 7th cervical vertebrae; the head and neck incline toward the healthy side; the malposed vertebra protrudes and shows marked tenderness and resistance to pressing; attempts to assume a normal posture or turn the head and neck are impossible because of squeezing pain; spasm of tendons and muscles at the injured area.

Therapeutic Principle: Reposition, relax spasm, dredge and promote the flow of Vital Energy and Blood, nourish and consolidate Tendons and joints.

Principal Measure: Rub Fengchi (GB 20) with joined hands; pull, push and knead the neck; pluck, vibrate and knock the neck to reposition it. During the procedure, you should hear a snapping sound. Be sure to avoid over-stretching.

Subordinate Measure: Pinch and grasp Jianjing (GB 21) and the major tendon behind the neck; nip and knead Lieque (Lu 7) and Weizhong (UB 40); pinch and grasp the spine.

2. Tendon spasm and malposition of articulations

Signs & Symptoms: The head and neck incline toward the healthy side, or stretch and incline forward rigidly; other signs and symptoms are basically the same as those in the previous entry. When the head and neck are forced to assume their normal position, there is serious pain which radiates along the pathway of the injured Tendinomuscular Meridian.

Principal Measure: Pinch and grasp Fengchi (GB 20); pull, push and knead the neck; pluck, vibrate and knock the neck; pull up the neck; grab and grasp with Eagle's Talons; push, pinch and grasp the neck.

Subordinate Measure: Grasp Jianjing (GB 21); press and push the clavicular fossae; nip and knead Lieque (Lu 7), Hegu (LI 4) and Weizhong (UB 40).

Stiff neck

This describes aching neck, wryneck and restricted motion after sleep.

Etiology: Stiff neck is often caused by neck strain, an uncomfortable pillow, or an attack of Wind-Cold.

Diagnosis & Treatment

1. Vital Energy stagnation and Blood stasis

Signs & Symptoms: Usually involves protracted aching of the neck or frequent relapses into neck pain. The head and neck incline to the affected side and can be turned or moved only with difficulty; if passively bent to the healthy side, the pain is aggravated but still tolerable.

Therapeutic Principle: Relax Tendons and muscles, relieve spasm and pain, dredge Meridian and Collaterals, activate Blood, eliminate stasis.

Principal Measure: Pull the neck, pinch and grasp the neck, pull up the neck.

Subordinate Measure: None.

2. Blockage from Wind-Cold

Signs & Symptoms: Spasm and stiffness of Taiyang Tendinomuscular Meridian of the Foot at the nape, involving the back; weighty pain, difficulty in turning; desire for warmth, aversion to Wind-Cold.

Therapeutic Principle: Warm Meridian, dredge Collaterals, expel Wind, disperse Cold, relax Tendons, ease joints, eliminate blockage.

Principal Measure: Twist the neck; pull the neck; pull, push and knead the neck; pluck, vibrate and knock the neck; push the back with pinching and grasping (principally the back branches of Taiyang Tendinomuscular Meridian of the Foot and Yangming Tendinomuscular Meridian of the Hand).

Subordinate Measure: Rub Fengchi (GB 20) with joined hands; twist Tianying (Ashi point) with the fingers; pinch and grasp Jianjing (GB 21), Weizhong (UB 40), Chengshan (UB 57) and Kunlun (UB 60).

Cervical spondylosis

This is a type of retrograde, slowly-developing osteo-degeneration. It involves hypertrophic changes in the cervical vertebrae and degeneration of the intervertebral disks, resulting in a variety of clinical syndromes. This occurs commonly in people over 45 years of age. According to TCM, it is caused by Deficiency of Liver-Kidney Energy and malnutrition of Tendons, joints and bones.

Etiology: Vital Energy stagnation and Blood stasis at the neck due to strain; blockage of Vital Energy and Blood due to attack of Cold evil; Deficiency of Liver-Kidney Energy due to weakness and senility. Ultimately, there will be adhesion and rigidity.

Diagnosis & Treatment

1. Strain

Signs & Symptoms: Protracted neck pain or indisposition, or recurring stiff neck; symptoms aggravated after overwork or on wet days; spasm and stiffness of cervical muscles; wryneck, difficulty in turning.

Therapeutic Principle: Relax Tendons and muscles, relieve spasm and pain, dredge and promote the flow of Vital Energy and Blood, lubricate and ease joints.

Principal Measure: Pinch and grasp cervical vertebrae; press and knead the side of the neck; pull, push and knead the neck; pluck, vibrate and knock the neck; deep-press the spine with kneading and revolving.

Subordinate Measure: Grasp Jianjing (GB 21), knead Tianzong (SI 11) and Quyuan (SI 13), grasp Tianliao (TW 15) and Jianwaishu (SI 14), all on both sides.

2. Blockage caused by Cold evil

Signs & Symptoms: Weighty pain at the nape and back, aversion to cold; the pain may be alleviated by warming. There is adhesion and rigidity of the cervical tendons and muscles and difficulty in turning. Visible roughness of skin, sparseness of hair.

Therapeutic Principle: Expel Wind, disperse Cold, warm Meridians, dredge Collaterals, regulate and promote the flow of Vital Energy and Blood, soften Tendons, ease joints.

Principal Measure: Rub the sides of the neck with joined hands; pinch and grasp the cervical vertebrae; twist the neck; pluck, vibrate and knock the neck; push the back with pinching and grasping, scratch the back.

Subordinate Measure: Pinch and grasp Weizhong (UB 40), Chengjin (UB 56), Chengshan (UB 57), Kunlun (UB 60) and Taixi (K 3), all on both sides.

3. Deficiency of Liver-Kidney Energy

Signs & Symptoms: Pain and numbness at the nape and back; heavy sensation in the head; occipital headache; stickiness and stiffness of the cervical vertebrae; flaccidity, atrophy and feebleness of the tendons and muscles of the neck; numb limbs, dizziness, insomnia.

Therapeutic Principle: Warm the Middle Warmer, invigorate Vital Energy, nourish Liver-Kidney, strengthen Tendons and joints.

Principal Measure: Twist the neck; pull, push and knead the neck; pluck, vibrate and knock the neck; pluck Collaterals with knocking and scratching; deep-press the spine with kneading and revolving; strengthen the waist by rolling and rubbing; relax the chest by pressing and kneading; push the abdomen with round-rubbing and revolving; Taiji round-rub the abdomen.

Subordinate Measure: Grasp Yingu (K 10), Zhubin (K 9), Jiaoxin (K 8), Dazhong (K 4), Sanyinjiao (Sp 6), Ququan (Liv 8), all on both sides.

Injuries to the back and waist

Inflammation of the trapezius muscle

This is a soft tissue injury in the area of the back and shoulder. Adult women and people who engage in high activity with both arms often suffer from this disorder.

Etiology: Taiyang Tendinomuscular Meridian of the Foot travels along the back, and its left and right branches touch the spine from both sides, terminating at the occiput. Another branch connects with Jianyu (LI 15). Overexertion, strain or attack of Cold-Dampness may cause this injury. In time, spasm and pain along this Tendinomuscular Meridian may develop into rigidity of the back, stiff neck and weighty sensation in the shoulder.

Diagnosis & Treatment

1. Vital Energy stagnation and tendon adhesion

Signs & Symptoms: Sudden onset of sharp, tearing pain at the back and shoulder, as if being pulled when the neck or arm is moved. Stringy spasm and nodular structures may be felt at Lingtai (GV 10), where tenderness is most pronounced. Other tender points are Yuzhen (UB 9), Dazhui (GV 14), Shendao (GV 11), Zhiyang (GV9), Dazhu (UB 11), Fengmen (UB 12), Jueyinshu (UB 14) and Dushu (UB 16).

Therapeutic Principle: Eliminate stagnation and stasis, dredge and promote the flow of Vital Energy and Blood, relax Tendons and muscles, relieve spasm and pain.

Principal Measure: Pull, push and knead the neck; pluck, vibrate and knock the neck; twist the neck; push the back with pinching and grasping; deep-press the back with kneading and revolving; pluck Collaterals with knocking and scratching.

Subordinate Measure: Knead Xinshu (UB 15), Geshu (UB 17), Ganshu (UB 18), Danshu (UB 19), Pishu (UB 20), Weishu (UB 21), Shenshu (UB 23), Weizhong (UB 40) and Kunlun (UB 60), all on both sides.

2. Blood stasis and tendon adhesion

Signs & Symptoms: Stringy spasm and pain of tendons and muscles along the spine. As the condition progresses, they become rigid and hardened. There is difficulty in bending the waist, turning the head or moving the arms; anxiety about protracted sitting or lying down. In serious cases, there may be a heavy feeling in the chest, heaving of sighs, occipital headache, dizziness and somnolence.

Therapeutic Principle: Divide Tendons, rectify joints, relax the chest, ease respiration, dredge Meridians, activate Collaterals, dissipate stasis, relieve pain.

Principal Measure: Deep-press the back with kneading and revolving; push the back with pinching and grasping; pluck Collaterals with knocking and scratching; strengthen the waist by rolling and rubbing; grasp the abdomen with pinching and jerking; knead the leg with rotating and rubbing; relieve the chest by dotting and vibrating; relax the chest by pressing and kneading.

Subordinate Measure: Knead Dazhui (GV 14), Shenzhu (GV 12), Lingtai (GV 10), Zhongshu (GV 7) and Mingmen (GV 4) with the fingers.

Injury to costovertebral joints

Intercostal neuralgia often arises in cases of injury to the costovertebral joints, with wandering pain along the ribs. However, this is not a true intercostal neuralgia — its actual cause is the injury to or malposition of costovertebral joints.

Etiology: Overexertion in stretching or wrenching of the waist, bruising of the front wall of the chest, or even coughing and sneezing may be the causes of this disorder.

Diagnosis & Treatment

Signs & Symptoms: The 4th - 7th (especially 4th and 5th) ribs are most liable to injury; stabbing or tearing pain wanders and radiates along intercostal spaces; deep-pressing or stabilizing the injured joints may alleviate the pain; breathing, turning the body and coughing all aggravate the pain; often the patient presses his/her chest to minimize motion from respiration.

Therapeutic Principle: Divide Tendons, rectify joints, dredge stasis, relieve spasm and pain, relax the chest, rectify Vital Energy.

Principal Measure: Deep-press the spine with kneading and revolving; push and wipe to divide the ribs; relax the chest by pressing and kneading; pluck Collaterals with knocking and scratching; revolve the spine and back with the forearm; relieve the chest by dotting and vibrating.

Subordinate Measure: Revolve Huantiao (GB 30) with the elbow; revolve Fengshi (GB 31) with the forearm; nip and knead Yanglingquan (GB 34), Yangjiao (GB 35) and Xuanzhong (GB 39).

Injury to the back and the waist

The back and the waist are important areas of the body where Vessel and Tendinomuscular Meridians pass by, connect with each other and attach to internal organs. They are the pivot of most physical activity and susceptible to injury, resulting in such problems as stiffness and pain in the lumbar and lumbosacral regions, and thighs.

Etiology: Tendinomuscular Meridians and spinal joints may be injured by falling, quick movement, bruising, wrenching or sprain, especially in older and weaker people with Deficient Kidney Energy, and with slack tendons and joints.

Diagnosis & Treatment

1. Stiffness and pain in the lumbar region from injury to Foot Taiyang Tendinomuscular Meridian (sacrospinalis muscles)

Signs & Symptoms: Pain and spasm in the muscles and tendons of the back and waist, extending from nape to buttocks; preferred posture is with hip joints flexed and waist straight, propping the upper body with arms on thighs; squatting is difficult and motion is restricted. Tenderness at Qihaishu (UB 24), Dachangshu (UB 25), Guanyuanshu (UB 26), Xiaochangshu (UB 27), Yaoshu (GV 2) and Yaoyangguan (GV 3).

Therapeutic Principle: Relax Tendinomuscular Meridians, relieve spasm and pain, dredge Meridians, activate Collaterals, regulate and promote the flow of Vital Energy and Blood.

Principal Measure: Push the back with pinching and grasping; deep-press the spine with kneading and revolving; pluck Collaterals with knocking and scratching; jerk and pull to relax the waist; strengthen the waist by rolling and rubbing; twist to restore the waist.

Subordinate Measure: Knead and grasp Xinshu (UB 15), Geshu (UB 17), Ganshu (UB 18), Pishu (UB 20), Shenshu (UB 23), Weizhong (UB 40), Kunlun (UB 60) and Taixi (K 3), all on both sides.

2. Stiffness and pain in the lumbar region from injury to a branch of Foot Taiyang Tendinomuscular Meridian (latissimus dorsi)

Signs & Symptoms: Spasm and pain in the waist extending from shoulder to buttocks; inability to bend, stretch or turn the body; when both arms are raised, lumbar pain becomes stabbing or tearing; tenderness at Eight Liao (UB 31-34, both sides), Shenshu (UB 23), Qihaishu (UB 24) and Dachangshu (UB 25); on palpation, there is stringy spasm of tendons and muscles along Tendon branches, and nodular structures may be felt on their surface.

Therapeutic Principle: Relax Tendinomuscular Meridians, relieve spasm and pain, dredge Meridians, activate Collaterals, regulate and promote the flow of Vital Energy and Blood.

Principal Measure: Arrange the waist back-to-back, bend and deep-press the knee to stretch the waist, pull the waist straight and obliquely, strengthen the waist by rolling and rubbing, jerk and drag to relax the waist, push the back with pinching and grasping, pluck Collaterals with knocking and scratching.

Subordinate Measure: Twist Tianying (Ashi point), Sanjiaoshu (UB 22), Yaoyangguan (GV 3), Mingmen (GV 4), Guanyuanshu (UB 26), Weizhong (UB 40) and Chengshan (UB 57) with the fingers.

3. Stiffness and pain in the lumbar region from injury to Foot Yangming Tendinomuscular Meridian (quadratus lumborum muscle)

Signs & Symptoms: Spasm and pain in the waist involving the hip joint and the side of the thigh; waist is bent toward the affected side and cannot turn or be straightened; tenderness at Jinsuo (GV 8), Zhongshu (GV 7), Jizhong (GV 6), Sanjiaoshu (UB 22), Shenshu (UB 23), Qihaishu (UB 24) and Zhishi (UB 52).

Therapeutic Principle: Relax Tendinomuscular Meridian, relieve spasm and pain, dredge Meridians, activate Collaterals, regulate and promote the flow of Vital Energy and Blood.

Principal Measure: Pull the waist with jerking and dragging, strengthen the waist by rolling and rubbing, push the back with pinching and grasping, pluck Collaterals with knocking and scratching, pull the leg with knocking and vibrating, knead the leg with revolving and pinching, knead the leg with rotating and round-rubbing.

Subordinate Measure: Knead Shenzhu (GV 12), Shendao (GV 11), Zhiyang (GV 9), Tianying (Ashi point), Eight Liao (UB 31-34, both sides), Weizhong (UB 40) and Chengjin (UB 56) with the fingers.

Myofibrositis of the back and waist

Clinical manifestations of the disorder are varied and complex because pathogenic factors, location, degree of seriousness and course of disease differ.

Etiology: Injuries to tendons and muscles due to quick movement, bruising, wrenching or strain; improper treatment; attack of Cold-Dampness; Deficiency of Liver-Kidney from age or weakness. Ultimately, tendons, muscles and joints may become flaccid or stiff.

Diagnosis & Treatment

1. Vital Energy stagnation and tendon adhesion

Signs & Symptoms: Stiffness, aching, feebleness and indisposition of the back and waist; insomnia from intolerable weighty pain brought on by extended bed rest; symptoms worst on waking, alleviated by activities of the day, but overexertion brings serious pain.

Therapeutic Principle: Dredge the flow of Vital Energy, relax Tendinomuscular Meridians.

Principal Measure: Push the back with pinching and grasping; deep-press the back with kneading and revolving; strengthen the waist by rolling and rubbing; pluck Collaterals with knocking and scratching; roll the leg with knocking and vibrating; knead the leg with rotating and round-rubbing; drag the leg with plucking and grasping; pad the popliteal fossa and flex the knee, stretch and rock the ankle.

Subordinate Measure: Revolve Chengfu (UB 36) with the elbow, grasp Weizhong (UB 40), revolve the popliteal fossa with the forearm, pinch and grasp Kunlun (UB 60) and Taixi (K 3), all on both sides.

2. Blood stasis and tendon adhesion

Signs & Symptoms: Spasm, pain and stiffness in the back and waist; inability to bend forward or look up; the pain becomes localized and increased when turning; spinal joints stick up and become rigid; palpation demonstrates stringy spasm of tendons and muscles; deep colored urine, constipation, abdominal distension and indisposition.

Therapeutic Principle: Resolve stasis, dredge Collaterals, relax Tendons and muscles.

Principal Measure: Pinch and grasp the back, deep-press the back with kneading and revolving; scratch the back; push the back with pinching and grasping; strengthen the waist by rolling and rubbing; bend and deep-press the knee to stretch the waist; pull the waist straight and obliquely; rock the knee to twist the hip; pad the popliteal fossa to flex the knee; stretch and rock the ankle, pinch and grasp Six Meridians of the Foot.

Subordinate Measure: Dot Mingmen (GV 4), Yaoyangguan (GV 3) and Yaoshu (GV 2); nip and grasp Ququan (Liv 8), Yanglingquan (GB 34), Weizhong (UB 40), Kunlun (UB 60), Xingjian (Liv 2) and Dadun (Liv 1), all on both sides, all reducing.

3. Adhesion of tendon from Cold-Dampness

Signs & Symptoms: Weighty stiffness and pain in the lumbar region with difficulty in bending forward or looking up; stiffness of tendons and muscles in the back and waist with a heavy sensation; symptoms aggravated after overwork or on wet days; desire for warmth, aversion to cold; inability to sit or lie down for extended periods of time, or to walk extended distances.

Therapeutic Principle: Relax Tendons and muscles; regulate and promote the flow of Vital Energy and Blood, disperse Cold, eliminate Dampness, dissipate stasis, relieve pain.

Principal Measure: Strengthen the waist by rolling and rubbing; revolve Shenshu (UB 23) and Zhishi (UB 52) with the forearm; restore the waist back-to-back; pull the waist straight and obliquely; pull the waist with jerking and dragging; push the back with pinching and grasping; deep-press the spine with kneading and revolving; pluck Collaterals with knocking and scratching; drag the leg with plucking and grasping; pull the leg with knocking and vibrating.

Subordinate Measure: Revolve Yinmen (UB 37) with the forearm; grasp Weiyang (UB 39), Fuyang (UB 59), Chengshan (UB 57), Feiyang (UB 58), Yangfu (GB 38) and Kunlun (UB 60), all on both sides.

4. Pain and stiffness in the lumbar region from Kidney Deficiency

Signs & Symptoms: Soreness of the back and waist with muscular atrophy and feebleness; serious weighty pain when bending forward or looking up; pressing alleviates symptoms; cold limbs, lassitude, clear urine, loose stool.

Therapeutic Principle: Regulate and promote the flow of Vital Energy and Blood, warm the Middle Warmer, invigorate Kidney, soften Tendons, rectify joints.

Principal Measure: Revolve the back with the forearm, push the back with pinching and grasping, pluck Collaterals with knocking and scratching, strengthen the waist by rolling and rubbing, revolve Shenshu (UB 23) and Zhishi (UB 52) with the forearm, rock the knee to twist the hip joint, roll the leg with revolving and pinching, knead the leg with rotating and round-rubbing, pinch and grasp the Three Yin Meridians of the Foot, pinch and grasp the Three Yang Meridians of the Foot.

Subordinate Measure: Nip and knead Weizhong (UB 40), Chengjin (UB 56) Chengshan (UB 57), Taixi (K 3) and Kunlun (UB 60), all on both sides, all invigorating.

Injury to minor articulations of the lumbar vertebrae

This is often seen in young and middle-aged people, and is easily misdiagnosed as prolapsed disk. Its clinical manifestations are acute stiffness and pain in the lumbar region accompanied by leg pain.

Etiology: Malposition of the lumbar vertebral joint or injury to related tendons and muscles. Governor Vessel Meridian is in charge of the lumbar vertebrae, and the leg pain may be classified as that of Taiyang, Yangming and Shaoyang Tendinomuscular Meridians of the Foot according to their pathways.

Diagnosis & Treatment

1. Injury to joint and Vital Energy stagnation

Signs & Symptoms: Deep, crushing pain at the injured spot; stringy spasm of related tendons and muscles with reluctance to move; the waist bends towards the unaffected side and cannot be straightened; coughing or relaxing of the waist aggravates pain; the spinal process of the injured vertebra is resistant to pressing. On knocking and shaking examination, the lateral vibration of the injured vertebra is strongest. Leg pain will appear if symptoms persist for 3-5 days.

Therapeutic Principle: Reposition, dredge to promote the flow of Vital Energy, relax Tendons, resolve stasis, relieve pain.

Principal Measure: Jerk and drag to relax the waist, bend and deep-press the knee to stretch the waist, restore the waist back-to-back, twist circularly to restore the waist, resolve stasis to strengthen the waist, push the back with pinching and grasping, deep-press the back with kneading and revolving, pluck Collaterals with knocking and scratching, rock the knee to twist the hip joint, drag the leg with plucking and grasping, pull the leg with knocking and vibrating.

Subordinate Measure: Revolve Shenshu (UB 23), Zhishi (UB 52), Weizhong (UB 40), Kunlun (UB 60) and Taixi (K 3) with the forearm, all on both sides.

2. Malposition of joints and Blood stasis

Signs & Symptoms: Lumbar spasm and pain involving the leg, possibly to the shank; the waist bends towards the unaffected side, buttocks protrude toward the affected side; reluctance to move; standing up can only be done with help and support; stepping forward is impossible because of serious spasm in the waist and leg; it is difficult to lie in a supine posture; the spinal process of the malpositioned vertebra is resistant to pressing. In knocking and shaking examination, there is a feeling of distension and hardness, and the vibrating reaction is weakened. There is abdominal distension with a weighty sensation, and constipation.

Therapeutic Principle: Reposition, dredge Meridians and Collaterals, activate Blood, resolve stasis, regulate Tendinomuscular Meridians.

Principal Measure: Twist to restore the waist, arrange the waist back-to-back, pull the waist straight and obliquely, strengthen the waist by rolling and rubbing, pull the waist with jerking and dragging, deep-press the back with kneading and revolving, pad the popliteal fossa to flex the knee, pull the leg with knocking and vibrating, drag the leg with plucking and grasping.

Subordinate Measure: Revolve Huantiao (GB 30), nip Zusanli (St 36), grasp Chengjin (UB 56) and Chengshan (UB 57), pinch Kunlun (UB 60) and Taixi (K 3), all on both sides.

Prolapse of the lumbar intervertebral disk

Lumbar pain and stiffness and neuralgia of the hip are produced by this disorder. It is often seen in young and strong males.

Etiology: Injury due to overexertion or outside force. Tendinomuscular and Vessel Meridians are obstructed by the protruding disk, causing spasm and pain in the waist and leg. Ultimately, this condition can lead to numbness and atrophy of tendons and muscles.

Diagnosis & Treatment

Signs & Symptoms: Inability to stand upright because of serious crushing pain, the waist bends toward the unaffected side, standing is impossible without help and support, symptoms may be alleviated by lying on the side. Leg pain appears gradually, on one side, involving the back side of the buttock, the thigh and sometimes the ankle. Leg pain is aggravated by movement of the waist.

Therapeutic Principle: Divide Tendons, rectify joints, dredge obstruction, promote the flow of Vital Energy and Blood, resolve stasis, relieve pain.

Principal Measure: Jerk and drag to relax the waist, bend and deep-press the knee to stretch the waist, arrange the waist back-to-back, scratch the back, strengthen the waist by rolling and rubbing, revolve Huantiao (GB 30) with the elbow, nip and grasp Yanglingquan (GB 34), roll the leg with revolving and pinching, knead the leg with rotating and round-rubbing, nip and grasp the Three Yang Meridians of the Foot, whirl Tianying (Ashi point) with the finger.

Subordinate Measure: Pinch and grasp Weizhong (UB 40), Chengshan (UB 57), Zusanli (St 36), Juegu (GB 39) and Kunlun (UB 60).

Massage the healthy side once for each 3 massages to the affected side. Revolve Huantiao (GB 30) with the elbow until a warm sensation is felt.

Lumbosacral strain

This is often found in middle-aged patients, especially females. It is the result of repeated onset of acute or chronic injury to the lumbosacral joints and their peripheral soft tissues.

Etiology: Constitutional weakness, improper nursing after delivery, overwork, strain, attack of Cold-Dampness. In time, there is flaccidity of tendons and stiffness of joints. Hard work can bring on relapse.

Diagnosis & Treatment

Signs & Symptoms: Vague weighty pain in lumbosacral region; tenderness at Yaoyangguan (GV 3), Guanyuanshu (UB 26) and Shangliao (UB 31); stiffness in the waist; restricted motion of the hip joint; inability to carry weight on the back. In serious cases, walking is difficult; symptoms are aggravated by change of weather, menstruation, or bending the waist for extended periods of time.

Therapeutic Principle: Divide Tendons, rectify joints, dredge Meridians, activate Collaterals, resolve stasis, relieve pain, soften Tendons, ease joints.

Principal Measure: Revolve Eight Liao (UB 31-34, both sides) with the forearm, revolve Huantiao (GB 30) with the elbow, roll with hands and revolve with the forearm, strengthen the waist by rolling and rubbing, pluck Collaterals with knocking and scratching, rock the knee to twist the hip joint, jerk and drag the leg to relax the waist.

Subordinate Measure: Nip and knead Weizhong (UB 40), Chengshan (UB 57), Kunlun (UB 60), Taixi (K 3) and Sanyinjiao (Sp 6), all on both sides.

Injury to the sacroiliac joint

This often occurs in women who have had multiple births and in young men.

Etiology: The various tendons around the sacroiliac joint are relaxed and flaccid in women who have had multiple births, and in young men who are physically active. Therefore, this joint is susceptible to injury during overflexing of the hip joints or improper turning of the body. According to TCM, this joint connects with the Shaoyang Tendinomuscular Meridian of the Foot.

Diagnosis & Treatment

Signs & Symptoms: Swelling and pain at the sacroiliac; bent waist with buttocks protruding toward the injured side; attempts to stand up bring squeezing localized pain; turning the trunk and bending the hip is restricted; the patient walks with difficulty; tenderness at Xiaochangshu (UB 27), Pangguangshu (UB 28) and Zhonglushu (UB 29). When the ala ilii are pressed toward each other, there is sharp pain at the injured region.

Therapeutic Principle: Reposition, soften Tendons, ease joints, resolve stasis, relieve pain.

Principal Measure: Jerk and drag to relieve the waist, bend and deep-press the knee to stretch the waist, revolve Eight Liao (UB 31-34, both sides) with the forearm, strengthen the waist by rolling and rubbing, rock the knee to twist the hip joint, roll the leg with revolving and pinching, knead the leg with rotating and round-rubbing.

Subordinate Measure: Knead Tianying (Ashi point), Xiaochangshu (UB 27), Pangguangshu (UB 28), Zhonglushu (UB 29), Baihuanshu (UB 30), Weizhong (UB 40) and Sanyinjiao (Sp 6) with the fingers.

Injuries to the buttocks

Traumatic syndrome of the piriformis muscle

This refers to buttock and leg pain (dry neuralgia of the hip) caused by direct or indirect injuries to the piriformis muscle.

Etiology: Shaoyang Tendinomuscular Meridian of the Foot connects with the sacral bones. It may be injured by improper adduction or intorsion of the thigh, or by strain from lateral bending of the waist, resulting in swelling and pain of the piriformis. In time, there is obstruction of Tendinomuscular and Vessel Meridians, and leg pain develops.

Diagnosis & Treatment

1. Tendon spasm and Vital Energy stagnation

Signs & Symptoms: Spasm and pain in the buttock after injury, restricted motion of the hip. In time, symptoms gradually extend along the side of the thigh and the shank, and may be intolerable. There may be tearing pain accompanied by cramps. In serious cases, there is a feeling of weight in the chest, anxiety and insomnia.

Therapeutic Principle: Relax Tendons and muscles, dredge and promote the flow of Vital Energy and Blood, relieve spasm and pain.

Principal Measure: Revolve both buttocks (principally Huantiao [GB 30]) with the forearm; revolve the lumbosacral region with the forearm; pinch and grasp the Three Yang Meridians of the Foot; revolve the leg with the elbow and dot it; chop the leg with both hands; roll, clap and knock the leg with the hands.

Subordinate Measure: Dot Fengshi (GB 31), Ququan (Liv 8), Yangling-quan (GB 34) and Yangjiao (GB 35).

For each 3 massages on the injured side, do one on the other side.

2. Tendon adhesion and Blood stasis

Signs & Symptoms: Spasm and pain in the buttocks after injury; swelling, hardness or nodular structures may be felt by palpation; reluctance to move because of intolerable pain generated along the Shaoyang Tendinomuscular Meridian of the Foot. Symptoms are often aggravated at night; feeling of weight in the chest, anxiety, dry stool, constipation. Leg pain sometimes extends along the Taiyang Tendinomuscular Meridian of the Foot, since this may be involved at the connecting spot by adhesion.

Therapeutic Principle: Relax Tendons and muscles, dredge Meridians and promote the flow of Vital Energy and Blood, resolve stasis, dissipate nodules, relieve spasm and pain.

Principal Measure: Revolve Huantiao (GB 30) with the elbow, revolve the lumbosacral region with the forearm, revolve the leg with the elbow and dot it, roll the leg with revolving and pinching, knead the leg with rotating and round-rubbing, rock the knee to twist the hip joint, stretch and rock the ankle.

Subordinate Measure: Whirl Fengshi (GB 31), Zusanli (St 36) and Waiqiu (GB 36) with the thumbs.

Massage the healthy side once for each 3 massages to the injured side.

Bruised coccyx

Etiology: Usually due to direct impact by sudden sliding or falling, and the injured coccyx is pushed in. In children, the coccyx is not fully developed, and the injury is usually mild, but in adults, the condition may be serious, making the person unable to either sit or to lie in bed.

Diagnosis & Treatment

Signs & Symptoms: Swelling, distension and weighty pain at the space between the coccyx and the sacrum; spasm of related tendons and muscles; palpation reveals angular dislocation of the coccyx, or a floating effect; the injured area is resistant to pressing. Symptoms are aggravated when the patients sits or is supine; the waist is bent without ability to stand straight or walk freely; difficulty in defecation due to pain.

Therapeutic Principle: Reposition, activate Blood, resolve stasis, relieve spasm and pain.

Principal Measure: Repositioning a coccygeal malposition or fracture is difficult, especially stabilization after the reposition. However, some techniques may be used: whirl an area above the fracture with the thumbs; revolve the waist, the buttocks and the sacral area with the forearm; dot the waist and the spine; pinch the spine. Techniques should be performed gently.

Subordinate Measure: Dot Yaoshu (GV 2), Yaoyangguan (GV 3), Mingmen (GV 4), Xuanshu (GV 5), Jizhong (GV 6), Zhongshu (GV 7), Zhiyang (GV 9) and Dazhui (GV 14), all gently.

Traumatic arthritis of the hip joint

This is often seen in teenagers.

Etiology: The hip joint is a type of Void Aperture in TCM, and is rich in Energy and Blood. It is easily injured by falling, sudden movement, or impact, resulting in swelling, localized pain, and restricted motion.

Diagnosis & Treatment

Signs & Symptoms: Stringy spasm of muscles in the buttocks; tenderness at Huantiao (GB 30); swelling and protrusion at Zuwuli (Liv 10) and Yinlian (Liv 11), which is resistant to pressing. In patients with twisting of tendons and muscles, the feet are misaligned and they are reduced to hobbling; patients with tendon spasm walk on tiptoe; patients with joint stickiness walk sideways with protruding buttocks. In serious cases, the hip joint stays flexed and cannot be straightened. There is reluctance to move, because of the sharp pain produced.

Therapeutic Principle: Divide Tendons, rectify joints, activate Blood, resolve stasis, relieve spasm and pain.

Principal Measure: Rock the knee to twist the hip joint, revolve the waist with the forearm, pull the waist straight and obliquely, grasp the abdomen with lifting and jerking, push the abdomen with round-rubbing and revolving, pull the leg with knocking and vibrating, drag the leg with plucking and grasping, roll the Three Yin Meridians of the Foot with the hands.

Subordinate Measure: Revolve Huantiao (GB 30) with the elbow; nip Yanglingquan (GB 34), Zusanli (St 36), Diji (Sp 8), Lougu (Sp 7), Gongsun (Sp 4) and Sanyinjiao (Sp 6).

Injuries to the knee

Traumatic synovitis of the knee joint

This is an injury to the synovial membrane from outside force or from strain, resulting in the retention of blood and fluid within the knee joint, accompanied by swelling, pain and restricted motion.

Etiology: The knee joint is a type of Void Aperture in TCM. When it is injured, there is stagnation and retention of Vital Energy, Blood and fluids. In time, stickiness, adhesion of tendons and muscles, and rigidity of the joint may occur.

Diagnosis & Treatment

1. Vital Energy stagnation in joint Aperture

Signs & Symptoms: Relaxation and feebleness of the knee joint; swelling and fullness around the patella, which floats up and down on palpation; localized glossy paleness; swelling and pain or discomfort at the popliteal fossa, difficulty in flexion and extension.

Therapeutic Principle: Divide Tendons, rectify joints, dredge Meridians and promote the flow of Vital Energy and Blood, eliminate stagnation and stasis.

Principal Measure: Pull and grasp Weixia (approx. 1 Body Inch below Weizhong [UB 40]), nip and grasp the knee joint, press and round-rub the patella, pad the popliteal fossa and bend the knee, rock the knee to twist the hip joint, drag the leg with plucking and grasping, pull the leg with knocking and vibrating.

Subordinate Measure: Nip and grasp Xiguan (Liv 7), Liangqiu (St 34), Dubi (St 35), Zusanli (St 36) and Jiexi (St 41), all on both sides.

2. Blood stasis in joint Aperture

Signs & Symptoms: Hardened swelling and protrusion around the patella, with an aerated sensation on palpation; the patella floats but cannot be shifted; the local spot is warm, moist and of dim complexion; various tendons in the popliteal fossa are stiff and hardened; the knee remains straight; reluctance to move.

Therapeutic Principle: Relax Tendons, rectify joints, dredge Meridians and ease joint Aperture, activate Blood, resolve stasis.

Principal Measure: Nip and grasp Lianqiu (St 34), nip and grasp the knee joint, jerk and drag the leg, dot Ququan (Liv 8), revolve the popliteal fossa with the forearm, pull the leg with knocking and vibrating, knead the knee with rotating and round-rubbing, revolve Biguan (St 31) with the forearm.

If the swelling caused by bleeding within the joint continues to develop, laceration of large Vessel Collaterals should be taken into account. Carry out careful observation and differential diagnosis. Proceed very carefully.

3. Joint stickiness

Signs & Symptoms: Diffused swelling around the knee joint; no obvious floating sensation of the patella on palpation; localized pain and discomfort; fasciae are thick and rough; the knee joint is relaxed and feeble; there is difficulty in flexion and extension. Symptoms are intermittent.

Therapeutic Principle: Relax Tendons and muscles, dredge Meridians and promote the flow of Vital Energy and Blood, clear and open joint Apertures, lubricate and ease the joint.

Principal Measure: Pad the popliteal fossa and flex the knee joint, rock the knee to twist the hip joint, stretch and rock the ankle, jerk and drag the leg, drag the leg with plucking and grasping, roll the leg with revolving and pinching, knead the leg with rotating and round-rubbing.

Subordinate Measure: Pinch and grasp Lianqiu (St 24) and Yinshi (St 33); nip Zusanli (St 36), Yinlingquan (Sp 9), Dubi (St 35) and Inner Xiyan (Ex-LE 2).

If the knee joint is straight and rigid, or is bent and cannot be straightened; or, on palpation, the tendons around the joint are stiff or the patella is fixed and cannot be moved, consider the following measures.

Therapeutic Principle: Draw apart to slacken the joint, dredge joint Apertures, relax Tendons and muscles, promote the flow of Vital Energy and Blood.

Principal Measure: Weighty Flood-gate bending method, dot the popliteal fossa and flex the knee joint, jerk and drag the leg, pull the leg with knocking and vibrating, roll the leg with revolving and pinching, knead the leg with rotating and round-rubbing, pound the kneecap with open fists.

Subordinate Measure: Dot Lianqiu (St 34), Ququan (Liv 8), Yanglingquan (GB 34) and Shangjuxu (St 37); pinch and grasp Diji (Sp 8) and Sanyinjiao (Sp 6).

Injury to the medial collateral ligament of the knee joint

The tearing of the medial collateral ligament produces swelling and pain at the medial condyle of the tibia, and restriction of movement.

Etiology: The medial collateral ligament connects with the Three Yin Tendinomuscular Meridians of the Foot. Injury is usually caused by wrenching or hyperextension of the leg, or bruising of the knee when it is adducted. There is lengthening and spasm of the tendons, swelling and pain in the joint, and restriction of movement.

Diagnosis & Treatment

1. Tendon lengthening

Signs & Symptoms: The knee joint is unstable, inclining toward abduction; the patient cannot stand or walk, the knee remains straight and cannot be flexed; swelling and pain at the medial condyle of the tibia which is resistant to pressing, reluctance to move; obvious tenderness at Xiguan (Liv 7), Ququan (Liv 8), Yingu (K 10) and Inner Xiyan (Ex-LE 2). In serious cases, there may be swelling due to blood retention.

Therapeutic Principle: Relax Tendons and muscles, protect injured tendons, consolidate joints, dredge Meridians and promote the flow of Vital Energy and Blood, dissipate stasis, relieve pain.

Principal Measure: Revolve Biguan (St 31) with the forearm, bend and deep-press the knee, pull the leg with knocking and vibrating, pinch and grasp the muscles of the shank, pound the kneecap with open fists, drag the leg with plucking and grasping, rectify the leg.

Subordinate Measure: Dot Futu (St 32), Yinshi (St 33), Liangqiu (St 34) and Xiyan (Ex-LE 2); nip and grasp Zusanli (St 36) and Shangjuxu (St 37); knead Xiguan (Liv 7), Ququan (Liv 8), Yingu (K 10) and Inner Xiyan (Ex-LE 2).

2. Tendon spasm

Signs & Symptoms: Spasm forces the knee joint into a straight position which cannot be flexed, reducing the patient to hobbling; abduction of the shank brings sharp pain; swelling at the area where Taiyin Tendinomuscular Meridian of the Foot connects with the joint; nodules may be felt on spastic tendons.

Therapeutic Principle: Relax Tendons and muscles, dredge Meridians and promote the flow of Vital Energy, activate Blood, resolve stasis, draw apart to slacken the joint.

Principal Measure: Revolve the popliteal fossa with the forearm, rock the knee to twist the hip joint, rectify the leg, pound the kneecap with open fists, roll the leg with revolving and pinching, knead the leg with rotating and round-rubbing, pad the popliteal fossa and flex the knee.

Subordinate Measure: Knead and pinch Xiguan (Liv 7), Dubi (St 35), Ququan (Liv 8), Yingu (K 10), Zusanli (St 36), Gongsun (Sp 4), Sanyinjiao (Sp 6) and Weizhong (UB 40); rotate the knee joint.

Injury to the lateral collateral ligament of the knee joint

Trauma at the lateral condyle or tearing of the lateral collateral ligament produces localized swelling and pain and restricted motion.

Etiology: The fibula connects with the Shaoyang Tendinomuscular Meridian of the Foot. Wrenching the knee, or bruising the knee when it is abducted and the shank adducted, may injure the lateral collateral ligament. Swelling, spasm and pain may also involve the side of the shank.

Diagnosis & Treatment

1. *Injury to the branching point of the Shaoyang Tendinomuscular Meridian of the Foot*

Signs & Symptoms: Swelling and pain at the side of the knee, resistant to pressing; spasm and nodules discernible on palpation; when the shank is adducted, pain radiates along the side of the fibula to the top of the foot; the knee joint flexes only minimally.

Therapeutic Principle: Divide Tendons, rectify joints, activate Blood, resolve stasis, relieve spasm and pain.

Principal Measure: Pound the kneecap with open fists, drag the leg with plucking and grasping, pull the leg with knocking and vibrating, revolve the popliteal fossa with the forearm, chop the leg with both hands, rectify the leg, pinch and grasp the Six Meridians of the Foot.

Subordinate Measure: Nip and grasp Biguan (St 31), Zuwuli (Liv 10), Yinshi (St 33), Yinlingquan (Sp 9), Zusanli (St 36), Jiexi (St 41) and Sanyinjiao (Sp 6), all on both sides.

2. *Injury to branching point of Yangming Tendinomuscular Meridian of the Foot*

Signs & Symptoms: Swelling and protrusion at the lateral condyle of the fibula, resistant to pressing; bending the knee is restricted by severe pain; spasm and pain radiate along the side of the shank to the ankle.

Therapeutic Principle: Divide Tendons, rectify joints, activate Blood, resolve stasis, relieve spasm and pain.

Principal Measure: Roll the leg with revolving and pinching, knead the leg with rotating and round-rubbing, pound the kneecap with open fists, pinch and grasp the Six Meridians of the Foot, revolve the popliteal fossa with the forearm, knock and clap the leg, rectify the leg.

Subordinate Measure: Nip and knead Zusanli (St 36), Yinlingquan (Sp 9), Yingu (K 10) and Jiexi (St 41), all on both sides.

Epiphysitis of the tibial tubercle (Surfer's knots)

This is often seen in children and teenagers, and is characterized by swelling, hyperplasia, protrusion of the tibial tubercle, and restricted knee joint motion.

Etiology: Children and teenagers move about a lot and are susceptible to injury. Additionally, their Kidney Energy is Deficient and their Tendons and bones are not of full strength.

Diagnosis & Treatment

Signs & Symptoms: Localized swelling and pain at the tibia beneath the patella, resistant to pressing; slight localized heat and dim complexion; broken fragments may be felt on palpation; squatting or bending the knee is difficult, and there is reluctance to run or jump.

Therapeutic Principle: Relax Tendons, activate Blood, resolve stasis, relieve pain.

Principal Measure: Press and round-rub the knee, rock the knee to twist the hip joint, twist the popliteal fossa with the fingers, revolve the front of the thigh (principally Futu [St 32]) with the forearm, knead the side of the shank.

Subordinate Measure: Revolve Huantiao (GB 30) with the elbow; revolve Biguan (St 31), Futu (St 32), Yinshi (St 33), Yanglingquan (GB 34), Yangjiao (GB 35) and Sanyinjiao (Sp 6) with the forearm, all on both sides.

Injury to the popliteal muscle

This is often seen in teenagers and is characterized by swelling and pain at the popliteal fossa, inability to straighten the knee, and hobbled motion.

Etiology: The popliteal fossa is rich in Vital Energy and Blood. Taiyang Tendinomuscular Meridian of the Foot passes through this area and connects to the knee at its back. Jumping, climbing or bruising may injure the popliteal muscles.

Diagnosis & Treatment

1. Vital Energy stagnation and tendon spasm

Signs & Symptoms: The knee joint is flexed and can only be extended with serious pain. Tendons and muscles in the popliteal fossa are stringy and tense, resistant to pressing; the patient hobbles on tiptoe; attempts to step higher cause intolerable pain; symptoms may retreat during exercise or movement, but return when the patient is at rest.

Therapeutic Principle: Relax Tendons and muscles, dredge Meridians and promote the flow of Vital Energy and Blood, relieve spasm and pain.

Principal Measure: Rock the knee to twist the hip joint; round-rub the knee with the hands; nip and grasp the knee joint; pinch and grasp tendons and muscles around the knee; roll the inner side of the shank with the hand; nip and grasp the outside of the shank; knock, clap, pound and chop the back of the shank.

Subordinate Measure: Dot Chengjin (UB 56) and Chengshan (UB 57), nip Zusanli (St 36), pinch Diji (Sp 8), nip and knead Kunlun (UB 60) and Taixi (K 3).

2. Blood stasis and joint stickiness

Signs & Symptoms: Swelling, fullness and hardening of the popliteal fossa with marked tenderness; the knee is extended and cannot be flexed; the patient stands on tiptoe, hobbling in motion if able to walk at all; reluctance to move; fragments may be felt on tendons in the popliteal fossa.

Therapeutic Principle: Relax Tendons and muscles, dredge Meridians, activate Collaterals, promote the flow of Blood, resolve stasis, relieve spasm and pain.

Principal Measure: Knead and pinch the popliteal fossa; pinch the calf; pad the popliteal fossa and flex the knee; nip and grasp the space of the knee joint; rock the knee to twist the hip; knock, clap, pound and chop the back of the shank.

Subordinate Measure: None.

Traumatic dislocation of the patella

The patella is held and stabilized by the tendon of the quadriceps muscle, which terminates at the tibial tubercle through the patellar ligament. Normally, it is at the patellar surface of the femur, but under outside force, it may be shifted laterally. While this type of injury is uncommon, it is occasionally seen in teenagers.

Etiology: The patella is linked with the Yangming Tendinomuscular Meridian of the Foot which connects to the fibula. Lateral dislocation may result from falling, impact or violent wrenching of the knee.

Diagnosis & Treatment

Signs & Symptoms: Abnormal contour of the knee, which is slightly flexed and stiff; movement is restricted by pain; inability to stand; stringy spasm of Yangming Tendinomuscular Meridian shows from the knee up to Futu (St 32).

Therapeutic Principle: Reposition, divide Tendons, rectify joints, relieve spasm and pain.

Principal Measure: (Reposition of the knee) Stand on the affected side of the patient, who is supine. Pad the foot under the knee joint to relieve pain and spasm. Grip both sides of the upper part of the dislocated patella with the thumb and index finger of one hand, holding the thigh with your palm. Grip both sides of the lower patella with the thumb and index finger of the other hand, pressing firmly against the shank with the palm. Withdraw the padded foot from beneath the knee and deep-press the knee with both hands, while pushing and plucking the patella to the center line. As the knee joint straightens, the patella returns to its normal position. After this, round-rub the knee joint with the hands, knead the popliteal fossa with the fingers, roll the front of the thigh with the hands, pinch and grasp tendons and muscles along the medial of the thigh.

Subordinate Measure: Revolve Biguan (St 31), Futu (St 32), Yinshi (St 33) and Liangqiu (St 34) with the forearm; nip Dubi (St 35), Zusanli (St 36) and Jiexi (St 41).

After this reduction, if there is swelling in the joint from blood retention, refer to treatment of Blood stasis in Traumatic synovitis of the knee joint.

Patellar dislocation may reoccur and be habitual due to relaxation or flaccidity of tendons and joints from constitutional weakness. In this case, use the following approach.

Therapeutic Principle: Regulate and promote the flow of Vital Energy and Blood, relax Tendons, ease joints, nourish and strengthen Tendons and muscles.

Principal Measure: Nip and grasp the periphery of the knee joint, round-rub the knee with the hands, pinch the Six Meridians of the Foot (principally Yangming Tendinomuscular Meridian).

Subordinate Measure: Same as above.

There is wide variation in pathologic changes to the knee joint, but their therapeutic methods differ only slightly. However, when the swelling of the knee is remarkable, management should be carefully considered. In this situation, it is best to avoid local manipulation, careless bending or deep-pressing, or violent jerking and stretching.

Traumatic myofascitis of the gastrocnemius muscle

This is often seen in males 40-60 years old. There is swelling and pain of the muscles at the back of the shank after injury, and motion is restricted.

Etiology: Taiyang Tendinomuscular Meridian of the Foot passes along the back of the leg and buttocks. When the calf is over-stretched by strenuous climbing on tiptoe, or injured by direct impact, there will be Vital Energy stagnation and Blood stasis. In time, tendons and muscles become sticky and stiff.

Diagnosis & Treatment

1. Vital Energy stagnation and tendon spasm

Signs & Symptoms: Sudden onset of stabbing or tearing pain at the gastrocnemius with any exertion on the Taiyang Tendinomuscular Meridian of the Foot. Presently, spasm and pain in the tendons and muscles will appear, and is resistant to pressing. The knee is flexed and cannot be extended, and the patient cannot walk. Nodular structures appear on the spastic tendons.

Therapeutic Principle: Dredge Meridians and promote the flow of Vital Energy, activate Collaterals, relax Tendons, relieve spasm and pain.

Principal Measure: Manipulate along the pathway of the Taiyang Tendinomuscular Meridian of the Foot; pinch the calf, pound the leg with open fists and grasp the leg; pound, chop and round-rub the leg; roll the leg with the hands and clap the leg; revolve the leg with the forearm with pinching and grasping; chop the leg with both hands; rectify the leg.

Subordinate Measure: Pinch and grasp Kunlun (UB 60), Chengshan (UB 57), Chengjin (UB 56), Heyang (UB 55), Weizhong (UB 40), Weiyang (UB 39), Fuxi (UB 38), Yinmen (UB 37) and Chengfu (UB 36).

2. Blood stasis and tendon stiffness

Signs & Symptoms: Sudden onset of sharp or tearing pain when the patient tightens the gastrocnemius muscle with any force, leaving numbness and discomfort after relaxation. Symptoms present themselves gradually: swelling and hardening of the injured area, resistance to pressing; the knee remains flexed and cannot be extended; tendons and muscles become stiff and hardened; local complexion becomes dull; surface blood vessels become visible; symptoms are more serious at night, and prevent peaceful sleep.

Therapeutic Principle: Relax Tendons and muscles, dredge Meridians and promote the flow of Vital Energy and Blood, resolve stasis, relieve pain.

Principal Measure: Pinch the calf; rock the knee to twist the hip joint; knead the leg with rotating and round-rubbing; roll the leg with revolving and pinching; pull the leg with knocking and vibrating; pad the popliteal fossa and flex the knee; drag the leg with plucking and grasping; chop the leg with joined hands; knock, clap and pound the leg.

Subordinate Measure: Pinch and grasp Chengfu (UB 36), Weizhong (UB 40), Heyang (UB 55), Fuyang (UB 59), Chengjin (UB 56), Chengshan (UB 57) and Kunlun (UB 60).

Injuries to the ankle

Injury to the Achilles tendon (Tendo calcaneus)

This may be classified as laceration or tenosynovitis of the Achilles tendon.

Etiology: Taiyang Tendinomuscular Meridian of the Foot joins the heel and connects with Chengshan (UB 57) and the knee joint. If it is hyperextended, laceration may occur at the heel or at Chengshan (UB 57), lengthening the tendon with swelling and pain. Extended hiking may also injure this tendon, and lack of proper treatment may lead to tendon stickiness.

Diagnosis & Treatment

1. Tendon lengthening

Signs & Symptoms: Mostly seen in adults; sudden onset of sharp pain at the Achilles tendon, followed by gradually developing swelling and pain; movement of the ankle is restricted, hobbling the patient; palpation may reveal nodular structures or gaps.

Therapeutic Principle: Activate Blood, resolve stasis, relieve spasm and pain.

Principal Measure: Pinch and grasp the Achilles tendon; pinch the calf; knead the leg with rotating and round-rubbing; roll the leg with revolving and pinching; pad the popliteal fossa and flex the knee; knock, clap and chop the leg.

Subordinate Measure: Pinch and grasp Chengshan (UB 57) and Chengjin (UB 56); pull and grasp Weizhong (UB 40); revolve Yinmen (UB 37) with the forearm; knead Shenshu (UB 23), Pishu (UB 20), Xinshu (UB 15) and Feishu (UB 13) with the fingers, all on both sides.

N.B. If the Achilles tendon is torn, massage is ineffective, and it must be treated surgically.

2. Tendon stickiness

Signs & Symptoms: Mostly seen in children and young females; swelling, aching and discomfort of the heel; feebleness; fear of the area being pressed or squeezed. In time, there will be spasm and pain, and tumescence and thickness may be felt; movement produces a frictional noise; the patient is hobbled.

Therapeutic Principle: Relax Tendons and muscles, dredge Meridians and promote the flow of Vital Energy and Blood, resolve stasis, relieve spasm.

Principal Measure: Rock the knee to twist the hip joint, pad the popliteal fossa and flex the knee, knead the leg with rotating and round-rubbing, pinch the calf, roll the leg with revolving and pinching, pluck Collaterals with knocking and scratching (principally the heel).

Subordinate Measure: Pinch and grasp Kunlun (UB 60), Taixi (K 3) and Chengshan (UB 57); pull and grasp Weizhong (UB 40); revolve Yinmen (UB 37) with the forearm.

Epiphysitis of the heel

This is commonly seen in juveniles and is the result of deficient blood supply due to injury.

Etiology: The heel bears the weight of the whole body and is the place where Taiyang Tendinomuscular Meridian of the Foot joins and connects. It may be injured by jumping, running or strain. Ultimately, stagnated Vital Energy and suffused Blood will condense and adhere at that spot.

Diagnosis & Treatment

Signs & Symptoms: Swelling, pain and tenderness, reddening and protrusion at the back of the heel; roughness and thickness of local tendons may be felt by palpation; movement of the ankle is restricted; the heel is resistant to pressing on both sides; the patient cannot stand for any extended period, and walks holding the heel up to avoid contact with the ground.

Therapeutic Principle: Divide Tendons, stroke bones, dredge Collaterals, activate Blood, resolve stasis.

Principal Measure: Pinch the calf, pad the popliteal fossa and flex the knee, stretch and jerk the ankle, knead the leg with rotating and round-rubbing, roll the leg with revolving, pinching and grasping, pull the leg with knocking and vibrating, drag the leg with plucking and grasping, pluck Collaterals with knocking and scratching (principally at the heel).

Subordinate Measure: Knead Pushen (UB 61), Kunlun (UB 60), Taixi (K 3), Fuliu (K 7), Chengshan (UB 57), Weizhong (UB 40) and Diji (Sp 8) with the fingers; pinch and grasp Xuehai (Sp 10) and Jimen (Sp 11).

Treatment of the Five Sense Organs

Tinnitus

This is frequently encountered, and is characterized by a subjective impression of hearing sound (usually described as ringing or tinkling) which interferes with normal hearing. It is closely related to the functional state of Liver, Gall Bladder and Kidney Meridians, and may be characterized as Deficiency or Excess.

Etiology: Harassment of Clear Aperture by weak Fire due to Deficiency of Kidney Yin; flaming up of Liver-Gall Bladder Fire from emotional depression; adverse uprising of Phlegm-Fire from accumulation of Dampness in Middle Warmer.

Diagnosis & Treatment

1. Depletion of Kidney Yin

Signs and Symptoms: The tinnitus is like the continuous, shrill chirping of cicadas; more serious at mid-day than at night; it can be stopped by pressing the ears with the fingers; dizziness, soreness, and weakness of the waist and knees. *Tongue:* red with minimal fur. *Pulse:* thready, rapid.

Therapeutic Principle: Nourish Yin, retrieve Yang.

Principal Measure: Stroke and caress the head, deep-press the spine with kneading and revolving, strengthen the waist by rolling and rubbing, push the abdomen with round-rubbing and revolving.

Subordinate Measure: Rub Ermen (TW 21), Tinggong (SI 19) and Tinghui (GB 2); push the helix; nip Yifeng (TW 17); push the mastoid; knead Daying (St 5) and Sanyinjiao (Sp 6); rub Yongquan (K 1).

2. Flaming up of Liver-Gall Bladder Fire

Signs and Symptoms: Sudden onset of tinnitus like a rushing stream; most serious before noon; pressing the ear with the fingers aggravates it; headache, short temper, irritability; symptoms increase when angry. *Tongue:* red with yellow fur. *Pulse:* stringy, rapid.

Therapeutic Principle: Reduce Fire, ease the Clear Aperture.

Principal Measure: Stroke and caress the head, pinch and grasp Fengchi (GB 20), push the back with pinching and grasping, push and wipe to divide the ribs.

Subordinate Measure: Knead the helix; rub Ermen (TW 21), Tinggong (SI 19) and Tinghui (GB 2); nip and knead Dadun (Liv 1) and Xingjian (Liv 2); revolve Huantiao (GB 30) with the elbow; nip Yanglingquan (GB 34); roll the Three Yang Meridians of the Foot.

3. Adverse uprising of Phlegm-Fire

Signs and Symptoms: The tinnitus varies from being like the sound of cicadas to a total inability to hear external sound; heaviness in the chest; excessive expectoration with bitter taste in mouth; impeded urination and defecation. *Tongue:* yellow, greasy fur. *Pulse:* stringy, slippery.

Therapeutic Principle: Harmonize Stomach, diminish Turbidity.

Principal Measure: Relieve the chest by dotting and vibrating, push and wipe to divide the ribs, press the abdomen with deep-pressing and kneading, stroke and caress the head.

Subordinate Measure: Rub Ermen (TW 21), Tinggong (SI 19) and Tinghui (GB 2); push the helix; Beat Heaven's Drum; nip Yifeng (TW 17), Fenglong (St 40) and Zuqiaoyin (GB 44); push Yongquan (K 1).

Earache (otalgia)

This indicates ear pain without draining pus.

Etiology: Accumulation of Liver-Gall Bladder Heat which harasses the ear; Shaoyang and Taiyang Meridians are obstructed by exogenous Wind-Heat.

Diagnosis & Treatment

1. Accumulation of Liver-Gall Bladder Heat

Signs and Symptoms: Intolerable pressing pain in the ear; localized swelling and redness; often accompanied by tinnitus; dizziness; restricted motion of the lower jaw; bitter taste in mouth; dry throat; diminished sensitivity to sound; fever, irritability, short-temper. *Tongue:* red with yellow fur. *Pulse:* stringy, rapid.

Therapeutic Principle: Clear and reduce Liver Fire.

Principal Measure: Stroke and caress the head; open Passes and dredge Apertures; nip and grasp Fengchi (GB 20); pluck, vibrate and knock the neck; grasp Jianjing (GB 21).

Subordinate Measure: Knead area between Fengchi (GB 20) and Quepen (St 12); dot and deep-press Ermen (TW 21), Tinggong (SI 19) and Tinghui (GB 2); knead the helix, Beat Heaven's Drum; revolve Huantiao (GB 30) with the elbow; nip Yanglingquan (GB 34); push Yongquan (K 1).

2. Invasion of exogenous Wind-Heat

Signs and Symptoms: Pain, itching and redness on the periphery of one or both ears; symptoms milder in the morning, more serious at night; tinnitus, cough, headache, distended feeling in the eye, stuffed nose; symptoms may extend to the cheek; aversion to wind, weariness, lassitude. *Tongue:* red with thin yellow fur. *Pulse:* superficial, rapid.

Therapeutic Principle: Expel Wind, detoxify evils.

Principal Measure: Open Passes and dredge Apertures; pluck, vibrate and knock the neck; push and wipe to divide the ribs; revolve Huantiao (GB 30) with the elbow.

Subordinate Measure: Push the helix, Ermen (TW 21), Tinggong (SI 19), and Tinghui (GB 2); push from Yifeng (TW 17) to Quepen (St 12); nip Quchi (LI 11) and Hegu (LI 4); rub Yongquan (K 1).

Suppurative blepharitis

This is classified as suppurative blepharitis of the upper lid and the lower lid, characterized by marked swelling and redness of the palpebral conjunctiva.

Etiology: This is usually caused by combat between Wind and Heat at the eyelid, or the accumulation of Dampness-Heat in Spleen-Stomach from overeating of fatty and pungent foods.

Diagnosis & Treatment

1. Combat between Wind and Heat

Signs and Symptoms: Diffuse swelling, redness, pain and hardening of the eyelid, which is resistant to pressing; profuse discharge and tears. In serious cases, there may be swelling of the face and scalp; fever, aversion to cold, anxiety and restlessness. *Tongue:* thin white fur. *Pulse:* superficial, rapid.

Therapeutic Principle: Clear Heat, detoxify evils.

Principal Measure: Knead and deep-press Jingming (UB 1), Taiyang (Ex-HN 4), Hegu (LI 4) and Quchi (LI 11). Knead the pupil: the patient is supine with both eyes closed. After dressing the eyes with a piece of sterilized gauze, knead and press the pupil gently and slowly through the gauze and the eyelid, taking care not to drag or shift the gauze. Work on each pupil 5-10 minutes.

Subordinate Measure: Nip and knead Zanzhu (UB 2), Fengchi (GB 20), Yangbai (GB 14), Sibai (St 2) and Yintang (Ex-HN 2).

2. Accumulation and obstruction of Dampness-Heat

Signs and Symptoms: Redness, burning, itching and pain of the eyelid and cheek; may be complicated by rubella, oozing skin ulcers and erosion; heaviness in the head and limbs, weariness and lassitude; feeling of weight in the chest; poor appetite; difficult urination with deep-colored urine. *Tongue:* yellow, greasy fur. *Pulse:* soft, floating, rapid.

Therapeutic Principle: Clear Heat, eliminate Dampness.

Principal Measure: Stroke and caress the head, knead Fengfu (GV 16) with the fingers, knead and grasp Fengchi (GB 20), pinch and grasp Jianjing (GB 21), relax the chest by pressing and kneading, push and wipe to divide the ribs, press the abdomen with deep-pressing and kneading, roll the leg with revolving and pinching.

Subordinate Measure: Nip and rectify the base (or both bases) of the thumb nail 3-5 times, nip Twelve Jing (Well) Points, rub Yongquan (K 1).

In treating this disorder, when there is a sty which is about to fester, stab at that place with a sterilized, three-sided needle. After the pus has been drained off, knead and deep-press Jingming (UB 1), Taiyang (Ex-HN 4), Quchi (LI 11) and Hegu (LI 4).

Myopia

There are two types of myopia — congenital and acquired.

Etiology: Congenital myopia is caused by an Excess of Yin Energy and a Deficiency of Yang Energy. Acquired myopia is caused by adverse uprising of Liver Fire due to depletion of Kidney Water, reading or working with poor lighting, or Deficiency of Vital Energy and Blood after illness.

Diagnosis & Treatment

Generally speaking, congenital myopia cannot be cured by treatment, but the acquired type may be corrected by massage.

Signs and Symptoms: (Acquired myopia) protruding eyeballs, poor distance vision and squinting; dryness, tiredness and distension of eye after periods of watching; aching and discomfort around the eyebrows.

Therapeutic Principle: Nourish Liver-Kidney, supplement Essence, benefit Blood.

Principal Measure: Stroke and caress the head, open Passes and dredge Apertures, knead and grasp Fengchi (GB 20), dot Fengfu (GV 16), nip points around the eyes, push and wipe to divide the ribs, strengthen the waist by rolling and rubbing.

Subordinate Measure: Nip and knead the major thenar mound at Yuji (Lu 10), Yemen (TW 2), Hegu (LI 4), Sanyinjiao (Sp 6) and Yanglingquan (GB 34).

Epiphora

This indicates excessive, uncontrollable lacrimation, or excessive lacrimation caused by wind. It may be classified as cold or hot. Cold epiphora is aggravated in winter and is difficult to manage. Hot epiphora is generally accompanied by signs and symptoms of external ocular injury. Shedding of tears because of emotional changes is not involved here.

Etiology: Cold epiphora is often caused by Deficiency of both Liver-Kidney and Essence-Blood, depletion of Vital Energy and Blood due to Liver depression, or attack of exogenous Wind. Hot epiphora is often caused by the flaming up of Fire, originating from depression of Liver Energy, or from pungent and rich diets, or from exogenous Wind-Heat.

Diagnosis & Treatment

1. Cold epiphora

Signs and Symptoms: Commonly seen in older people with Blood Deficiency, also epiphora caused by wind, without redness or swelling of the eyes. In its early stage, it is relieved in summer and aggravated in winter. Ultimately, the season will make no difference. Vision is constantly blurred. *Tongue:* pale with white, moist fur. *Pulse:* deep, slow.

Therapeutic Principle: Nourish Blood, disperse Cold.

Principal Measure: Stroke and caress the head, open Passes and dredge Apertures, nip Baihui (GV 20), knead and grasp Fengchi (GB 20), push the back with pinching and grasping, pluck Collaterals with knocking and scratching, push the abdomen with round-rubbing and revolving, lift and grasp Jianjing (GB 21).

Subordinate Measure: Knead Dagukong (Ex UE 5) (the space between the bone tips at the middle segment of thumb when the thumb is bent); the Xiaogukong (Ex UE 6) (at the tip of the second segment of the little finger, while it is bent); nip Zusanli (St 36).

2. Hot epiphora

Signs and Symptoms: Redness and swelling of the eyes, aching at night; photophobia; tears are sticky and turbid with a hot sensation; short-temper, irritability, insomnia, bitter taste in mouth, and dry stool. *Tongue:* red with yellow fur. *Pulse:* stringy.

Therapeutic Principle: Clear and reduce Liver Fire.

Principal Measure: Open Passes and dredge Apertures, nip and knead points around the eye, nip and grasp Fengchi (GB 20), dot Fengfu (GV 16) with the fingers, push and wipe to divide the ribs, press the abdomen with deep-pressing and kneading, lift and grasp Jianjing (GB 21), deep-press the spine with kneading and revolving, pinch the arm with nipping and kneading, roll the leg with revolving and pinching.

Subordinate Measure: Nip and knead the middle finger at the back end of its second segment, knead Sanyinjiao (Sp 6) and Zulinqi (GB 41), rub Yongquan (K 1).

Toothache

This does not include those caused by decay.

Etiology: Accumulation of Heat in the Stomach from pungent diet, constitutional dominance of Yang, attack of Wind-Heat or Wind-Cold, flaming up of Deficient Fire due to depletion of Kidney Yin.

Diagnosis & Treatment

1. Stomach Heat

Signs and Symptoms: Distending toothache involves the head and loose tooth; swelling, redness, pain and putrefaction of the gum; hot and foul breath; thirst and a desire for cold drinks; possible swelling and pain of the lip, the tongue or the cheek; constipation, deep-colored urine. *Tongue:* red with yellow fur. *Pulse:* full, rapid.

Therapeutic Principle: Clear Stomach, reduce Fire.

Principal Measure: Relax the chest by pressing and kneading, grasp the abdomen with lifting and grasping, push the abdomen with round-rubbing and revolving, stroke and caress the head, knead points around the mouth with the fingers.

Subordinate Measure: Nip Hegu (LI 4), Jiache (St 6), Zusanli (St 36), and Neiting (St 44); knead the lower jaw from Chengjiang (CV 24) to Tinghui (GB 2).

2. Wind-Cold

Signs and Symptoms: Toothache accompanied by twitching, aversion to cold, desire for hot drinks without thirst, breath is normal. *Tongue:* pale red with thin white fur. *Pulse:* superficial, tense.

Therapeutic Principle: Expel Wind, disperse Cold.

Principal Measure: Stroke and caress the head; nip Baihui (GV 20); grasp Fengchi (GB 20), lift and grasp Jianjing (GB 21), knead Tinggong (SI 19), Tinghui (GB 2) and Yifeng (TW 17).

Subordinate Measure: Nip Taichong (Liv 3) and Xingjian (Liv 2), push and knead the cheek from Renzhong (GV 26) or Chengjiang (CV 24) to Jiache (St 6).

3. Wind-Heat

Signs and Symptoms: Toothache with redness, swelling and distending pain of the gum; the pain is aggravated by chewing; desire for cold drinks, aversion to heat; also, swelling, hotness and pain in cheek; thirst accompanied by sore throat, fever, headache. *Tongue:* red tip with thin white or slightly yellow, dry fur. *Pulse:* superficial, rapid.

Therapeutic Principle: Expel Wind, clear Heat.

Principal Measure: Open Passes and dredge Apertures, lift and grasp Fengchi (GB 20), pinch the arm with nipping and kneading, knead and grasp to relax the throat.

Subordinate Measure: Nip Neiguan (Per 6), Waiguan (TW 5), Zusanli (St 36) and Neiting (St 44).

4. Kidney Deficiency

Signs and Symptoms: Vague, intermittent toothache; loose teeth; redness at cheekbones and lips; dry throat, palpitation, anxiety, insomnia; soreness of waist and knees. *Tongue:* red without fur. *Pulse:* thready, rapid.

Therapeutic Principle: Invigorate Kidney, benefit Essence.

Principal Measure: Stroke and caress the head, strengthen the waist by rolling and rubbing, pluck Collaterals with knocking and scratching, relax the chest by pressing and kneading, roll the arm with pushing and grasping, roll the abdomen with knocking and vibrating, knead the leg with rotating and round-rubbing.

Subordinate Measure: Nip Hegu (LI 4) and Lieque (Lu 7); knead Zusanli (St 36), Sanyinjiao (Sp 6) and Taixi (K 3); rub Yongquan (K 1).

Pharyngitis

This is characterized by dryness, swelling, pain and a feeling as if there were a foreign body in the throat. Often complicated by nasal inflammation.

Etiology: Attack of exogenous Wind-Heat; flaming up of Deficient Fire due to Deficiency of Lung Yin; uprising of accumulated Stomach Heat.

Diagnosis & Treatment

1. Stomach Heat

Signs and Symptoms: Redness, dryness, swelling and pain of the pharynx and the gums; halitosis, longing for drinks; burning pain in stomach; belching with putrid odor, regurgitation of acid, constipation, deep-colored urine. *Tongue:* crimson with greasy yellow fur. *Pulse:* slippery, rapid.

Therapeutic Principle: Clear Heat, ease the throat.

Principal Measure: Relieve the chest by dotting and vibrating, knead and grasp to relax the throat, grasp the abdomen with lifting and grasping, pinch the arm with nipping and kneading.

Subordinate Measure: Knead Tiantu (CV 22) with a bent finger, knead Qishe (St 11), push the neck from Lianquan (CV 23) to Tiantu (CV 22).

2. Deficiency of Yin

Signs and Symptoms: Dryness and itching of throat with a dim red color, hoarse voice, thirst, lack of saliva, dry cough with minimal sputum. *Tongue:* red with thin fur. *Pulse:* thready, rapid.

Therapeutic Principle: Nourish Yin, reduce Fire.

Principal Measure: Relax the chest by pressing and kneading, push and wipe to divide the ribs, pinch the arms with nipping and kneading, push the abdomen with round-rubbing and revolving, knead and grasp to relax the throat, rock and deep-press to initiate vocalization, lift and grasp Jianjing (GB 21).

Subordinate Measure: Knead Yunmen (Lu 2); knead Tiantu (CV 22) with a bent finger; nip Hegu (LI 4); knead Renying (St 9), Zusanli (St 36) and Sanyinjiao (Sp 6).

Globus hystericus

This is also called obstruction of the larynx. The patient feels as if the throat is blocked by a lump of some sort, that cannot be dislodged, but which has no effect on eating or drinking.

Etiology: Vital Energy stuffiness in the larynx from emotional depression; adhesion of Phlegm in the throat due to diminished function of Spleen.

Diagnosis & Treatment

1. Adverse uprising of Liver Energy

Signs and Symptoms: Intermittent sensation of foreign body in the throat, anxiety, irritability, fullness in the rib cage, belching; emotional agitation intensifies symptoms. *Tongue:* thin fur. *Pulse:* stringy.

Therapeutic Principle: Relieve depression, rectify Liver Energy.

Principal Measure: Relieve the chest by dotting and vibrating, push and wipe to divide the ribs, roll the arm with pushing and grasping, roll the abdomen with knocking and vibrating, roll the leg with revolving and pinching, revolve Huantiao (GB 30) with the elbow, knead and grasp to relax the throat.

Subordinate Measure: Nip Hegu (LI 4), Neiguan (Per 6) and Jianshi (Per 5); dot Tiantu (CV 22) with a bent finger.

2. Adhesion of Phlegm

Signs and Symptoms: Intermittent sensation of foreign body, sticky Phlegm adheres to the throat and cannot be expelled, feeling of congestion and weight in the chest and rib cage, hiccups, nausea, poor appetite. *Tongue:* thick, greasy fur. *Pulse:* soft, floating, slippery.

Therapeutic Principle: Resolve Phlegm, ease the throat.

Principal Measure: Dot Fengfu (GV 16) with the fingers, nip and grasp Fengchi (GB 20), relieve the chest by dotting and vibrating, push and wipe to divide the ribs, push the abdomen with round-rubbing and revolving, grasp the abdomen with lifting and grasping, push the back with pinching and grasping, knead and grasp to relax the larynx.

Subordinate Measure: Nip Neiguan (Per 6), Waiguan (TW 5), Jianshi (Per 5) and Zusanli (St 36).

Aphonia

This is also called sudden loss of the voice and is often complicated by dryness, harshness, pain and discomfort in the throat, and weak or hoarse voice.

Etiology: Aphonia may be classified as the Deficient and the Excess. Excess aphonia is usually caused by an attack of exogenous evils; stagnation of Liver Energy at the larynx due to emotional depression, or stagnation of Heart-Spleen Energy from mental strain; restriction and contraction of the vocal cord due to fright, rage, grief, etc. Deficient aphonia is usually caused by depletion of Lung Energy and loss of body fluids from prolonged singing, loud speaking, or shouting.

Diagnosis & Treatment

1. Attack of Wind-Cold

Signs and Symptoms: Sudden onset, sore throat with constricted sensation accompanied by an aversion to cold, fever, stuffy nose, clear nasal discharge. *Tongue:* pale with thin white fur. *Pulse:* superficial, tense.

Therapeutic Principle: Relieve the external, disperse Cold, ventilate Lung Energy, ease the throat.

Principal Measure: Open Passes and dredge Apertures; nip and grasp Fengchi (GB 20); knead Fengfu (GV 16) with the fingers; pluck, vibrate and knock the neck; rock and deep-press to initiate vocalization.

Subordinate Measure: Nip Shousanli (LI 10), Waiguan (TW 5), Yuji (Lu 10) and Shaoshang (Lu 11).

2. Attack of Wind-Heat

Signs and Symptoms: Aphonia with swelling, pain and dryness of throat; pain increase during swallowing; thirst, desire for drinks, fever, mild aversion to wind. *Tongue:* red with yellow fur. *Pulse:* superficial, rapid.

Therapeutic Principle: Expel Wind, clear Heat, dredge Apertures, ease the throat.

Principal Measure: Stroke and caress the head, open Passes and dredge Apertures, relieve the chest by dotting and vibrating, push and wipe to divide the ribs, knead and grasp to relax the larynx, rock and deep-press to initiate vocalization, revolve Huantiao (GB 30) with the elbow, rub Yongquan (K 1).

Subordinate Measure: Nip Quchi (LI 11), Neiguan (Per 6), Yuji (Lu 10) and Shaoshang (Lu 11).

3. Sudden aphonia

Signs and Symptoms: Speaking without sound, emotional depression, lassitude, symptoms increase in anger or agitation. *Tongue:* thin, greasy white fur. *Pulse:* stringy, rapid or deep, uneven.

Therapeutic Principle: Relieve depression, rectify Liver Energy, tranquilize the mind, relax the larynx.

Principal Measure: Stroke and caress the head, open Passes and dredge Apertures, knead Fengfu (GV 16) with the fingers, knead and grasp Fengchi (GB 20), lift and grasp Jianjing (GB 21), relieve the chest by dotting and vibrating, push and wipe to divide the ribs, press the abdomen with deep-pressing and kneading, knead and grasp to relax the larynx, rock and deep-press to initiate vocalization, pinch the arm with nipping and kneading.

Subordinate Measure: Nip and knead Hegu (LI 4), Zhigou (TW 6), Yangjiao (GB 35) and Foot-Tonggu (UB 66); rub Yongquan (K 1).

Inflammation of the throat

This refers to swelling, redness and pain in the throat accompanied by difficulty in swallowing and hoarseness. It corresponds to pharyngitis or sore throat.

Etiology: Attack of Wind-Heat or Wind-Cold due to weakness of defense mechanism, careless daily life or sudden change of weather; flaming up of Deficient Fire due to depletion of Yin and Blood from overwork or mental strain.

Diagnosis & Treatment

1. Attack of Wind-Heat

Signs and Symptoms: Initially, there is dryness, heat, reddening of the throat and difficulty in swallowing. Later, there is swelling, burning pain, hoarseness and sticky, yellow sputum accompanied by fever, aversion to wind, headache, cough, constipation and deep-colored urine. *Tongue:* red with yellow fur. *Pulse:* superficial, rapid.

Therapeutic Principle: Clear Heat, ease the throat, eliminate swelling, relieve pain.

Principal Measure: Open Passes and dredge Apertures, knead Fengfu (GV 16) with the fingers, lift and grasp Fengchi (GB 20) and Jianjing (GB 21), relieve the chest by dotting and vibrating, knead and grasp to relax the larynx, rock and deep-press to initiate vocalization.

Subordinate Measure: Nip and knead Shousanli (LI 10), Quchi (LI 11), Hegu (LI 4) and Waiguan (TW 5).

2. Attack of Wind-Cold

Signs and Symptoms: Initially, difficulty in swallowing, pain, harshness and redness of the throat. Later, swelling and pain in the throat, feeling of fullness in the chest, cough, labored breathing, thin white sputum accompanied by clear nasal discharge, headache, fever, and a desire for warmth with an aversion to cold. *Tongue:* pale with white fur. *Pulse:* superficial, tense.

Therapeutic Principle: Relieve the external, expel Wind, resolve stasis, ease the throat.

Principal Measure: Stroke and caress the head, open Passes and dredge Apertures, nip and grasp Fengchi (GB 20), lift and grasp Jianjing (GB 21), knead and grasp to relax the larynx, rock and deep-press to initiate vocalization, relieve the chest by dotting and vibrating, pinch the arm with nipping and kneading.

Subordinate Measure: Grasp Hegu (LI 4) and Zhigou (TW 6), rub Yongquan (K 1).

3. Depletion of Yin and Blood

Signs and Symptoms: Slight swelling and redness of the throat; harshness and pain when swallowing; symptoms more intense at night; all accompanied by dryness of the larynx and the tongue, heat at palms and soles of feet, listlessness and weariness. *Tongue:* red without fur. *Pulse:* thready, rapid.

Therapeutic Principle: Invigorate Kidney, nourish Yin, foster Blood, reduce Fire.

Principal Measure: Lift and grasp Fengchi (GB 20), knead Fengfu (GV 16) and Dazhui (GV 14) with the fingers, push the back with lifting and grasping, relieve the chest by dotting and vibrating, push and wipe to divide the ribs, knead and grasp to relax the larynx, rock and deep-press to initiate vocalization, lift and grasp Jianjing (GB 21).

Subordinate Measure: Knead Quchi (LI 11); grasp and knead Hegu (LI 4), Zusanli (St 36) and Sanyinjiao (Sp 6); push Yongquan (K 1).

Bleeding gums

Etiology: Accumulation of Stomach-Intestine Heat due to habitual ingestion of rich, pungent foods or liquor; flaming up of Deficient Fire due to depletion of Kidney Yin.

Diagnosis & Treatment

1. Stomach Heat

Signs and Symptoms: Swelling, pain and redness of the gums; profuse bright red bleeding; foul breath; fever, thirst and constipation. *Tongue:* red with greasy yellow fur. *Pulse:* full, rapid.

Therapeutic Principle: Clear Stomach, reduce Fire.

Principal Measure: Knead and grasp Fengchi (GB 20), lift and grasp Jianjing (GB 21), relax the chest by pressing and kneading, grasp the abdomen with lifting and grasping, push the abdomen with round-rubbing and revolving, revolve Huantiao (GB 30) with the elbow.

Subordinate Measure: Knead Xuehai (Sp 10) and Zusanli (St 36), nip and knead Neiguan (Per 6) and Waiguan (TW 5).

2. Depletion of Kidney Yin

Signs and Symptoms: Loose teeth without swelling or redness of the gums, minimal bleeding of pale red color, diminished ability to taste, normal breath odor, dizziness, tinnitus, heat at the palms and soles of the feet, soreness and weakness at the waist and knees. *Tongue:* pale red with minimal fur. *Pulse:* thready, rapid.

Therapeutic Principle: Nourish Yin, reduce Fire.

Principal Measure: Pluck, vibrate and knock the neck, push the back with pinching and grasping, strengthen the waist by rolling and rubbing, knead the leg with rotating and round-rubbing, stroke and caress the head, push the abdomen with round-rubbing and revolving, lift and grasp Jianjing (GB 21).

Subordinate Measure: Knead Taixi (K 3) and Dazhong (K 4), rub Yongquan (K 1).

Injury to the temperomandibular joint (TMJ)

This is characterized by pain and snapping during movement of the jaw, and is often seen in young and middle-aged people.

Etiology: Usually, this injury is caused by improper chewing, attack of Wind-Cold, or malnutrition of tendons and muscles due to Deficiency of Liver-Kidney or Vital Energy and Blood.

Diagnosis & Treatment

Signs and Symptoms: Pain and swelling at the affected side of the jaw, restricted opening of the mouth, loss of strength in chewing accompanied by pain and snapping. If the cause is depletion of Liver-Kidney Yin, the tendons and joints on both sides will be slack, inhibiting the chewing motion, and the snapping is more pronounced. There is also dizziness and tinnitus.

Therapeutic Principle: Soften Tendons, ease joints, relieve spasm and pain.

Principal Measure: Rectify the joint. The patient may sit upright in a chair or supine, with a relaxed body. Press against the upper incisors with a thumb and the lower incisors with the index finger of the same hand, and gradually open the mouth. At the same time, knead Xiaguan (St 7), Jiache (St 6), Tinghui (GB 2) and the joint gap of the affected side with the fingers of the other hand, until tendons and the joint are relaxed.

Subordinate Measure: Revolve Huantiao (GB 30), grasp Weizhong (UB 40), nip Sanyinjiao (Sp 6), all on both sides.

Runny nose with turbid discharge

If this sort of discharge flows back into the throat, there will be continual spitting.

Etiology: Attack of Wind-Cold or Wind-Heat based on hidden fever from Deficiency of Lung Energy.

Diagnosis & Treatment

1. Wind-Cold

Signs and Symptoms: Continuous clear nasal discharge, stuffy nose, frequent sneezing; occasionally the discharge flows backward, causing continual spitting; loss of sense of smell. Symptoms are aggravated by cold weather, and often accompanied by fever without sweating, and headache. *Tongue:* pale with thin white fur. *Pulse:* superficial, tense.

Therapeutic Principle: Expel Wind, disperse Cold, ventilate Lung Energy, dredge Apertures.

Principal Measure: Open Passes and dredge Apertures, knead and grasp Fengchi (GB 20), knead Fengfu (GV 16) and Dazhui (GV 14) with the fingers, relieve the chest by dotting and vibrating, pull the arm with rotating and rectifying.

Subordinate Measure: Knead Yingxiang (LI 20), Yifeng (TW 17) and Fengfu (GV 16); grasp Waiguan (TW 5) and Hegu (LI 4).

2. Wind-Heat

Signs and Symptoms: Continuous nasal discharge, dry nasal cavity, sore throat, violent sneezing, stuffy nose, swelling and redness of anterior nostrils. In time, nasal discharge becomes thick, yellowish and difficult to clear; a backward flow of this causes spitting; distending pain at forehead and eyebrows, loss of sense of smell; fever, aversion to wind; headache, dizziness, cough, perspiration. *Tongue:* red with white fur. *Pulse:* superficial, rapid.

Therapeutic Principle: Expel Wind, clear Heat, ease Lung Energy, dredge Apertures.

Principal Measure: Stroke and caress the head; knead Fengfu (GV 16) and Dazhui (GV 14) with the fingers; pinch and grasp Fengchi (GB 20); press and push the clavicular fossa; relax the chest by pressing and kneading; push and wipe to divide the ribs; pluck, vibrate and knock the neck.

Subordinate Measure: Knead Yingxiang (LI 20) and Fengchi (GB 20), grasp Hegu (LI 4) and Quchi (LI 11).

Nosebleed

This refers to spontaneous nosebleed without trauma, often seen in teenagers, especially in spring or autumn in dry climate.

Etiology: Attack of Wind-Heat on nasal Collaterals, accumulation of Heat in Spleen and Stomach rises up and scorches Yang Collaterals of the nose.

Diagnosis & Treatment

1. Lung Heat

Signs and Symptoms: Pain, heat and dryness of nasal cavity; bleeding of bright red blood; swelling, pain and redness of the throat; thirst; short, dry cough, perspiration, aversion to wind. *Tongue:* red with white fur. *Pulse:* superficial, rapid.

Therapeutic Principle: Expel Wind, clear Lung Heat.

Principal Measure: Open Passes and dredge Apertures, knock the fontanel with the hands, relax the chest by pressing and kneading, push and wipe to divide the ribs, revolve Huantiao (GB 30) with the elbow, nip and knead Hegu (LI 4).

Subordinate Measure: Knead Fengchi (GB 20); knead Tiantu (CV 22) with a bent finger; pluck, vibrate and knock the neck; nip Shaoshang (LI 11) and Yongquan (K 1).

2. Stomach Heat

Signs and Symptoms: Pain and dryness in the nasal cavity; profuse, bright red bleeding; halitosis, sore throat, desire for drinks, constipation, deep-colored urine, varied appetite. *Tongue:* red with yellow fur. *Pulse:* full, rapid.

Therapeutic Principle: Relax bowels, induce appetite and digestion, clear Heat, cool Blood.

Principal Measure: Stroke and caress the head, knock the fontanel with the hands, lift and grasp both ears, push and wipe to divide the ribs, press the abdomen with deep-pressing and kneading, revolve Huantiao (GB 30) with the elbow.

Subordinate Measure: Grasp Shousanli (LI 10), Hegu (LI 4) and Shaoshang (Lu 11); knead Zusanli (St 36).

Dislocation of the mandibular joint

This is usually caused by improper activities of the lower jaw or by outside force. The mouth cannot be opened or closed.

Etiology: Excessively wide mouth opening, impact, etc.; relaxation of related tendons due to age or Deficiency of Liver- Kidney Energy.

Diagnosis & Treatment

1. Joint malposition

Signs and Symptoms: The mouth remains slightly opened with spasm, aching and distension of the mandibular joint. The jaw cannot be moved either way, and the patient is unable to speak. The process of the joint shifts forward and the joint space is widened. There is stringy spasm of tendons and muscles, tenderness, and resistance to pressing at the joint.

Therapeutic Principle: Soften Tendons, relieve spasm, reposition.

Prescription: The patient may sit upright or lie in a supine posture. Massage Jiache (St 6), Xiaguan (St 7) and Daying (St 5) with techniques such as kneading, pushing, pressing, pulling, etc., until there are sensations of soreness, distension and numbness at the mandibular joint. After this, deep-press the lower jaw heavily near the malposed part downwards and back. This will usually reposition the joint. After that, knead and rub the periphery of this joint with the thenar mound until a warm sensation is felt. You may also incorporate pinching and grasping Fengchi (GB 20) and nipping and kneading Hegu (LI 4) to relieve pain.

2. Single dislocation

Signs and Symptoms: The patient's face deviates toward the healthy side with a slightly opened, uncloseable mouth; occasional salivation; impaired speech; depression at Tinghui (GB 2); protrusion beneath the cheekbone; spasm of the buccinator muscle.

Prescription: Stand by the affected side of the patient, who sits upright or lies in a supine position. Stabilize the patient's head with one hand. With the other hand, insert the thumb into the patient's mouth to deep-press the molars of the affected side, while holding and supporting the jaw with the other fingers. (Bandage your thumb with a piece of antiseptic gauze to protect it from being bitten.) Have the patient relax his/her jaw, press the jaw down forcefully to stretch the joint and force it to return to its normal position. After this, knead Tinggong (SI 19), Tinghui (GB 2), Shangguan (GB 3), Jiache (St 6) and Xiaguan (St 7) with the fingers, then round-rub these points with the palms. Additionally, pinch and grasp Fengchi (GB 20) until a warm sensation is perceived.

3. Double dislocation

Signs and Symptoms: The jaw is dropped, and the opened mouth cannot be closed; continuous salivation, impaired speech, protrusion at both cheeks, depressions at both Tinghui (GB 2).

Prescription: The patient should be supine with the head stabilized. Push and knead both cheeks with the fingers, and have the patient relax as much as possible. Insert both thumbs slowly into the patient's mouth and press them to the lower molars on both sides (wrap your thumbs in antiseptic gauze to protect them from being bitten). Deep-press Lianquan (CV 23) with both middle fingers, and hold and support both sides of the lower jaw with the remaining fingers. Using both thumbs simultaneously, press the jaw back and down forcefully. When the joint space has been widened, make an effort to lift the upper jaw with both middle and index fingers. This should complete the repositioning. After this is done, knead both Tinggong (SI 19), Tinghui (GB 2), Jiache (St 6), Shangguan (GB 3) and Xiaguan (St 7) with the fingers to relax the tendons and joints, and to relieve pain. Advise the patient that hearty laughter, vigorous chewing and such may cause re-dislocation of the jaw.

Appendixes

Massage for athletes

Massage for athletes is an important part of sports medicine. The ability to take into account the different physiological requirements of various sports and gymnastic events, and understand the different constitutions and neural types of athletes, has become a specialty. In this section, we integrate Traditional Chinese massage with the fundamental principles of current athletic anatomy, physiology and medical science, and recommend those measures which have been proven simple and effective.

Massage before competition

This is aimed at tranquilizing the mind, strengthening muscles, improving the dexterity of joints and the flexibility of tendons, and keeping the athlete in good form.

Prescription for a sound sleep

Indications: Palpitation, anxiety, restlessness, insomnia, loss of appetite, profuse spontaneous perspiration, elevated pulse rate and blood pressure.

Requirements: 30 minutes before competition, let the athlete lie supinely in a quiet room with soft illumination, good ventilation and a comfortable temperature. Have the athlete relax with closed eyes, attention concentrated, and breath regulated. Manipulate briskly for 10-15 minutes. The massage should be gentle, fluent, rhythmic and successive.

Procedure: Vibrate Baihu (GV 20) and Yintang (Ex-HN 2). Gather in all five fingers of each hand close to each other, with their tips aligned, like a plum flower. Press the tips to selected points, and quiver the fingers slightly, making the applied force penetrate into each point, until a warm sensation may be felt. Stroke and caress the head, knock Baihu (GV 20) gently until the athlete falls asleep.

Prescription for tranquilization

Indications: Distractedness, mental stress, confusion, accelerated rate of respiration, elevated blood pressure.

Requirements: 20 minutes before competition, let the athlete lie in a soft, comfortable bed. Manipulate gently and slowly for 5-10 minutes both prone and supine.

Procedure: Stroke and caress the head, push the back with pinching and grasping, deep-press the spine with kneading and revolving, pull the waist with rolling and rubbing, knead the leg with rotating and round-rubbing.

Prescription for refreshing

Indications: Mental depression, timidness, weariness, loss of strength before competition.

Requirements: 15 minutes before competition, let the athlete lie supinely in a soft bed. Manipulate energetically and rapidly for 5-10 minutes.

Procedure: Open Passes and dredge Apertures; stroke and caress the head; pull, push and knead the neck; pinch the arm with nipping and kneading; roll the leg with revolving and pinching.

Massage during competition

This is aimed at improving the athlete's mental state, relieving muscular fatigue, spasm, rigidity of joints, and maintaining good form.

Prescription for eliminating fatigue

Indications: Weariness, muscular aches with trembling, spasm and stiffness of joints.

Requirements: Combined treatment should be employed to massage the entire body of the athlete, and lay stress on the fatigued parts according to the characteristics of the sport. Generally, the massage lasts 10-15 minutes, with moderate exertion.

Procedure: Pinch the arm with nipping and kneading, roll the arm with pushing and grasping, deep-press the spine with kneading and revolving, push the back with pinching and grasping, pull the waist with jerking and dragging, strengthen the waist by rolling and rubbing, pull the leg with knocking and vibrating, roll the leg with revolving and pinching.

Subordinate Measure: Nip Jianyu (LI 15), Quchi (LI 11), Laogong (Per 8), Yangchi (TW 4), Yangxi (LI 5); press and knead Huantiao (GB 30) and Weizhong (UB 40); nip Zusanli (St 36), Kunlun (UB 60) and Juegu (GB 39).

Massage after competition

This is aimed at promoting the mental and physical recovery of the athlete after competition through a sound sleep or rest. It is well known that massage can relieve fatigue, as well as relax tendons, muscles and joints.

Prescription for relaxing Meridians

Indications: Dizziness, heaviness in the head, listlessness, weariness, lassitude, aching and loss of strength in limbs, loss of appetite, restless sleep.

Requirements: Have the athlete bathe, then lie in a soft bed to rest and breathe deeply for 3-5 minutes. Manipulate forcefully but slowly for 30-60 minutes.

Procedure: Relieve the chest by dotting and vibrating, relax the chest by pressing and kneading, push the abdomen with round-rubbing and revolving, press the abdomen with deep-pressing and kneading, push the back with pinching and grasping, deep-press the spine with kneading and revolving, strengthen the waist by rolling and rubbing, pluck Collaterals with knocking and scratching, roll the leg with revolving and pinching, knead the leg with rotating and round-rubbing.

Subordinate Measure: Nip Neiguan (Per 6), Zusanli (St 36), Weizhong (UB 40) and Sanyinjiao (Sp 6).

Prophylaxis and treatment of disorders in sports competition

Abdominal pain from exercise

This is most likely to occur at the epigastrium or around the navel during a heel-and-toe walking race, long-distance or marathon race. It often interferes with the athlete's ability to finish the event.

Etiology: Deficiency of Heart and Lung Energy due to insufficient training and adaptation. In violent sports, there is sudden loss of body fluids and impediment of the Energy Mechanism, resulting in disharmony of Spleen and Stomach; blockage of the flow of Vital Energy and Blood; or Blood stasis in internal organs due to their bumping or jostling.

Diagnosis & Treatment

1. Disharmony between Spleen and Stomach

Signs & Symptoms: Initially, there is pain and a feeling of fullness in the epigastric region. Later, frequent vomiting and hiccupping; pain becomes serious and the area around the navel may be involved; a desire for being pressed; resting may alleviate symptoms.

Therapeutic Principle: Disperse and rectify Liver Energy.

Prescription: Relieve the chest by dotting and vibrating, push and wipe to divide the ribs, push the abdomen with round-rubbing and revolving, press the abdomen with deep-pressing and kneading, grasp the abdomen with lifting and jerking.

2. Blood stasis in Liver and Spleen

Signs & Symptoms: Vague pain around the navel; feeling of fullness, distension and weight in the rib cage. As it progresses, there is stabbing or tearing pain involving both the rib cage and the abdomen. Symptoms may be alleviated by pressing, leaning or resting, but they cannot be eliminated in this manner.

Therapeutic Principle: Activate Blood, relieve stasis.

Principal Measure: Relieve the chest by dotting and vibrating, relax the chest by pressing and kneading, push and wipe to divide the ribs, press the abdomen with deep-pressing and kneading, Taiji round-rub the abdomen.

Subordinate Measure: Nip Neiguan (Per 6), revolve Huantiao (GB 30) with the elbow, nip Zusanli (St 36).

3. Impediment and blockage of Energy Mechanism

Signs & Symptoms: Constricting pain at both sides of the rib cage with a feeling of fullness and weight; respiration restricted as it triggers pain. Progressively, there will be dry throat and mouth, continuous running pain along the back and rib cage, and frequent hiccups.

Therapeutic Principle: Relieve spasm, rectify Energy.

Principal Measure: Relax the chest by pressing and kneading, push and wipe to divide the ribs, press the abdomen with deep-pressing and kneading, push the abdomen with round-rubbing and revolving, deep-press the back with kneading and revolving.

Subordinate Measure: Nip Neiguan (Per 6), Yanglingquan (GB 34), Zusanli (St 36) and Weizhong (UB 40).

Kinetic syncope

The athlete faints suddenly, during competition, then quickly regains consciousness.

Etiology: Sudden depletion of Vital Energy, Blood and body fluids, such as would be caused by excessive perspiration, over-tiredness or emotional strain, based on Spleen-Stomach Deficiency.

Diagnosis & Treatment

Signs & Symptoms: Pale complexion, profuse sweating; sudden fainting with cold limbs, rough breathing. After regaining consciousness: weariness, loss of strength, thirst, desire for drinks. *Tongue:* pale with thin fur. *Pulse:* deep, faint.

Principal Measure: Open Passes and dredge Apertures, stroke and caress the head, relieve the chest by dotting and vibrating, relax the chest by pressing and kneading, push and wipe to divide the ribs, grasp the abdomen with lifting and jerking, roll the abdomen with knocking and vibrating.

Subordinate Measure: If there is dizziness and headache, nip Baihu (GV 20), Quchi (LI 11), Hegu (LI 4) and Lieque (Lu 7). If there is vomiting and hiccups, nip Neiguan (Per 6) and Zusanli (St 36) together.

Prophylaxis: If there is pale complexion, profuse sweating and unstable gait, remove the athlete from competition.

Principal Measure: Stroke and caress the head, open Passes and dredge Apertures.

Subordinate Measure: Nip Fengchi (GB 20), Neiguan (Per 6), Waiguan (TW 5) and Lieque (Lu 7).

Traumatic chest and rib cage pain

This is often seen in grueling or violent competitions, such as ball games and weight lifting.

Etiology: Spasm and pain of tendons and muscles at the chest and rib cage from tugging, sudden motion, wrenching or uncoordinated activity; injury from impact, squeezing or pressure; obstruction of Vessel Collateral by overexertion or holding the breath.

Diagnosis & Treatment

1. Damage to Vital Energy

Signs & Symptoms: Wandering pain and distension at the chest and rib cage with restricted respiratory movement. Initially, onset of pain is sudden and intense and may be alleviated by exercise, although excessive exercise aggravates symptoms; later, the condition progresses, including emotional depression and loss of appetite.

Therapeutic Principle: Disperse and rectify Liver Energy.

Prescription: Relieve the chest by dotting and vibrating, push and wipe to divide the ribs, push the abdomen with round-rubbing and revolving, grasp the abdomen with lifting and jerking, push the back, deep-press the spine with kneading and revolving, relax the chest by pressing and kneading.

Have the patient stand. Deep-press both Yanglingquan (GB 34). After prickling sensations appear, have the patient bend forward and back from the waist, 10-15 times each way. Deep-press both Zusanli (St 36), and after the prickling sensations appear, have the patient again bend forward and back from the waist, 10-15 times each way. Deep-press Ganshu (UB 18) and Zhangmen (Liv 13) on the opposite side, and after the prickling sensations appear, have the patient turn the body right and left 10-20 times each direction. Finally, deep-press Renzhong (GV 26), and after the prickling sensations appear, have the patient cough 10-15 times to vibrate the chest and rib cage.

2. Damage to Blood

Refer to Section 1, Internal Medicine, "Chest Pain".

Kinetic patellar strain

This is often seen in basketball, volleyball, high diving and high jumping.

Etiology: Injury to tendons from impact, jumping, strain, etc.; attack of Wind-Cold.

Diagnosis & Treatment

Signs & Symptoms: Initially, vague pain or aching at the upper knee, with slackening of the knee joint; the person bends the knee intermittently for relief. Gradually, the symptoms become more intense, and there is stabbing pain during flexion and extension, especially after exercise; ultimately there is atrophy and slackening of tendons and muscles, roughening of the patellar edge, serious tenderness, aversion to cold, and reluctance to move.

Therapeutic Principle: Activate Blood, resolve stasis, soften Tendons, rectify joints.

Principal Measure: Push and knead the Six Meridians of the leg, grasp and revolve the patella, rotate the knee, pad the popliteal fossa and flex the knee, knead the popliteal fossa, roll the leg.

Subordinate Measure: Pluck the joint space, dot and knead Heding (Ex-LE 1) and the inner and outer Dubi (St 35).

Kinetic tibialgia (Shinsplints)

This is also called fatigue tibialgia, and is characterized by swelling and pain at the lower end of the tibia. The patient's motion is restricted.

Etiology: The supply of Vital Energy and Blood to the lower shank is minimal, since the muscles are lean and the skin is thin in that area. Kinetic tibialgia is usually caused by excessive or improper exertion, outside force, or an attack of Wind-Cold-Dampness.

Diagnosis & Treatment

Signs & Symptoms: Initially, aching and discomfort in the lower shank, then pitting edema and pain along the length of the tibia, with symptoms increasing. Palpation reveals spasm of Tendon Collaterals on both sides of the shank with band-like or nodular structures. The injured area is resistant to pressing. Symptoms are milder by day, more serious at night, especially after work. Motion of the leg is restricted.

Therapeutic Principle: Activate Blood, dissipate stasis, relieve spasm and pain.

Principal Measure: Push Six Meridians of the leg, roll the leg, pinch the Achilles Tendon, knead the inner shank from Yinlingquan (Sp 9) to Taixi (K 3) with the fingers.

Subordinate Measure: Nip and knead Shenshu (UB 23), Weizhong (UB 40), Chengshan (UB 57) and Zusanli (St 36).

Kinetic cramping of the calf

This is also called spasm of the calf and may occur during or after competition. It is frequently seen in long-distance runners and swimmers.

Etiology: Insufficient warm-up, depletion of body fluids due to profuse perspiration, over-fatigue, attack of Wind-Cold-Dampness.

Diagnosis & Treatment

Signs & Symptoms: Sudden onset of intolerable cramp in the calf which may last varying amounts of time; the athlete cannot stand up; the cramp may recur, sometimes from careless motion; when it passes, the calf aches and is exhausted, resistant to pressing.

Therapeutic Principle: Relax Tendons, dredge Collaterals, relieve spasm and pain.

Principal Measure: During the spasm, pull the big toe and bend it backward to stretch the tendons and relax the spasm; pinch the Achilles tendon; knead the popliteal fossa; roll the leg; pinch the calf.

Subordinate Measure: Knead Shenshu (UB 23) and Ganshu (UB 18), grasp Yanglingquan (GB 34) and Zusanli (St 36), knead Chengshan (UB 57), grasp Kunlun (UB 60).

Common kinetic trauma

Refer to Section 4, Trauma.

Self-massage for personal hygiene

Massage for personal hygiene means to massage yourself with your own hands, and thereby improve your condition of health or treat your own disease. Of course, techniques should be chosen according to your own physiological or pathological conditions and therapeutic requirements. Good effects can only come for practicing self-massage over a long period of time, so the development of proficiency in self-massage for personal hygiene occupies an important place in the health care of the Chinese people.

Self-massage is in the category of active hygiene, which is comprised of a variety of different schools and exercises. We recommend those effective measures in common use according to traditional theories of Yin-Yang, Five Elements, Yin and Yang organs, and Meridians. In addition, the valuable experiences of senior doctor Gu Daifeng are also included in this section.

Through the practice of self-massage, those who are healthy may consolidate that health to prevent disease; those who are diseased may convalesce; those who are weak may become stronger; and those who are aged may extend their lifespan.

Characteristics of self-massage

A wide variety of diseases may be treated and prevented. All people may benefit from self-massage — young and old, male and female, healthy or sick, with organic or functional diseases — as long as their hands are functional.

Self-massage is convenient, safe, and economical. Most of the techniques can be done anywhere at any time, without restrictions of condition or circumstance.

It is easy to learn and do, as long as you can remember the location and functions of related points, and can master common techniques.

Good effects can definitely be achieved, if you practice properly and with perseverance.

Guidelines for self-massage

Resolve: It is important to carry out self-massage with a cheerful frame of mind. It is not just an exercise of action — it is mental and physical training. In order to achieve maximum results with minimum effort, it is important to maintain good spirits. It is difficult to see how a mentally-depressed person could obtain any benefits from self-massage.

Confidence: Be confident in your success and your perseverance. It is not useful to "go fishing for three days and dry the nets for two" because effects cannot be consolidated. It takes a long time to cure a serious or lingering ailment, or to achieve good health and longevity. "Constant effort brings certain success."

Scientific regimen: Plan your sessions. Don't massage yourself immediately after meals, when hungry, or when you have an urge to urinate or defecate. Women should not overdo massage during menstruation or pregnancy. Techniques, herbal preparations and amount of force applied should be chosen carefully. After self-massage, rest and wash the body with a towel dipped in warm water. Fingernails should be kept trimmed.

Environment: Self-massage should be done in a clean room with a comfortable temperature. Keep away from wind as if you were "taking shelter from arrows," because "Wind is the first and foremost factor to cause various diseases." This is especially true for the aged and the weak.

Avoid over-fatigue: Even more important is to control sexual intercourse when on a regimen of self-massage. When virility is improved through strengthening the Yang, do not dissipate the good results you have achieved through sexual indulgence. Otherwise, your efforts will be wasted.

Moderate living: Adequate rest, particularly sound sleep; reasonable nutrition with good dietary habits; walking, slow running, or other gymnastic exercises — all these are critical to your health. Self-massage is not a panacea — in treating certain diseases, medical therapy should be followed concurrently.

Preparation for self-massage

The best way is to be naked in a room by yourself. If it is cold, wear an unlined garment or cover yourself with a thin blanket. Regardless of the posture you choose according to the areas to be massaged, relax your entire body, with the area being massaged the most relaxed.

Breathe evenly and concentrate your mind. After assuming an appropriate posture, breathe naturally. In time, try to learn to breathe abdominally, at the same time ridding yourself of distracting thoughts and concentrating your attention on the region of Dantian. If this is difficult to achieve, don't force yourself, and don't even take pains to achieve it. It is easier just to think "relaxation" when inhaling and "tranquilization" when exhaling, and remain calm and relaxed for 3-5 minutes. When you begin to practice breathing, start with short sessions and gradually prolong the exercise.

Have your various herbal preparations ready for use. When it is hot and you are inclined to perspire, prepare and apply talcum powder to decrease the friction. When it is cold and your skin is dry, a small amount of Vaseline or glycerine may be useful. If you are suffering from headache and dizziness, you may choose Menthae Water and Essential Balm to clear Wind evil. For joint pain, Turpentine is useful; for abdominal pain, Ginger Juice.

Routine of self-massage

1. Routine of massage

A. Posture: Whichever posture you use, the back and the waist should be on the same axis.

Supine: Suitable for massage of the head and face, the neck, the chest and the abdomen.

Lying on the side: For massage of the flank, the waist and the buttock.

Sitting on a stool: All parts of the body.

B. Manipulations: They should be done in a soft, circular fashion, sustained and even, gentle without being superficial, heavy without becoming stagnant.

Force applied: Change gradually, from mild to heavy and from heavy to mild.

Speed: Change gradually from slow to fast and fast to slow.

Depth: Change gradually from shallow to deep and deep to shallow.

Direction: Invigorating and Strengthening: Counter to the direction of the Meridians, rotate clockwise, working inward, softly and gently for a longer time.

Reducing and Clearing: Along the direction of the Meridians, rotate counter-clockwise, moving outward, strenuously and heavy for a shorter time.

C. Techniques: They should be done in a relaxed and tranquil condition. The procedure is as follows:

Scope: From the spot to the line, from the line to an entire area.

Sequence: From the entire body to a local area, and from a local area to the entire body.

2. Routine of exercise

Exercise should be carried out leisurely and freely. Respiration should co-operate with intention. All the parts of the body which are movable should perform linear and rotary motions along all possible directions.

To improve health and promise longevity, we emphasize massage of the entire body. To cure disease and relieve discomfort, focus massage on the local area. The theory of "take the tender spot as the point" is applicable and should be incorporated with the theory of Meridians.

Exercise should be practiced after self-massage, until you feel sensations of soreness, numbness, slight aching and comfortable fatigue. Choose and perform them according to your own abilities. Neither half-hearted muddling nor exhausting fatigue is appropriate.

Proficiency in self-massage for personal hygiene

The sequence of self-massage is determined by the motor regularity of the human body and the theory of Meridians. Exercises of different parts of the body should be done in the following order: hands, arms, head, neck and nape, chest, rib cage, waist, legs, feet, abdomen, external genital organs. Each part may also be exercised alone.

When beginning a specific massage, manipulate slowly and gently in a wide area to induce adaptation of the local area. After this, choose the points more swiftly and vigorously. Finally, gradually decrease the scope and the force, and finish the massage slowly.

Various techniques are recommended as follows.

Techniques for the hand

The hand is the most active part of the body. It is also the origin and terminus of the Three Yin and Three Yang Meridians of the Hand. Therefore, functional changes of internal organs are closely related to the activities of the hand

1. Rub and wash hands

Concentrate your mind. Rub both palms together until you perceive a warm sensation. Then, rub the back of each hand with the palm of the other. Then, wash one hand with the other (stroking along longitudinal, transverse and revolving directions) until you achieve reddening, heat, glossiness and a feeling of distension, and do the same with the other hand.

2. Nip and knead the points of hands

With the tip of one thumb, nip and knead the points of the other hand: Taiyuan (Lu 9), Daling (Per 7), Shenmen (H 7), Laogong (Per 8), Yangxi (LI

5), Yangchi (TW 4), Yanggu (SI 5), Hegu (LI 4), Zhongzhu (TW 3), Shaoshang (Lu 11), Shangyang (LI 1), Zhongchong (Per 9), Guanchong (TW 1) and Shaoze (SI 1). Finally, nip Shixuan (Ex-UE 9) forcefully on both hands. Nip each point 3-6 times to obtain an aching sensation.

3. Rectify fingers along Meridians

Rectify the fingers of each hand with the other. Drag and stroke each finger 3 times. Then hold the thumb and each finger of the hand securely and tug them 3 times to slacken finger joints. Finally, twist each finger joint 3 times to obtain sensations of distension and numbness.

4. Clench fists and extend fingers

Sit upright and relax your mind. Place both hands in front of you at chest height, and stare at the fingers. Begin with the thumb — extend and straighten each finger forcefully in sequence, then bend them in and clench them forcefully one by one. After you complete 3 rounds, extend and straighten all 10 fingers, and press the palms forward as far as possible, then clench your fists firmly 3 times. Stop and rest for a while, relax your fingers, then twist and rock your wrists.

Effects: These exercises can make your fingers nimble and your wrists flexible. By dredging the Three Yin and Three Yang Meridians of the Hand, Vital Energy and Blood are regulated and harmonized, especially those within the internal organs and upper limbs. These techniques may prevent and treat numbness, coldness, and chilblain of the fingers, as well as tremors, stiffness, pain and loss of strength in the fingers after stroke, including senile dermal plaque or nevus. In addition, these exercises are indicated for such disorders as common cold, vomiting, dizziness, toothache, sore throat, insomnia, loss of memory, heart disease, or arthritis of the shoulder.

Techniques for the arms

There are three important joints in the upper limbs, whose range of motion is the widest of the body — the shoulder, elbow and wrist. The Six Meridians of the Hand pass through them. These techniques are aimed at easing joints and activating Collaterals.

1. Rub and bathe the arms

Press one hand closely against the other inner wrist, and rub the inner arm along the Three Yin Meridians of the Hand from the wrist to the armpit. Then, starting at the tip of the shoulder, rub the outside of the arm along the Three Yang Meridians of the Hand down to the back of the hand. Repeat this several times until you feel sensations of warmth and distension in the arm. You may use one-way rubbing and bathing, with the direction of motion chosen according to the principle of invigoration and reduction (invigoration = against the direction of the Meridian; reduction = along with the direction of the Meridian). You may also use back-and-forth rubbing.

2. Nip and grasp the three joints

Nip and grasp the following points strenuously, using the thumb, index and middle fingers.

A. Around the wrist joint: Taiyuan (Lu 9), Lieque (Lu 7), Yangchi (TW 4), Daling (Per 7), Neiguan (Per 6) and Waiguan (TW 5).

B. Around the elbow joint: Quchi (LI 11), Shaohai (H 3), Chize (Lu 5) and Shousanli (LI 10).

C. Around the shoulder joint: Jianyu (LI 15), Jianliao (TW 14), Jianjing (GB 21), Bingfeng (SI 12), Binao (LI 14), Taijian (lift the shoulder) and Jubi (raise the arm), (new points).

You may also incorporate pinching, kneading, knocking and dotting. Continue until you feel sensations of soreness, numbness and distension.

3. Spread the arms

Stand or sit up with a calm and relaxed mind. To start, cross both arms to hold the tips of the opposite shoulders with your hands; bend the arms and pull the shoulders in, the tighter the better. Then stretch your arms straight out to expand your chest, keeping all three joints in a straight line; or, stretch your arms forward and to the side with palms pushing outwards at no more than shoulder height. These are called transverse or horizontal arm stretches. Bend your elbows with the wrists raised and raise your hands to support the heavens, or imitate the actions of holding on to the top of a wall; or crook your arms as if rolling something up and swing your arms as if you are cracking whips. These are called longitudinal or vertical arm stretches. Bend both arms forward and back (slanting or oblique arm stretches). Straighten both arms, and, with the shoulders as the pivots, make circles forward and backward. These are called circular arm stretches. Choose these techniques according to your own condition, and be careful to practice them slowly and smoothly.

Effects: These are effective in lubricating and easing joints, warming and dredging Meridians. Locally, they may prevent and treat numbness, pain, paralysis of the arm, arthritis of the shoulder, tennis elbow, and cervical spondylosis. Systemically, they may prevent and treat common cold, vomiting, stomach ache, nausea, insomnia, mental distraction, heart disease, bronchitis and hemiplegia.

Techniques to benefit the brain

The brain is the residence of intelligence and the most important part of the body. It communicates with various Vessels and Yang Meridians. These techniques should be considered one series.

1. Push the forehead and comb the hair

Bend both hands in a natural position. Press each thumb pad to each Taiyang (Ex-HN 4), and the remaining fingers on both eyebrows (four to each side). With your fingers slightly separated, push both hands energetically up along the scalp to comb the hair. During this technique, push and rub the forehead, the top of the head and the occipital area successively with both thenar mounds and the heels of the hands. When both thumbs reach Fengchi (GB 20), collect the other fingers gradually in toward the index fingers, and push and rub the scalp from Baihu (GV 20) to Fengfu (GV 16) and Dazhui (GV 14).

2. Rub ears and wipe eyes

Turn the wrists of both hands and cup your palms over your ears, pressing your fingers to Fengchi (GB 20). Leading with the little fingers, rub from Fengchi (GB 20) transversely across the ears and the eyes to the midline, keeping pressure with the fingertips. The other fingers and both thenar mounds follow across. When the tips of the middle fingers stop at Jingming (UB 1), the ring and little fingers will be at the nose, the index fingers at the eyes, and both thumbs will press Quanliao (SI 18).

3. Wipe the nose and wash the face

Press the middle fingers (with other fingers following) to rub and wipe the nose downward along both sides. Then, with the palms, rub both cheeks, and the mouth and the lower jaw, as if you were washing your face.

In summary, here is the sequence: Eyes and forehead — comb hair and rub head — crown to occiput — Dazhui (GV 14) — turn wrist and rub ears — wipe eyes — wipe nose — wash face — join the palms at the lower jaw.

Before beginning, you should be at ease, relaxed and quiet of mind. During the technique, focus attention without distraction. On completion, close your eyes and rest for a while.

4. Nip and knead principal points

One to five fingers may be used simultaneously to nip and knead. The most commonly chosen points are as follows:

Forehead: Taiyang (Ex-HN 4), Yintang (Ex-HN 2), Yangbai (GB 14).

Head: Shenting (GV 24), Shangxing (GV 23), Baihu (GV 20), Touwei (St 8), Tianchong (GB 9), Naohu (GV 17), Yuzhen (UB 9), Fengfu (GV 16), Fengchi (GB 20).

Face: Xiaguan (St 7), Ermen (TW 21), Yifeng (TW 17), Tongziliao (GB 1), Quanliao (SI 18), Jingming (UB 1), Yingxiang (LI 20), Renzhong (GV 26), Chengjiang (CV 24).

Effects: These are effective in benefiting the brain, refreshing the mind and improving looks. Locally, they may prevent and treat headache, migraine, listlessness, dizziness, dreaminess, insomnia, hair loss, grey hair, tinnitus, nasal obstruction, blurred vision, facial plaque, nevus, acne and wrinkles. Systemically, they may prevent and treat paralysis and numbness of limbs, deafness, aphasia, hypertension and facial paralysis.

Techniques for improving vision

The eyes are the external Aperture of the Liver and the confluent areas of Yang Meridians and Vessel Collaterals. These exercises may promote the flow of Vital Energy and Blood, eliminate mental fatigue and improve vision.

1. Press and knead the periocular area

Make open fists with both thumbs slightly bent. Press and knead the points around the eyes with the thumb joints. The sequence is as follows: Jingming (UB 1), Zanzhu (UB 2), Chengqi (St 1), Sibai (St 2), Sizhukong (TW 23), Tongziliao (GB 1) and Taiyang (Ex-HN 4). In this exercise, proceed from the center outwards with appropriate pressure, each point to be done a minimum of 6 times. Then press and knead the eyeballs clockwise and counter-clockwise along the edge of the sockets, again for a minimum of 6 times, with the pads of the middle and index fingers, until you feel a sensation of warmth and distension. When you're done, close your eyes and rest for a while.

2. Pinch and wipe the eyebrows and the eyes

Close both eyes. Pinch both eyebrows from Yintang (Ex-HN 2) to Sizhukong (TW 23) with the pads of the thumb and index finger of both hands (or pinch each eyebrow with both hands) until you feel warmth and distension. Then, with your hands open, press and deep-press both Taiyang (Ex-HN 4) with the thumbs. At the same time, bend your two index fingers tightly into hook-shapes (knuckle joint straight), and use the middle segments to scrape and wipe the eyebrows from both Zanzhu (UB 2) to both Taiyang (Ex-HN 4). Afterwards, scrape and wipe the eyeballs and lower eye sockets from the center outward to Taiyang (Ex-HN 4) with them. Repeat until you feel warmth, distension and coziness.

3. Three methods for eye training

Stand up with a relaxed and clear mind; deep-press the lower abdomen softly with one hand on top of the other. Practice the following exercises:

A. Revolve eyes in all six directions: Open your eyes and stare up, down, right and left. Then look from left to up, from up to right, from right to down, and from down to left. Then rotate your gaze in the opposite direction. Repeat for a total of 6 cycles, going for maximum field of vision. Be careful not to turn or move your neck. In the beginning, if it will be helpful, use your finger as a guide to the visual line.

B. Open your eyes as widely as possible, gaze as far as you can, and focus your mind, as if you had no body. If you feel tired, close your eyes and begin again.

C. Close your eyes to rest your mind. After doing the two previous exercises, keep your eyes half or mostly closed, retaining just a thread of vision, and notice the tip of your nose. Listen calmly to your own breathing, or focus your attention on Qihai (CV 6) or Dantian for about 10 minutes.

Effects: These are effective in clearing Liver Fire, improving vision, and for refreshment. They may prevent and treat headache, dizziness, amblyopia, myopia, hyperopia, strabismus, presbyopia, pterygium, trichiasis and other eye disorders.

Techniques for ventilating the nose

The nose is the external Aperture of the Lung and is connected with the Yangming Meridian. Ventilating the nose may improve respiration and strengthen the defense mechanism of the body.

1. Press and knead the periphery of the nose

Clench one or both open fists with the thumb(s) bent. Press and knead the following points with the thumb joint until you feel sensations of aching, numbness and distension: Yintang (Ex-HN 2), Shangen (Bridge of the nose), Suliao (GV 25); both Yingxiang (LI 20) and Heliao (LI 19); Renzhong (GV 26). These points may also be nipped with the fingers.

2. Push and rub the bridge of the nose

The hand is held the same as above. Push and rub both sides of the nose energetically, back and forth, from Jingming (UB 1) and Chengqi (St 1) to Yingxiang (LI 20) and Dicang (St 4). Move the hands along the same direction or alternately up and down, until the skin is reddened and you feel sensations of warmth and distension.

3. Pinch and grasp the external nares

Place the tip of your index finger on Suliao (GV 25) and pinch and grasp both nares with the thumb and middle finger. Pinch and grasp 100 times, co-ordinating the technique with your respiration. It is normal to have nasal discharge. Lifting and grasping the nares may be also done with this technique.

Effects: These techniques are effective in improving the sense of smell and easing the ventilation of Lung Energy. They may prevent and treat the common cold with sniffling, stuffy nose, nosebleed, sinusitis, deficient sense of smell, atrophic rhinitis, and facial paralysis.

Techniques for improving hearing

The ear is the external Aperture of the Kidney, and is closely related to various Meridians and internal organs as has been shown by oto-acupuncture therapy.

1. Sweep and rub the ears

Bend both arms with the hands naturally straightened. Touch the tips of your thumbs to the earlobes with the other four fingers close to the auricles. Sweep and rub the auricles back and forth with the fingers by swinging your wrists. Continue until you feel a sensation of warmth.

2. Nip points and pull ears

With the tips of the thumbs or other fingers, nip and knead Shuaigu (GB 8) and Jiaosun (TW 20) above the ear; Qubin (GB 7), Heliao (TW 22), Ermen (TW 21), Tinggong (SI 19) and Tinghui (GB 2) in front of the ear; Yifeng (TW 17) and Yixia (below Yifeng) below the ear; and Wangu (GB 12) and Fengchi (GB 20) behind the ear. Continue until you feel sensations of aching and distension. Then nip and knead the upper and lower conchae and the helix until you feel mild pain. After a pause, pinch the auriculae from both sides and stroke them with the thumb and index finger (or bent index and middle finger) forward, back, up and down, 6 times in each direction.

3. Beat Heaven's Drum

There are three methods of performing this technique:

A. Open ears with both fingers: Straighten the index finger of each hand, with other fingers bent and the palms facing forward. Insert your index fingers into your earholes and spin them 180 degrees 3 times, then pull them out quickly and suddenly. You should hear a "Ba-ba" sound while pulling your fingers out. Repeat for a total of 3-6 times.

B. Squeeze ears with palms: Raise your shoulders and press the center of your palms close to the earholes, with the tips of your middle fingers at Fengfu (GV 16), and the other fingers at your head and nape to stabilize the palms. Squeeze both ears by pressing and loosening palms successively and energetically. The movement of the palms is driven by the wrists and elbows, with relaxed shoulders. To begin, go slowly, then fast to achieve a humming sound. Squeeze a minimum of 30 times.

C. Cover ears and knock head: Press your palms close to your ears, with the center of the palm tight against the earhole. Stabilize your hands with your thumbs and little fingers. Knock the occipital area or Naohu (GV 17), Fengfu (GV 16) and Yamen (GV 15) with the other three fingers, either working as one, or separately, in turn. A "Dong, dong" sound should be heard during the knocking, as if a drum is being beaten.

Effects: Effects are similar to those of oto-acupuncture. Locally, they may prevent and treat deafness, tinnitus, chilblain of the ear, and other disorders within the ear. They may also improve hearing. Systemically, they may prevent and treat common cold, stiff nape, dizziness, eye pain, toothache, facial paralysis and hemiplegia.

Techniques inside the mouth

The mouth and the lips are the opening of the Spleen; teeth are the surplus of bones and belong to the Kidney. The gums connect with the Yangming Meridians of the Hand and the Foot; and the tongue is the opening of the Heart, and also connects with Collaterals of Liver and Spleen Meridians. Saliva moistens and benefits the Five Yin Organs. Relying on the health and sturdiness of the tongue and teeth, digestion is promoted, pronunciation is eased, vitality is strengthened and the face is beautified.

These techniques consist of methods for stabilizing teeth, easing the tongue, and swallowing saliva.

1. Techniques for stabilizing teeth

A. Grinding the teeth in a closed mouth: Relax yourself with a peaceful mind. Keep the upper and lower teeth close together. First, grind strenuously at the molars, then gradually shift forward until your are grinding at the incisors. Practice this technique repeatedly, either on one side or both, until you feel an aching and distension at the cheeks, and you notice an increase in saliva.

B. Knocking the teeth in a closed mouth: Relax yourself with a peaceful mind. Close your mouth loosely. Knock the upper teeth with the lower, rhythmically, with a *ka, ka* sound. The knocking may be symmetrical or diagonal, mild or heavy. Frequency should go from slow to rapid. Continue until you feel numbness and distension at the gums, and an increase in saliva.

2. Techniques for easing the tongue

A. Churning the Tongue: Relax, with a peaceful mind. Close your mouth loosely. Lick the upper and lower gums in a circle outside the teeth, repeatedly, as if stirring something in a pot, until you feel numbness and distension at the tongue and cheeks, and the mouth is full of saliva. This is also called *The Red Dragon Disturbs the Sea*.

B. The tongue holds up the palate: Relax your mind and both cheeks. Close your mouth and press your tongue up to the hard palate. It is best to focus on Dantian while doing this.

3. Technique of swallowing saliva

Grind your teeth, bulge out your cheeks and churn your tongue to stimulate saliva. When it fills the mouth, swallow it energetically in three or more separate parts repeatedly. You should hear a *Gu, gu* sound while swallowing. During this technique, it is best to imagine the saliva being swallowed into the lower abdomen.

Effects: These techniques sober the mind, moisten dryness, improve chewing and the digestive function, promote detoxification and immunization. Specifically, they may prevent and treat toothache or wobbly teeth; swelling, pain, bleeding or atrophy of the gums; dryness or ulceration of the tongue; deviation or paralysis of the tongue; dizziness, vexation or dry stool.

Techniques for relaxing the neck

The neck holds up the head, and connects with the chest and internal organs, as well as the shoulders and arms. The Conception Vessel Meridian travels along its midline at the front, and the Governor Vessel Meridian along the midline at the back. The Three Yang Meridians of the Hand and Foot travel along its sides. These techniques may relax the neck and ease the throat.

1. Knead and grasp the front of the neck

Make a loose fist and press the index finger across Chengjiang (CV 24). Knead Lianquan (CV 23) with the tip of the thumb, and knead Tiantu (CV 22) with the bent middle finger of the other hand. Manipulate simultaneously until you feel numbness and distension. Then, knead and grasp both sides of the neck, laying stress on the front. Knead and grasp the following points according to their Meridian distribution, outward from the center, and from top to bottom: Renying (St 9), Shuitu (St 10), Qishe (St 11), Futu (LI 18), Tianding (LI 17), etc. Finally, stroke, rub, pinch and lift both sides of the neck alternately with each hand, from the sides to the center, and from back to front, until you feel warmth and distension.

2. Press and rub the nape

Raise your shoulders, put both hands on your nape, and apply force through your middle fingers, assisted by the others. Press and deep-press the nape from Fengfu (GV 16) to Dazhui (GV 14), along the spinal processes of the cervical vertebrae. Then, interlace your fingers at the base of the skull and press the heels of your hands to both Fengchi (GB 20). Press and rub them strenuously to achieve a warm sensation.

3. Relax the neck along six directions

Stretch your neck forward, backward, right and left as far as it will go; then turn it clockwise and counter-clockwise. This should be done slowly, with the neck relaxed. Avoid holding your breath or continuing if there is any difficulty.

Effects: These are effective in easing the throat, relaxing the neck, dredging the Energy Mechanism, and relieving spasm. They may prevent and treat swelling and pain of the throat, asthma, hiccups, coughing, vomiting, gagging, hoarseness, stiff neck, cervical spondylosis; also headache, vertigo and numbness caused by disorders of the cervical vertebrae.

Techniques for relaxing the chest and rib cage

Heart and Lung reside in the chest, and Liver and Gall Bladder are in charge of the rib cage where Jueyin and Shaoyang Meridians of the Foot travel. The chest and rib cage connect with the neck, head, abdomen and the waist. Exercises to these areas may treat disorders of the throat as well as the intestinal tract.

1. Push and rub the clavicular fossae

Place the pad of the thumb on Tiantu (CV 22); stretch the index and middle fingers side by side, applying force primarily through the pad of the middle finger, and push and rub the clavicular fossae strenuously back and forth on one side. Work alternately with both hands until you feel distension and pain.

2. Press and knead important points

Press and knead the following points individually or simultaneously with the fingers or the thenar mound: Yunmen (Lu 2), Qihu (St 13), Huagai (CV 20), Yingchuang (St 16), Xiongxiang (Sp 19), Tanzhong (CV 17), Jiuwei (CV 15), Qimen (Liv 14) and Zhangmen (Liv 13). Of these, Tanzhong (CV 17) is the most important.

3. Rub and wipe along three directions

Bend the fingers of both hands into Eagle's Talons, apply force through the pads of the fingers, and rub and wipe vertically in a straight line from the throat to the chest to the epigastrium. Rub and wipe the chest and rib cage straight across from right to left and from left to right. Then rub and wipe the spaces between the ribs in a curve from the center outward. Do each technique 6 times. Don't hold your breath. You may also incorporate knocking softly and slowly with the fingers, hands or fists, but the knocking should be light and not too fast.

4. Spread the arms to expand the chest

Expand the chest by lifting and abducting your arms and swaying them backward. Coordinate your breathing. This may strengthen the physical abilities of the chest and improve cardiopulmonary functions.

Effects: These relax the chest, strengthen Heart, rectify and disperse Liver Energy, and benefit Spleen. They may prevent and treat chest pain, coughing or labored breathing; feelings of heaviness, distension or fullness in the chest and rib cage; disharmony between Liver and Stomach, heart diseases, bronchitis and chronic hepatitis.

Techniques to strengthen the waist and benefit Kidney

The waist is the seat of Kidney. Most Meridians pass through the waist, and the Belt Meridian runs around it. It carries the body's weight and is an important pivot to physical activity. Common symptoms are sensations of heaviness or weighty pain. Kidney is the foundation of all that is inborn, and is generally in a state of Deficiency, so it is often benefited by warming and invigorating.

1. Rub and roll Yaoyan (Ex-B 3)

Rub and roll both sides of the lumbar region of the spine, especially Shenshu (UB 23), with both hands or the back of both fists. Do this repeatedly from the level of the 12th rib to the iliac, until you feel warmth or slight perspiration. This may be incorporated with pressing and kneading (sitting posture). If you lie on one side, this can be done with one hand.

2. Knock and clap the lumbosacral region

Bend your arms behind your back, and knock or clap the waist along the lumbosacral area alternately with the back of the fist or the heel of the hand. Continue until you feel numbness, distension and aching.

3. Move the waist along the six directions

Stand naturally with a calm mind. Bend your waist forward and back, right and left, and twist it clockwise and counter-clockwise. It's important that your legs and buttocks be still, your respiration regular, your body relaxed, range of movement be wide, and you do the exercise slowly and according to your own ability.

Effects: These expel Wind, eliminate Dampness, strengthen the waist and spine, cultivate and consolidate the constitutional foundation, warm the waist and benefit Kidney. They may prevent and treat lumbago, weakness of the legs, lumbar sprain, strain or atrophy of lumbar muscles, neuralgia of the hip, hyperosteogeny, protruding disk, dissipation, enuresis, impotence, premature ejaculation, nephritis, prostatitis, neurasthenia, and irregular menstruation.

Techniques to strengthen legs and lighten feet

The leg has three joints — hip, knee and ankle. It bears the weight of the body and is in charge of moving the body's location. Six Meridians of the Foot travel along the leg. Generally speaking, joint pain, muscle pain and erratic movement of the leg are caused by Wind, Cold and Dampness. Strengthening the leg may ease the waist and eliminate many diseases. For example, if we massage the so- called *Longevity Point* (Zusanli [St 36]) unremittingly all year long, we can not only treat diseases of the legs, but Spleen and Stomach may also be invigorated. By practicing leg exercises, you can increase agility and nimbleness in walking and moving. In addition to varieties of *Standing like a Stake,* there are many types of leg exercises, such as kicking, bouncing and different ways of walking. To go into all the details is beyond the scope of this work.

1. Dot and grasp important points on Meridians of the Foot

Sit in a relaxed posture. Dot the important points on the legs with both middle fingers and grasp them with the fingers of both hands simultaneously on the same side, from above to below and from inner to outer. Determine your own level of exertion and manipulate each point 6 times.

Along the Yangming Meridian of the Foot, choose Biguan (St 31), Yinshi (St 33), Zusanli (St 36), Fenglong (St 40) and Jiexi (St 41); along the Shaoyang Meridian of the Foot, choose Huantiao (GB 30), Fengshi (GB 31), Yanglingquan (GB 34), Guanming (GB 37) and Qiuxu (GB 40). Then dot and grasp points of the inner side of the right leg with the left hand and the left leg with the right hand. Along the Taiyin Meridian of the Foot, choose Jimen (Sp 11), Xuehai (Sp 10), Yinlingquan (Sp 9), and Sanyinjiao (Sp 6); along the Jueyin Meridian of the Foot, choose Zuwuli (Liv 10), Yinbao (Liv 9), Ququan (Liv 8) and Xiguan (Liv 7). Along the Shaoyin Meridian of the Foot, choose Yingu (K 10), Zhubin (K 9) and Fuliu (K 7). Finally, grasp points along the Taiyang Meridian of the Foot after changing your posture and the position of the your legs. Choose Chengfu (UB 36), Yinmen (UB 37), Weizhong (UB 40), Chengjin (UB 56), Chengshan (UB 57) and Kunlun (UB 60).

2. Clasp and rub both legs

Place one hand on the outside of the leg below the ilium and the other at the groin, with finger tips facing each other. Clasp the leg with both hands and rub it forcefully downward to the ankle, then forcefully up to the base of the leg. You should feel warmth and distension. You may also clasp and rub both thighs and shanks separately.

3. Nip and knead both knees

While sitting, stretch both legs or bend them naturally. Hold your knees with the heels of the hands at both Heding (Ex-LE 1), the index and ring fingers at both Xiyan (Ex-LE 2) and the other fingers around the knee joint, as in the Eagle's Talons. Apply force through your fingertips, and nip and knead these spots by rocking your wrists with your elbows raised until you feel warmth, aching and distension under the patellae.

4. Pinch and lift the Achilles tendon

Sit and cross your legs, or squat or kneel on tiptoes with your heels facing up. Nip and knead both Achilles tendons several times. You should feel aching when done.

5. Rock ankles and rectify toes

Sit and cross your legs. Hold the bent knee in one hand and clasp the five toes with the other, palm to sole. Bend, stretch and drag the toes and rock the ankle in a circle, first clockwise, then counter-clockwise. Do this 6 times in each direction. Then bend the index and middle fingers together as pincers, and press each toe from both sides. Pinch, drag, stroke and rectify all of them, 6 times each. Repeat on the other foot.

6. Move the three joints of the leg

Stand steadily on one leg. Sway, kick, rock and twist the ankle, knee and hip joints of the other leg along the six different directions. Shift onto the other leg and repeat.

Effects: These techniques are effective to expel Wind, disperse Cold, activate Blood, dredge Meridians, lubricate and ease joints and relieve pain. Locally, they may prevent and treat pain, numbness, swelling, spasm, cramps, paralysis, feebleness or atrophy of the legs; also joint pain with a cold sensation, crane knee arthritis, swelling of the shank, vasculitis, phlebitis, or pain in the heel. Systemically, they may ease the waist, foster Kidney, harmonize Stomach and strengthen Spleen.

Techniques to warm Yongquan and benefit Yin

This consists of nipping, pinching toes and pushing, and rubbing the center of the sole of the foot, especially Yongquan (K 1). Toes are the place where the Three Yin and Three Yang Meridians of the Foot connect with each other, while Yongquan (K 1) is the starting point of the Shaoyin Meridian of the Foot. According to TCM, various parts of the sole, as those of the ear, are closely related to internal organs. This opinion has been upheld by current medical research.

1. Nip and pinch toes

Sit with crossed legs. Nip the tips of the toes with your thumb, beginning at the big toe and moving along. Then nip the joining part of red and white skin around each nail of the toes, until you feel pain and see redness. Then pinch each toe 6 times. Repeat on the other foot. You may also rectify the toes as part of this exercise.

2. Push and rub the center of the sole

Cross your legs or kneel with your soles facing up. Focus your attention at Yongquan (K 1). Push and rub the center of the sole along the length of the foot, from the arch to the tips of the toes; or push and rub it across with your thumb or the heel of your hand. Alternately, you may knead first, then push and rub as above. The speed and force you use should produce a scorching sensation. You might also choose to lie supinely, press the soles of the feet together, and rub them back and forth against each other until you feel the scorching heat. This technique also exercises the hip and knee. Generally, this technique is done before going to bed, after first having washed the feet.

Effects: These nourish Yin, reduce Fire, refresh the mind, dredge Apertures, clear Liver, benefit Kidney and drain Turbidity. Locally, they may prevent and treat numbness, coldness and edema of the foot, beriberi, anal fissures, chilblains, vasculitis and peripheral neuritis. Systemically, they may prevent and treat dizziness, palpitation, headache, fainting, epilepsy, loss of voice, stuffy nose, dissipation, insomnia, hypertension, and pharyngitis or laryngitis.

Round-rub the abdomen and revolve Dantian

Liver, Spleen and Kidney, along with Stomach, Intestine and Urinary Bladder, reside in the abdomen, where the Three Yin Meridians and Yangming Meridian of the Foot are closely related. Moreover, Conception Vessel Meridian is in charge of the abdomen, Belt Vessel Meridian binds it, and Vital Vessel Meridian originates there. Therefore, it is the stem of congenital endowment and the root of postnatal resources. In TCM, the upper abdomen indicates the area around Zhongwan (CV 12), middle abdomen indicates the area around the navel, Shaofu (young abdomen) indicates the areas beneath the rib cage or below the navel, and Xiaofu (little abdomen) is the lower abdomen or the region of Dantian. The abdomen belongs to Yin and needs to be warmed and cleared. During self-massage, the abdomen should be relaxed and your breathing should be coordinated with your manipulations. Don't hold your breath or bulge your belly.

1. Knead and round-rub the abdomen to clear it

Sit or lie supinely. Knead and round-rub the abdomen circularly with one or both hands alternately, using the navel as the center. For example, press your right hand to the upper abdomen, and proceed from upper abdomen to left Shaofu, then to Xiaofu, then to right Shaofu, then to upper abdomen, and then to the middle abdomen, finishing with the center of the palm pressing against Shenque (CV 8). This would be one round. The left hand works in the same fashion but in the opposite direction. Each hand should do a minimum of 10 rounds.

If you feel fullness and heaviness in both the chest and the abdomen, or beneath the rib cage, you may incorporate a method of pushing, rubbing and washing the chest. Push and rub from the chest or upper abdomen to the lower abdomen, passing through the middle abdomen; or knead and round-rub from the upper abdomen to Shaofu. In treating gastroptosis or Energy sinking of the Middle Warmer, the direction should be from the lower abdomen to the upper abdomen.

2. Dot and vibrate Shenque (CV 8)

Lie supinely. Dot and vibrate Shenque (CV 8) with your middle finger until you feel distension, numbness and quivering in the abdomen. Other important points of the abdomen may also be chosen according to conditions, such as Zhongwan (CV 12), Zhangmen (Liv 13), Tianshu (St 25), Qihai (CV 6) and Guanyuan (CV 4).

3. Pinch and lift the belly skin

Pinch and lift the belly skin with your thumb, index and middle finger from Jiuwei (CV 15) to the lower abdomen along the points of the Conception Vessel Meridian. Repeat for a total of 3 times. This may be incorporated with vibrating.

4. Revolve Dantian with one hand on another

Stand in a quiet environment after getting up in the morning, or lie in bed before going to sleep. Let your mind and body be relaxed and calm. Put the right hand over the left, with the Inner Laogong (Per 8) of one to the Outer Laogong of the other. Place the Laogongs over Qihai (CV 6). Deep-press the covered area in the following order 36 times clockwise and 36 times counter-clockwise:

Major thenar mound — heel of hand — minor thenar mound — finger pads — major thenar mound. You should feel warmth and distension in the lower abdomen. While doing this technique, focus your attention on this area, regulate your respiratory motion, and raise the anus each time in co-operation. When done, practice Techniques Inside the Mouth. When your mouth is full of saliva, swallow it in separate parts and imagine it reaching the lower abdomen. This exercise may be done independently of the others, and in time may improve your vitality and prolong your life.

Effects: These exercises strengthen Spleen and Stomach, regulate Vital and Conception Vessel Meridians, invigorate Kidney, rectify the womb, eliminate Dampness, depress the adverse uprising, adjust Vital Energy, conserve Blood, warm Yang, arrest collapse, benefit Essence and stimulate Vitality. Specifically, they may prevent and treat distension and fullness of the Stomach, stomach pain, diarrhea, constipation, indigestion, gastroptosis, gastric and duodenal ulcer, gastro-intestinal neurosis, chronic colitis, chronic hepatitis, hemorrhoids, fistula, rectocele, stranguria, enuresis, urinary incontinence, retention of urine, dissipation, involuntary seminal emission, impotence, premature ejaculation, dysmenorrhea, irregular menstruation or leukorrhea with or without bloody discharge.

Techniques to reinforce Kidney and strengthen Yang

This is primarily directed toward improving the function of male sexual organs. The penis (confluence of Tendons), scrotum and perineum are areas where Liver Meridian, Conception Vessel Meridian and Governor Vessel

Meridian meet and pass by. These techniques are suitable for the aged and middle-aged, and for those who suffer from hypogonadism. It is contraindicated for healthy, single men, since practice of this exercise will result in an upsurge of libido and penis erection. Under these circumstances, sexual intercourse should be avoided. Sexual indulgence can be harmful at that time. Better effects could be obtained by practicing *Sitting Still*, or other convalescent tranquilizing exercises along with this one. With the passing of time, these may improve health and promise longevity.

1. Revolve and knead the perineum

Sit up, expose your external genitals, relax your body and let your mind become peaceful. Press and shield Dantian with your left hand. Knead the perineum gently and slowly with the middle finger of the right hand, i.e., revolve your fingertip clockwise 36 times and counter-clockwise 36 times, until you feel distension, warmth and a slight numbness. Use appropriate force and speed. Concentrate your focus. This exercise is also effective in preventing and treating disorders of the rectum and anus if you practice rhythmic anus raising along with the technique.

2. Cup and prop the scrotum

Dot and press the base of the scrotum (close to the perineum) with the tip of the middle finger; cup, prop and rub the scrotum (testes) and the penis, to make them nestle closely in to the lower abdomen. Do this with both hands alternating for a minimum of 100 times, gradually increasing the force and speed until you feel distension, aching and warmth.

3. Pinch and roll the external genitals

Hold the testes in both hands; pinch and knead both testes separately with the thumb and index finger to the extent that aching is tolerable. Don't move too energetically. Then pinch and twist the penis from its base to its tip until you feel distension and aching while the penis is slightly erect. Finally, hold and press the penis and testes with both hands, applying force with the minor thenar mounds — roll them and shift your hands from the bottom to the top repeatedly. Determine the number of manipulations to practice according to your best judgment.

Effects: These exercises reinforce Kidney, strengthen Yang, benefit the brain and solidify Essence. They may prevent and treat impotence, prostatitis, hypogonadism, lumbago due to Kidney Deficiency, coldness in the abdomen, loose stool, rectocele, hemorrhoids, fistula, loss of memory or insomnia.

About the Editor

Sun Chengnan (1925-1991) was born into the tradition of Chinese medicine. A fourth-generation practitioner on his father's side and a ninth-generation practitioner via his maternal grandfather, he began practice in 1948. In 1953, he acknowledged Mi Wang Qishan of Shandong as his master, and established his own practice in the city of Dalian, attending to both traumatology and internal medicine.

In 1956, he became Doctor of TCM at the People's Hospital of Fushan County in Shandong, employing Tuina, acupuncture and moxibustion to treat all varieties of ailments.

From 1957 through 1959, he was a member of the Teaching and Research Group of Bonesetting and Tuina Advanced Studies School at Shandong College of TCM.

In 1960, he became director of the Shandong Hospital of TCM, also becoming a member of the standing council of the Shandong Branch of the Chinese Medical Association and director of the Shandong Tuina Association.

His expertise in treatment of back and joint trauma and disease, and his ability to relieve pain without drugs, using only Tuina and massage, became widely known, becoming international after his treatments of visiting foreign government officials and members of art and literary delegations from Europe.

Dr. Sun was a member of the All-China Reading and Editing Committee for Development of College Teaching Materials, and he conducted more than 20 training and lecture courses. He published 8 highly respected theses on medical topics, the best-known being *The Treatment of Lumbar Disc Protrusion with Tuina*. He was also directly involved in the research and development of such useful clinical aids as Anti-Hyperplasia Tablets and the Tuina Manipulator.

ACUPUNCTURE, MERIDIAN THEORY, and ACUPUNCTURE POINTS

by Li Ding

Meridian theory defines the network of channels and collaterals which distributes *qi* (vital energy), links organs and extremities, and enables the body to function. It is the guiding principle for all traditional Chinese medicine, especially acupuncture, massage, and qigong. This comprehensive text offers a lucid, organized approach to the fundamental concepts which acupuncturists and other TCM practitioners must master. The presentation of the acupuncture Points and their usage includes not only standard numbering, Chinese characters, and *pinyin*, but thoughtful English translations of Point names, a great aid in learning Points and comprehending their significance.

This is also a useful reference for experienced practitioners, as its systematic descriptions of Meridians, and the flow charts for each Meridian resolve many problems posed by conflicting information from other sources about complex aspects of the secondary Meridian branches.

Professor Li Ding, of Shanxi Medical College, serves on the Board of the All-China Society of Acupuncture and Moxibustion. He is author of ten previous books on acupuncture, moxibustion, and qigong.

$60.00   Cloth   ISBN 0-8351-2143-7   1992   414 pages   264 illustrations   charts

TREATING AIDS WITH CHINESE MEDICINE

by Mary Kay Ryan and Arthur S. Shattuck

Early in the AIDS epidemic, practitioners of Chinese medicine realized that this ancient healing art, based on enhancing the body's own functioning and ability to overcome illness, might offer unique resources in fighting a plague new to both Western and traditional Chinese medicine. This comprehensive handbook is the first to systematically present an overall framework for understanding and treating AIDS from the perspective of traditional Chinese medicine.

Includes sections on treating women, drug-addicted persons, and persons with hemophilia, and practical information about organizing clinics. While directed toward the practitioner of TCM, this book is also written for Western-trained doctors, healthcare workers, and others wishing to understand what TCM is, what it can and can't do for AIDS patients, and how to work with TCM practitioners.

The authors are co-founders and co-directors of AIDS Alternative Health Project and the Northside HIV Treatment Center in Chicago.

$29.95 Paper ISBN 1-881896-07-2 Available February 1994 300 pages illustrations charts